Special Research Unit 227 – Prevention and Intervention in Childhood and Adolescence

An interdisciplinary project of the University of Bielefeld

conducted by *Prof. Dr. Günter Albrecht, Prof. Dr. Peter-Alexis Albrecht, Prof. Dr. Otto Backes, Prof. Dr. Michael Brambring, Prof. Dr. Klaus Hurrelmann, Prof. Dr. Franz-Xaver Kaufmann, Prof. Dr. Friedrich Lösel, Prof. Dr. Hans-Uwe Otto, Prof. Dr. Helmut Skowronek*

Children at Risk: Assessment, Longitudinal Research, and Intervention

Edited by
Michael Brambring,
Friedrich Lösel,
Helmut Skowronek

Walter de Gruyter · Berlin · New York 1989

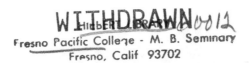

Michael Brambring
Professor of Psychology, University of Bielefeld

Friedrich Lösel
Professor of Psychology, University of Erlangen-Nürnberg

Helmut Skowronek
Professor of Psychology, University of Bielefeld

With 34 Figures and 67 Tables

Library of Congress Cataloging-in-Publication Data

Children at risk : assessment, longitudinal research, and intervention
/ edited by Michael Brambring, Friedrich Lösel, Helmut Skowronek.
XIV, 490 p. 17x24 cm. -- (Prevention and intervention in childhood and
adolescence : 7)
  Revised papers from a symposium held in 1987.
  Includes bibliographical references.
  ISBN 0-89925-592-2 (U.S.)
  1. Child psychiatry--Congresses. 2. Adolescent psychiatry-
-Congresses. 3. Mental illness--Risk factors--Congresses.
4. Mentally ill children--Longitudinal Studies--Congresses.
I. Brambring, Michael, 1943- . II. Lösel, Friedrich.
III. Skowronek, Helmut. IV. Series.
  [DNLM; 1. Adolescent Behavior--congresses. 2. Child Behavior
Disorders--congresses. 3. Handicapped-congresses. 4. Learning
Disorders--congresses. 5. Longitudinal Studies--congresses.
6. Risk Factors--congresses.   WS 350.6 C5355]
RJ499.C48889   1989
618.92'89--dc20
DNLM/DLC
for Library of Congress   89-23518
                                                              CIP

Deutsche Bibliothek Cataloging-in-Publication Data

**Children at risk: assessment, longitudinal research, and
intervention** / ed. by Michael Brambring ... - Berlin ; New
York : de Gruyter, 1989
  (Prevention and intervention in childhood and adolescence ; 7)
  ISBN 3-11-012134-4
NE: Brambring, Michael [Hrsg.]; GT

⊗ Printed on acid free paper

Printed in Germany
Printing: WB-Druck GmbH, Rieden am Forggensee / Binding: Lüderitz & Bauer GmbH, Berlin /
Cover Design: Hansbernd Lindemann, Berlin.

Preface

Most people would agree that large sections of the population in the Western industrialized countries are materially wealthy, even if the distribution of this wealth may reveal great differences. Opinions on how to evaluate this fact differ greatly depending on political attitudes. Critics point out that a high ecological, social, and psychological price is paid for this material wealth. There are, for example, indications that the material advances of society have not been accompanied by any corresponding improvement of mental health in childhood and adolescence. In some countries and problem areas, it has even been suggested that children and adolescents face an increase in social–emotional stress and problems in the domain of learning and achievement.

In the domain of physical disabilities, despite the improved medical care in these countries that has led to a reduction of the number of disabled children and adolescents in absolute terms, there has been an increase in the number of very seriously disabled and multihandicapped children.

For methodological reasons, it is impossible to obtain a reliable assessment of the exact number of children and adolescents with behavioral disorders, emotional problems, learning and achievement disorders, and physical disabilities. However, epidemiological estimations assume that between 10 and 20% of each cohort should be regarded as being either permanently or temporarily children at risk who require support and assistance. Prevention and intervention in children at risk is one of the most important tasks of society, particularly if we consider that the care of the next generation is an investment in the future. However, prevention and intervention can only succeed when we have a degree of understanding of the basic problems involved in the assessment, etiology, and course of endangered development. The important advances that can be observed in recent developmental psychopathology and developmental research on disabled children are largely due to improved assessment methods, more precise knowledge about causal and protective factors, and an increase in the number of longitudinal studies.

This is the background to the symposium organized by the Special Research Area 227: "Prevention and Intervention in Childhood and Adolescence" at the University of Bielefeld. The Special Research Area has been financed by the German Research Association (Deutsche Forschungsgemeinschaft) since 1986. It contains scientists from various disciplines who work together on basic and applied problems of prevention and intervention in childhood and adolescence.

The symposium was conducted toward the end of 1987 at the Interdisciplinary Research Center at Bielefeld University. The present volume brings together the revised papers. The papers are international, being written by experts from West Germany, Israel, Austria, Great Britain, Sweden, Holland, and the USA. At the same time, they are interdisciplinary and represent perspectives from psychiatry, psychology, pediatrics, educational science, and sociology. The authors work in different institutions and are committed to different theoretical directions. They deal with different age groups and with a breadth of disorders ranging from emotional problems, antisocial behavior, and criminality across learning disorders and dyslexia to visual disorders and other physical disabilities. Despite the great variety of the perspectives and problem areas brought together in this symposium, many *common interests* were revealed. This not only became clear during the personal exchange of opinions during the conference but also characterizes the papers presented in this volume:

1. They are committed to an empirical orientation in which there is a close relationship between the problems in pure research, applied research, and practice.

2. Individual disorders in childhood and adolescence are not regarded in isolation, but are presented as far as possible within the context of the entire bio–psycho–social development of young persons.

3. Emphasis is not only placed on risk factors and vulnerabilities in the sense of deficit models, but also on their interaction with those protective factors that can prevent or reduce the development of disorders.

The volumes is divided into four sections: The *first section* presents theoretical approaches, methods, and findings on epidemiology, classification, and assessment. Helmut Remschmidt discusses criteria and systems for adequate classification and reports on his large-scale studies on childhood and adolescent psychiatric epidemiology in the West German state of Hessen. Thomas Achenbach clarifies the need for an empirically based, standardized assessment of behavioral and emotional disorders and demonstrates the application of his internationally well-known Child Behavior Checklist. Frank Verhulst expands this approach transculturally by applying the Child Behavior Checklist in an epidemiological longitudinal study in Holland. Ursula Kastner-Koller and Pia Deimann address the general assessment of development in preschool children and report new findings on the traditional Bühler-Hetzer-Kleinkindertest at the Psychological Institute at Vienna. In a theoretical paper, Dietrich Eggert deals with the differences between a classification- versus intervention-oriented assessment and clarifies the characteristics of the latter with examples from his own inventories for the basic motor competencies necessary for learning in schools. Christian Klicpera also addresses learning and achievement problems and particularly those of learning to read. He reports on assessment studies in which the differentiation between initially poor and persistently poor readers appears to be particularly important. David Warren is concerned with the problems of assessing visually impaired children. Like Eggert, he pleads for an approach that is more closely oriented toward ipsative criteria than toward norms. In contrast, Michael Brambring's paper shows how a highly comparable multidimensional developmental assessment can be obtained even in severely handicapped (blind) children by differentiating between general and problem-specific sections of the instrument.

The *second section* presents studies on the development of children and adolescents with specific risk constellations and disorders. Emmy Werner reports from her longitudinal study on the Hawaiian island of Kauai that represents a milestone in the research on vulnerability and resiliency. While this author points to a great number of protective factors in the face of adversity, the data from the Mannheim epidemiological study from Wolfgang Tress, Gerhard Reister, and Lutz Gegenheimer particularly underline the stabilizing function of reference persons in early childhood. Friedrich Lösel, Thomas Bliesener, and Peter Köferl discuss the present state of invulnerability research and report the first findings from their Bielefeld study that confirm a series of hypotheses on resiliency while also indicating a series of problems that arise when trying to generalize across different operationalizations. David Farrington presents new findings from the Cambridge Study in Delinquent Behavior. On the one hand, the long-term predictive power of specific risk constellations is confirmed, while, on the other hand, differential courses of development become clear (e.g., late comers, desisters, persisters). In agreement with some of the papers in the first section, Renate Valtin uses a longitudinal study on the development of reading–writing difficulties to show that a variable–related viewpoint must be accompanied by a viewpoint that considers the entire person. In another theory –guided approach, Helmut Skowronek and Harald Marx present the concept, methods, and first findings of the Bielefeld Longitudinal Study on the prediction of reading–writing difficulties. One particular goal of this work is to screen risk children at preschool age.

Even though current developmental psychopathology views the longitudinal study as the best available method, the conceptual, methodological, and practical problems involved in this design are also becoming increasingly apparent. In the *third section* of this volume, Wolfgang Schneider illustrates a series of these problems with the example of the Munich longitudinal study on the genesis of individual competencies. Alexander von Eye deals with one specific, rarely considered but frequently present problem in longitudinal studies; that of non-existing data. His categorial data solutions will certainly be welcomed by re-searchers working in these fields. The paper from Theodor Ehlers and Herbert Rehmer addresses the question of person–related data integration in longitudi-nal studies. They use the Marburg study to illustrate a successful method using Latent Class Analysis.

As important as the diagnostic and course-related research into disorders and disabilities in childhood and adolescence is, its practical status is only gained through its relevance to the possibilities of prevention and intervention. The *fourth section* of the volume addresses this subject. Gerald Caplan reports on a model for primary prevention and crisis intervention in children of divorce that he has tested over many years. This model offers a conceptual framework and a concrete action program for a risk situation that has become, both qualita-tively and quantitatively, one of the most serious in modern industrial nations. How early, diagnostically based, and differentiated support measures can be successful even in severe physical disabilities is described by Theodor Hell-brügge with the Munich model of social–pediatric developmental rehabilitation. The general framework of a system of prevention and intervention for which both the foregoing papers illustrate specific starting points is presented by Friedrich Specht presents from a psychiatric perspective. A further, specific example of successful early intervention is provided by Gunnar Jansson in his studies on the early mobility training of blind children. Hans Brügelmann describes an educational psychological approach to reducing the risk of reading and writing problems that is based on a person- and context–related model. The work from Fritz Mattejat and Helmut Remschmidt is devoted to intervention in psychological disorders. They report a comparative evaluation of inpatient versus home treatment of children and adolescents in which family characteristics prove to be good predictors of a differential treatment success. Finally, Inge Seiffge–Krenke deals with how intensively adolescents experience psychological problems, which coping strategies they prefer, and which characteristics correlate with the willingness to enter counseling or therapy. The results suggest that there is a great need for such analyses of motivation to make psychosocial care services more acceptable to their clients.

The variety and concreteness of the examples and the "healthy mixture" of the conceptual considerations, empirical findings, and practical experience reports gave us and our colleagues at the Special Research Area the impression that we had learned a great deal. We hope that this experience will also be available to the readers of these texts. We wish to thank all the authors for the stimulating discussion during the symposium and for the high level of cooperation in producing this volume. It is thanks to them that our work was neither a burden nor went for a burton!

Helga Radtke, Petra Udelhoven, and Antje Waddington, were responsible for the typing. Jonathan Harrow translated several of the texts into English and gave us native speaker advice. Andreas Schale took care of the text processing and mounted the tables and figures. We thank them all for their help and also the German Research Association for its financial support.

The Editors

Contents

Part One

Diagnosis and Classification of Children with Behavioral Disorders and Handicaps

Epidemiology and Classification of Psychiatric Disorders in Childhood and Adolescence

Helmut Remschmidt

1. Introduction: Classification and Epidemiology

The aim of epidemiology is the study of the distribution of disorders in a population, "together with an examination of how the distribution varies with particular environmental or other circumstances" (Rutter, 1983). The usual way to carry out epidemiological studies is to count individuals with more or less clearly defined disorders and to look at all conditions which are statistically associated with the disorders in view.

Classification is a sorting process with the main principle of putting together objects, disorders, conditions, or relationships which have some traits in common but differ with respect to others. Classification of psychiatric disorders has always the goal of differentiating psychiatric conditions from each other according to defined criteria which always take into account similarity and dissimilarity of the object of classification. One way in which classification always progresses is to bring the objects, disorders, or behaviors which should be classified into a system. At the moment, two classification systems have been used widely: ICD–9, in child psychiatry in a multiaxial framework (Rutter et al., 1975; Remschmidt and Schmidt, 1986) and DSM–III (APA, 1980).

From these considerations, it is quite clear that epidemiological studies are not possible without valid and reliable classification systems, and the development of classification systems is not possible without epidemiology, which means the study of the distribution of disorders in different populations.

2. Classification: Methodological Problems and Results

During the last 15 years, many child psychiatrists and psychologists have become interested in the classification of psychiatric disorders in children and adolescents. In former times, there were a lot of reservations against all endeavors in the field of classification. People were afraid that individuality and specific and typical personality traits could disappear through the process of defining criteria and establishing rules for the diagnostic procedure. Several misunderstandings lay behind such opinions, one of the most important being that persons would be classified instead of disorders (or conditions).

Meanwhile, the question is no longer *if* classification is necessary and useful, but *how* classification should be made, and by what means the well-known classification systems can be improved.

2.1 Necessity of Classification

There are a lot of arguments for the necessity of classification. These arguments are important for very different scientific fields. In child psychiatry, classification of disorders is necessary for several reasons:

1. Progress in understanding psychiatric disorders to a great extent depends on the ability to differentiate behavior according to important categories (such as symptomatology, similarity, and dissimilarity of symptoms, age, developmental stage, etc.). Insofar, classification is a general requirement of all sciences.
2. Different disorders require different diagnostic procedures and different treatments.
3. A meaningful discussion between child psychiatrists from different countries is only possible if they have a clearly defined terminology.

2.2   Criteria for an Adequate Classification System

The criteria for an adequate classification of child psychiatric disorders have been summarized by Rutter (1965, 1977, 1985):

1. The classification must be based on facts and not on concepts, and it must be defined in operational terms.

2. The aim is to classify disorders or problems and not to classify children or adolescents as persons.

3. According to the development of children, "there should not be different classifications for different age periods, although there must be provision for disorders which arise only at a particular age".

4. The classification must be reliable, meaning that terms are used in the same way by different clinicians.

5. The classification must provide an adequate differentiation between disorders.

6. The classification must provide an adequate coverage so that important disorders are not omitted.

7. The differentiation should have a validity.

8. There should be logical consistency so that the system is based on a constant set of principles with a clear-cut set of precise rules.

9. The classification must convey information which is relevant to the clinical situation and which helps to make clinical decisions.

10. The classification must be practicable in ordinary clinical work.

For several years now, different child psychiatric classification systems have been used all over the world. There is a huge body of experience in the field of classification of child psychiatric disorders, and these endeavors have also stimulated progress in child psychiatry in several fields, for example, epidemiology, diagnostics, therapy, prevention, and rehabilitation.

2.3   Some Methodological Problems

Nevertheless, there are some methodological problems which should be mentioned in this context.

1. Problems of sampling: Empirically derived classification systems depend on samples of individuals and their disorders. In this field, errors are, of course, possible. An adequate classification system must be able to introduce disorders from several different samples, for instance, from clinical studies and epidemiological studies. In this connection, we have the problem of a "spectrum of psychopathology", reaching from doubtless psychopathological

states on to normality. Many studies have in this respect the problem of defining clearly the cut–off point that divides cases from normality or the "borderline field".

2. Selection of key variables (marker variables): Important for an adequate classification of psychiatric disorders in the selection of key variables that are typical for the disorder discussed. A good example for this problem is the hyperkinetic syndrome. There are different opinions as to whether hyperactivity, attention deficit, or impulsivity should be looked upon as the "key symptom". These differences are recognized in the classification of DSM–III. The system differentiates between attention deficit disorder with hyperactivity (314.01) and attention deficit disorders without hyperactivity (314.00) and distinguishes a third category: attention deficit disorders, residual type (314.80). In contrast, the multiaxial system, based on ICD–9, distinguishes the hyperactive syndrome with disturbance of activity and attention (314.0) from hyperkinesis with developmental delay (314.1) and hyperkinetic conduct disorders (314.2).

3. Complexity of the disorder: Classification systems always include disorders which differ according to their complexity. Classifications can be made on the level of symptoms or syndromes which may have different correlations with each other.

4. Etiology: The best classification system should be based on a clear etiology of the disorder. However, the history of classification systems shows that the aspect of etiology is no longer the central point of discussion. Several reasons are responsible for this development: On the one hand, the etiology of many child psychiatric disorders is not yet clear; on the other hand, there are only a few cases in which the etiology concerns only one factor. Most psychiatric disorders in children and adolescents are multifactorial in origin. The exclusion of etiological aspects, however, does not mean that etiology is not important. But it facilitates a discussion which is not overloaded by theoretical preoccupations.

5. Stability and change of psychopathological conditions: Another question concerns stability and change of psychopathological conditions over time, in at least two respects: (1) during the course of the development of the

individual child (individual perspective), or (2) over the centuries in relation to family, social, and cultural circumstances.

The perspective of individual development is, as we all know, included in the multiaxial system (ICD–9) and in DSM-III. The classification of psychosocial circumstances is included in the multiaxial system (5th axis), and there is a new proposal for the next version on the way.

6. Theoretical background of classification systems: The use of carefully defined and empirically based categories is substantial for all effective classification systems and a good basis for mutual understanding of child psychiatrists all over the world. But we also have to ask which theory lies behind the systems we are using. Is it possible to have classification systems without a theory, or at least, with a minimum of theoretical implications? There are a lot of problems in this respect, and I cannot go into details here. But let me mention two examples: Is it favorable to give up the concept of neurosis as has been done in DSM-III? Neurosis is, of course, a concept with many and different theories behind it. Is it useful and empirically based to create a new heading category called "pervasive developmental disorders", as has been done in DSM-III? What was the theory behind this? It may also be a danger to define holistic categories too quickly for very different conditions which have only a few features in common. If we do this, we might arrive at a more superficial thinking, leaving out the context and different etiologies.

7. Nosological entities to be classified: Another question has to do with the entities to be classified. Usually, we take into consideration the *individual* symptoms or characteristic features of the condition restricted to a disorder as manifested in a certain individual. But what about the *relationships* of this individual? Are they part of the condition or not? Should they be classified on an own axis? How stable are they? Can they be an important constituent of the diagnosis and classification? Of course, there are conditions such as school phobia which can be defined in terms of relationships, but does this model apply to all or to many other conditions?

This question, namely the classification of relationships, was a main topic of a symposium we had last year at the congress of the International Associa-

tion for Child and Adolescent Psychiatry in Paris, and there is a study
group working out a special proposal.

8. Classification and the body of knowledge: Finally, classification always
   depends on the body of knowledge concerning psychopathological conditions. If this knowledge becomes richer, it must have an influence on the
   definitions used and the rules for the classification process.

2.4   Different Systems of Classification

Classification systems in child psychiatry may be subdivided according to three
categories: one-dimensional systems, multiaxial systems of clinical origin, and
multidimensional classification systems resulting from statistical procedures.

One-dimensional systems

Examples for these systems are the International Classification of Diseases Nos.
8 and 9. In ICD-8 there were no special categories for child psychiatry. Insofar, this system was not adequate for the classification of psychiatric disorders
in children and adolescents. ICD-9 brought a remarkable progress concerning
several aspects: The classification of depression was better and more differentiated. Several child psychiatric disorders were included: typical psychosis of
childhood (ICD 299), disturbances of emotions specific to childhood and adolescence (ICD 313), hyperkinetic syndrome of childhood (ICD 314), specific
delays in development (ICD 315), adjustment reaction (ICD 109), and the not
very convincing category "special symptoms or syndromes not elsewhere classified" (ICD 307).

Nevertheless, the original ICD-9 system is a classification system for adults and
not for children.

Multiaxial classification systems of clinical origin

For many years now, it has been evident that one-dimensional classifications in
child psychiatry imply a very narrow approach to the process of diagnostics.
All clinicians know how important developmental factors, intelligence, and
psychosocial circumstances are for the clinical picture of child psychiatric

disorders. Bearing in mind these arguments, an international group under the chairmanship of Michael Rutter began to classify child psychiatric disorders in terms of a multiaxial approach. Meanwhile, there exists as an American counterpart the DSM–III which also uses a multiaxial approach and which is also derived from clinical experience. According to Spitzer (1980) and Cantwell (1980), the advances of DSM–III can be seen in the following aspects: (1) a good definition and description of psychiatric disorders; (2) a descriptive approach which is free from etiological preoccupations; (3) a comprehensive and systematic description of every disorder; (4) in the existence of standardized diagnostic criteria; and (5) in the multiaxial approach.

Both multiaxial systems have brought an important advance in the whole field of classification, and both systems have, of course, also weak points. One of them is, for instance, Category 307 (special symptoms or syndromes not elsewhere classified) which comprises such heterogeneous disturbances as stammering, anorexia nervosa, tics, stereotyped repetitive movements, specific sleep disorders, enuresis, encopresis, and psychalgia. A weak point of the DSM–III system is the absence of a special axis for intelligence factors. For other points of criticism, see Rutter and Shaffer (1980).

There are evaluation studies on both the multiaxial system and DSM–III. The results are very similar. They show that the agreement of experts in classifying global categories is fairly good, whereas the agreement diminishes when special subgroups have to be classified. On the whole, both systems can be looked upon as important steps in the direction of an empirically derived development of classification systems in child psychiatry.

Multidimensional classification systems derived from statistical procedures
Several attempts have been made to classify behavior disorders or behavior problems according to the results of multivariate statistical procedures. Most of these investigations are based on rating scales or on questionnaires concerning symptomatology of children. Within the procedure of classification, statistical methods such as factor analysis, cluster analysis, and discriminant analysis are used. Reviews concerning this approach to classifications were given by Quay (1979) and Achenbach (1980). The reviews derived from multivariate statistical approaches to classification come to very similar results which lead to the following dimensions of behavior (according to Quay, 1979): (1) Conduct

disorders, (2) symptoms of anxiety and withdrawal, (3) syndromes of immaturity, (4) socialized–aggressive disorders, (5) psychotic syndromes and autism, (6) syndromes of hyperactivity and hyperkinesis.

There is considerable evidence for the cross–cultural generality of conduct disorders and anxiety–withdrawal symptoms, whereas the generality of immaturity syndromes and socialized–aggressive disorders is less certain (Quay, 1979).

A comparison of these "dimensions of behavior" with the categories of the multiaxial system and DSM–III shows that both multiaxial classification systems derived from clinical experience do not cover all the behavior dimensions obtained with the statistical approach. It will be an important task for all research in the field of classification to bring together the results of these different methodological approaches. They differ not only concerning data collection, but also very often concerning sampling.

2.5   Training to Use Classification Systems

Some time ago, we carried out an evaluation study of the multiaxial classification system which at the same time aimed to evaluate the "training effect" of the system (Remschmidt et al., 1983). Twenty–one child psychiatrists with different lengths of experience in the field of child psychiatry had to classify 28 cases in two sessions with a 5–month training phase between the two sessions. The first session was without the use of the glossary, the training phase included the use of the glossary, and during the second session, the use of the glossary (which had been trained during the 5 months) was allowed. On the level of symptomatology, there was a high interrater agreement (of more than .85) concerning more "objective" items (e.g., encopresis, enuresis, drug abuse, delinquency, sexual deviations). The interrater agreement was lower with respect to items of a more subjective character (.34 – .38). The average agreement of the experts concerning the classification of the cases on the 1st axis was low (42,4%), and there was no substantial progress at the second session. But there were enormous differences with reference to different cases. For instance, there was a very high agreement (more than 90%) for a case of hyperkinetic syndrome and a very low agreement between experts concerning a case of a child with disintegrative psychosis. The reduction of the complexity of the classification process using only 3–digit ICD–codings led to a better interrater agreement. The scores were 53,5% in the first, and 62,6% during the second session. There were also remarkable differences in relation to different diagnoses with respect to this procedure.

Effect of the glossary: On the whole, the glossary had the effect of reducing the number of problem codings between the first and the second trial. A very interesting result concerning the glossary is the relationship between length of clinical practice in child psychiatry and a special rater score which is a measure of the adequacy of an expert's ratings. This rater score can be looked upon as a measure of the quality of the ratings. It was derived in the following way: The sum of the frequencies of all diagnoses was divided by the number of classified cases, the first case being doubled.

We found a low positive correlation before the knowledge of the glossary and a high negative correlation of the rater score with the length of clinical practice *after* the knowledge of the glossary.

There was a very clear difference between the first and the second session for the experts with a shorter clinical experience, which was not true for those with long (more than 6 years) clinical experience. These results show that there is a very good learning effect for those colleagues with a shorter length of clinical experience. This result applies to the 4–digit as well as to the 3–digit classification.

2.6 Continuities and Discontinuities, Stability, and Change of Diagnoses

Both epidemiology and classification have to face two other important facts:

1. Psychiatric disorders and age or developmental stage

Though there are different types of psychiatric disorders in children and adolescents, the same classification system should be used for the different age groups and different developmental stages (which are not the same).

We can distinguish at least three types of psychiatric disorders from childhood to adolescence and adulthood.

Type A: persistent disorders were described first by Rutter et al. (1970) as a result of the Isle-of-Wight Studies. They begin before the age of 10 years, occur predominantly in boys (sex ratio 2.1:1), and show a continuous course through adolescence to adulthood. To this type of disorder belong antisocial disturbances, personality disorders, some kinds of neuroses, and some cases of school phobia and depression.

Type B is very strongly characterized by developmental factors and by a reduction in frequency from childhood to adulthood. To this category belong some functional disorders such as enuresis, encopresis, hyperactivity, tics, one portion of the children usually called MCD-children, and also some neurotic reactions, especially animal phobias. These disorders usually come to an end during adolescence, and there is no continuity into adulthood. We can also call them nonpersistent psychiatric disorders.

Type C (new disorders) begin during adolescence in which they have their first manifestation. There are different opinions why their first manifestation lies in the phase of adolescence: Probably, the adolescent is − for the first time in his life − in a position to express his symptoms. On the other hand, it might be possible that, favored by biological and also by exogenous influences, genetic manifestations gain dominance. To this type of disorder belong depressive syndromes, compulsions, anorexia nervosa and bulimia nervosa, schizophrenia, and manic-depressive psychoses. These disorders with new manifestation during adolescence can clearly be differentiated from those of the persistent type (Rutter et al., 1970) because: (1) they occur more frequently in girls, (2) they show no connection with developmental delays or problems of education, and (3) they are not associated with family adversity or with a pathological family situation.

Finally, these disturbances show a very similar symptomatology to psychiatric disorders of adulthood. Concerning the sex relation, there occurs a change during puberty with a predominance of neurotic and depressive disorders and also adaptation reactions in girls, which is not true for schizophrenia.

2. Stability and change of diagnoses and the frequency of occurence

From the above-mentioned results, it is quite clear that psychiatric disorders in children and adolescents do not follow the same course from childhood to adolescence and adulthood. There may be changes of diagnoses over time and also different frequencies of occurence. To give two examples:

First, reading, writing, and spelling disorders are diagnoses that are made during childhood and, at the same time, show a very strong relationship to other psychiatric disorders in adolescence and adulthood. They are more frequent in boys than in girls and have a very strong relationship to antisocial behavior during adolescence and adulthood.

Second, the hyperkinetic syndrome, a typical diagnosis of early and middle childhood, shows a persistence in 40% of cases, whereas an improvement can be stated in 60%.

Coming back to the above-mentioned types, the majority belong to Type B, and 50% to Type A (persistent disorders). For those children in whom the symptomatology persists, there is a high risk of developing other psychiatric disorders in adolescence and adulthood (antisocial behavior, delinquency, drug dependency, and alcoholism).

Third, some disorders have become more frequent during the last decade, some less frequent. A good example for the first type are anorexia nervosa and bulimia. These syndromes show a remarkable rise in frequency in all Western civilized countries which is not true for the Far East, China, the Arabic world, and Eastern European countries.

3. Epidemiology: Methodological Problems and Results

3.1   Sampling: Field Samples and Clinical Samples

It is an aim of epidemiological studies to answer causal questions. But in many cases these studies are only able to establish statistical associations which cannot reach the level of causal relationships. Many people think that the only possible answer to causal questions lies in field samples. This is not true. Which sample you use depends on the question you have. Field samples, for instance, are appropriate to study the distribution of certain behaviors close to normality or disturbances of a certain severity but not calling for clinical help. Clinical samples, on the other hand, can answer questions in severe disorders, for instance, in schizophrenia or very severe anorexia nervosa. These conditions always come to a clinical institution if they reach a certain degree of severity. So field samples and clinical samples have mutual advantages and disadvantages. Further, there may be conditions which are important in field samples and not in clinical samples. A good example is the relationship of the family adversity index with psychiatric disturbances. In field samples, there is a strong relationship between the family adversity index and the degree of psychopathology. This is not true for clinical samples because clinical samples as such show a high degree of family adversity, and the relationship between a family adversity index and psychopathology is not established.

According to Rutter (1983), there are further misconceptions concerning epidemiological studies.

1. In order to give an epidemiological answer to causal questions, it is not necessary to carry out studies in the general population. It is sometimes more helpful to find special risk populations and to study the relevant questions in this special group.

2. Epidemiological answers do not per se lie in the study of very large numbers. It is sometimes better to study a smaller population which has been carefully selected with respect to a special question.

3. The power of epidemiological studies does *not* lie in the use of cross-sectional data. The most powerful results can be derived from longitudinal data, because stability as well as change are fundamental elements in psychiatric disorders, and you always have to check which influences are continuous and which are more prone to change in this continuity.

4. The strength of the epidemiological research strategy does not lie in "natural

situations" either. Epidemiological studies can successfully be combined with experimental and quasi-experimental designs.

5. Finally, psychiatric epidemiology is not restricted to the study of psychosocial factors as causal elements. It is very important to include data from different fields (e.g., biological factors, genetic dispositions, psychological factors, and also psychosocial influences).

3.2   Some Results in a Complete Clinical Population

Bearing in mind these methodological issues, I shall now present some results of an epidemiological cross-sectional study in a complete clinical population from three counties in the state of Hessen, covering a total population of 574,000 inhabitants. We were able to study all patients who came to clinical outpatient and inpatient institutions from July 1st, 1983 to June 30th, 1984. It was also possible to include the data of those patients who sought help outside of the three counties but who were living within these districts, by looking through the data of the relevant institutions outside of the three counties (districts). All patients had been documented according to the multiaxial classification system, and 62 outpatient institutions (among them 31 outside the model region), 4 child psychiatric inpatient units, and 4 institutions in the field of rehabilitation cooperated in this project. The project was supported by the federal government and the government of the state of Hessen over a period of 5 years.

Some general results of the study

The incidence Figures differed between the county of Marburg–Biedenkopf (283,000 inhabitants) and the neighboring counties of Waldeck–Frankenberg (155,000 inhabitants) and Schwalm–Eder–Kreis (181,000 inhabitants). The highest incidence was in Marburg–Biedenkopf (Fig. 1).

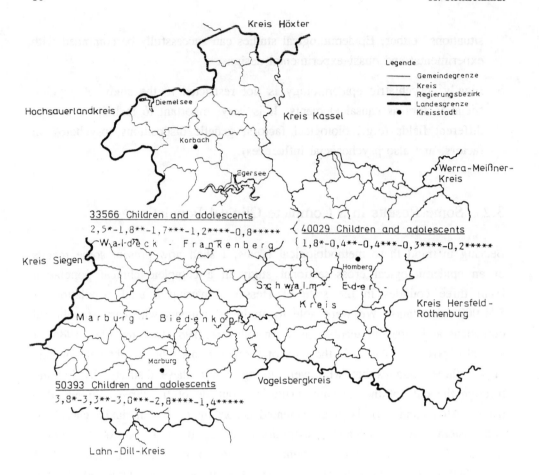

Notes

*   Users (children and adolescents) of the three counties, documentated in all institutions, coming from the three counties or from other regions outside

**   Outpatient users (children and adolescents) living inside the three counties

***   same as **, but special selection: disturbances on Axes 1, 2, and 4 or free description of psychiatric symptomes

****   same as **, but special selection: disturbances on Axes 1, 2, and 4

*****   same as **, but special selection: only disturbances on the 1st axis of the MAS (MAS = Multiaxial classification scheme for psychiatric disorders in childhood and adolescence)

Fig. 1:   Frequency of children and adolescents treated as outpatients as a percentage of the total population under 18 years

There were also remarkable differences concerning the inpatient treatment Figures. In Marburg– Biedenkopf, 15.5 patients per 10,000 inhabitants under 18 years had been treated in the inpatient units as compared to 11.3 and 7.5 in the neighboring counties. There was also a very high correlation between access to outpatient facilities and the duration of inpatient treatment. In regions with effective outpatient treatment facilities, the duration of inpatient treatment was about half as long compared to regions without effective outpatient facilities. The duration of inpatient treatment was at the same time also a function of distance. Patients from distant regions had to stay far longer in hospitals as inpatients than local patients.

Sex differences

We found the already established predominance of the male sex until puberty for several psychiatric disorders such as hyperkinetic syndrome, MCD, dyslexia, and conduct disturbances.

The relationship between conduct disturbances and neuroses or emotional disorders for boys and girls is shown in Fig. 2; the relationship between conduct disturbances and neuroses for social class in Fig. 3.

Concerning psychoses, there are no sex differences except the typical psychoses of childhood which are significantly more frequent in boys than in girls. These typical psychoses of childhood (autism and similar disturbances) do not change into adolescent or adult schizophrenia.

Clinical psychiatric syndrome

It is not possible to give all the results in detail here. I shall restrict myself to the global categories of neuroses and psychoses. Neurotic disturbances and emotional disorders are, as shown already, dependent on social class and intelligence. Fig. 3 shows their predominance in the higher social classes as well as their relationship to intelligence factors. The opposite picture can be shown for psychoses. There is a relationship to intelligence, but not to social class in our sample.

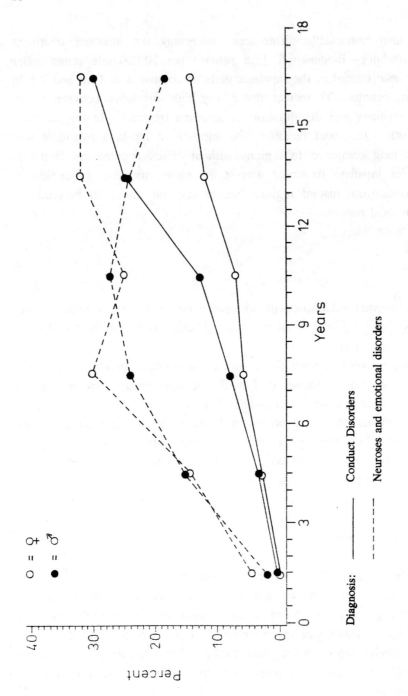

Fig. 2: Age- and sex distribution of conduct disorders and of neuroses and emotional disturbances in a total clinical population of children and adolescents from three counties

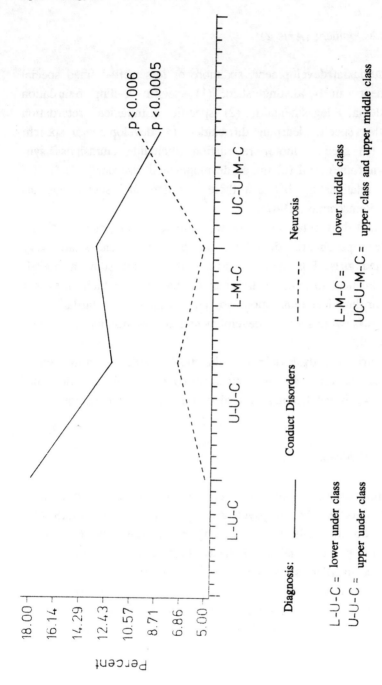

Fig. 3: Relationship between conduct disturbances and neuroses (and emotional disturbances) and social class in a total clinical population of children and adolescents

Specific delays in development (Axis 2)

According to the multiaxial development, six more or less well–defined special delays in development can be distinguished: (1) specific reading retardation (developmental dyslexia, "legasthenia"), (2) specific arithmetical retardation (dyscalculia), (3) other specific learning difficulties, (4) developmental speech/language disorder, (5) specific motor retardation (including clumsiness syndrome, dyspraxia syndrome), and (6) mixed developmental disorder.

There are different relationships between these disorders and social class as well as intelligence (Remschmidt, 1987).

There is a well–established relationship between these developmental disturbances and secondary psychiatric disorders, but the consequences are very different for boys and girls. For instance, boys with dyslexia show a statistically significant inclination to react with conduct disorders, which does not apply to boys with arithmetical retardation, speech and language retardation, or motor retardation. Girls with specific developmental delays do not react with conduct disorders at all.

On the other hand, girls with dyslexia and arithmetical retardation show significantly more emotional disorders and neurotic disturbances, while this does not apply to those with speech and language retardation and motor retardation.

Abnormal psychosocial situations

Fig. 4 shows the relationship between frequency of associated abnormal psychosocial situations and the clinical psychiatric syndrome of the MAS (1st Axis). Children who do not suffer from a psychiatric disorder have the lowest proportion of abnormal psychosocial situations in their families, whereas those suffering from conduct disorders show the highest proportion.

These results from a total clinical population do not definitely answer causal questions, but they can be used to stimulate special studies and also serve as a basis for longitudinal cohort studies which are already being carried out.

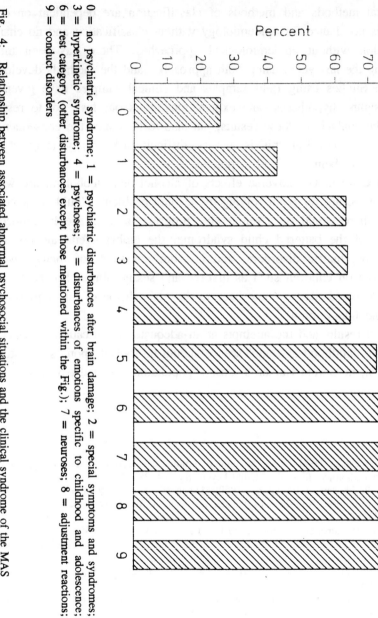

Fig. 4: Relationship between associated abnormal psychosocial situations and the clinical syndrome of the MAS

0 = no psychiatric syndrome; 1 = psychiatric disturbances after brain damage; 2 = special symptoms and syndromes; 3 = hyperkinetic syndrome; 4 = psychoses; 5 = disturbances of emotions specific to childhood and adolescence; 6 = rest category (other disturbances except those mentioned within the Fig.); 7 = neuroses; 8 = adjustment reactions; 9 = conduct disorders

4. Conclusions

Epidemiological methods and methods of classification are dependent on each other. There is no chance for epidemiology without classification and no chance for classification without epidemiological approaches. There has been much progress during the last years using both approaches and the methods developed in both areas. Studies using field samples and clinical samples have given us many new insights, hypotheses, and explanations. It is our task not to restrict ourselves to the analysis of these results, but also to introduce the consequences into everyday practice. But this is a very difficult task. Many insights and results are far from being realized in practice.

To give one example: The adverse effects of alcohol and alcoholism are well-established, but we are far from solving the alcohol problem. Could we succeed in doing this, there would be a remarkable progress in many fields: reduction of criminality, of the battered child syndrome, the embryo–fetal alcohol syndrome, many psychiatric disorders, and last but not least, of many adverse family influences on children such as divorce and sexual abuse. So, at the end of my paper, I would like to come back to the main theme of our symposium: "Prevention and Intervention".

Epidemiological results and the attempts at an adequate classification of psychiatric disorders in childhood and adolescence should be looked upon as milestones on the way to a, in Gerald Caplan's sense, "population–oriented psychiatry".

References

Achenbach, T.M. (1980): DSM–III in the light of empirical research on the classification of child psychopathology. Journal of Child Psychiatry, 19, 395–412.
APA (American Psychiatric Association) (1980): Diagnostic and statistical manual of mental disorders, 3rd edition. American Psychiatric Association, Washington DC.
Cantwell, D.P. (1980): The diagnostic process and diagnostic classification in child psychiatry – DSM–III. Introduction. Journal of Child Psychiatry, 19, 345–355.
Quay, H.C. (1979): Classification. In Quay, H.C., and Werry, J.S. (Eds.): Psychopathological disorders of childhood, 2nd edition. New York: Wiley & Sons.
Remschmidt, H. (1987): Was sind Teilleistungsschwächen? Monatsschrift für Kinderheilkunde, 135, 290–296.
Remschmidt, H., and Schmidt, M.H. (Eds.) (1986): Multiaxiales Klassifikationsschema für psychiatrische Erkrankungen im Kindes– und Jugendalter nach Rutter, Shaffer und Sturge, 2nd edition. Bern-Stuttgart-Toronto: Huber.

Remschmidt, H., Schmidt, M.H., and Göbel, D. (1983): Erprobungs- und Reliabilitätsstudie zum multiaxialen Klassifikationsschema für psychiatrische Erkrankungen im Kindes- und Jugendalter. In Remschmidt, H., and Schmidt, M.G. (Eds.): Multiaxiale Diagnostik in der Kinder- und Jugendpsychiatrie. Ergebnisse empirischer Untersuchungen. Bern–Stuttgart–Wien: Huber.

Rutter, M. (1965): Classification and categorization in child psychiatry. Journal of Child Psychology and Psychiatry, 6, 71–83.

Rutter, M. (1977): Classification. In Rutter, M., and Hersov, L. (Eds.): Child psychiatry. Oxford: Blackwell Scientific Publications.

Rutter, M. (1983): Epidemiological–longitudinal approaches to the study of development. In Schmidt, M.G., and Remschmidt, H. (Eds.): Epidemiological approaches in child psychiatry II. Stuttgart–New York: Thieme.

Rutter, M. (1985): Resilience in the face of adversity. Protective factors and resistence to psychiatric disorder. The British Journal of Psychiatry, 147, 598–611.

Rutter, M., and Shaffer, D. (1980): DSM-III. A step forward or back in terms of the classification of child psychiatric disorders? Journal of the American Academy for Child and Adolescent Psychiatry, 19, 371–394.

Rutter, M.L., Shaffer, D., and Sturge, C. (1975): A guide to a multi-axial classification scheme for psychiatric disorders in childhood and adolescence. London: Dept. of Child and Adolescent Psychiatry, Institute of Psychiatry.

Rutter, M., Tizard, J., and Whitmore, K. (1970): Education, health, and behavior. London: Longman.

Rutter, M., Tizard, J., Yule, W., Graham, P., and Whitmore, K. (1977): Epidemiologie in der Kinderpsychiatrie – die Isle of Wight Studien 1964–1974. Zeitschrift für Kinder- und Jugendpsychiatrie, 5, 238–279.

Spitzer, R.L. (1980): Classification of mental disorders and DSM-III. In Kaplan, H.J., Freedman, A.M., and Sadock, B.J. (Eds.): Comprehensive textbook of psychiatry. Baltimore: Williams & Wilkins.

Empirically Based Assessment of Child and Adolescent Disorders: Implications for Diagnosis, Classification, Epidemiology, and Longitudinal Research

Thomas M. Achenbach

1. Introduction

The basic diagnostic concepts for adult psychiatric disorders were established in the 19th century. In 1883, Emil Kraepelin assembled them into a classification system that continues to shape nosologies such as the World Health Organization's (1978) International Classification of Disease (ICD–9) and the American Psychiatric Association's Diagnostic and Statistical Manual (the DSM). Diagnostic categories for children's disorders are much more recent, however. Until 1968, the DSM offered only two categories specifically for childhood disorders. These were adjustment reaction of childhood and childhood schizophrenia. Since then, the second and third editions of the DSM — DSM–II and DSM–III — have added numerous new categories for childhood disorders. Yet, these categories are based neither on a lengthy clinical tradition nor on research diagnostic criteria such as those underlying some of the DSM's categories of adult disorders. The childhood categories are still quite tentative, reflecting a struggle to find better ways of thinking about childhood disorders.

Better methods for describing and grouping childhood disorders are needed to advance all aspects of efforts to help troubled children, including the identification of children in need of help, decisions about interventions, communication about individual cases, the training of professionals, and research on etiology, prognosis, and the efficacy of treatment.

Without a clear picture of children's problems, it is difficult to identify etiologies or to determine whether a child is improving or getting worse.

2. Empirically Based Assessment

To provide a more standardized basis for assessing children's problems and competencies, we have developed a general approach that we call empirically based assessment. I realize that the term "empirical" sometimes has a pejorative connotation, because it implies trial-and-error treatment that is not based on systematic theory or knowledge of underlying causes. However, because we know so little about the specific causes of most childhood disorders, it is seldom possible to diagnose or treat them in terms of underlying causes. Even when we know that there is an organic abnormality such as brain damage, it is unlikely to explain many aspects of a child's functioning. Instead, helping the child requires a detailed picture of how the child functions in various contexts, such as home and school. To find out how the child functions in these contexts, we need reports from people such as parents, teachers, observers, and the children themselves.

Our approach to assessment is empirical, *not* in the sense of being trial-and-error, but in the sense of being based on empirical data. The word "empirical" stems from the Greek word "empeiria", meaning experience. It is the experience of the people most involved with the child that we try to tap. Because children's behavior varies from one context and interaction partner to another, no one source of data can tell the whole story. Instead, we believe that it is essential to obtain standardized data from several sources. Even though there may be discrepancies between the different sources, these discrepancies can be as informative as agreements among them.

Multiaxial concepts offer useful guides to capturing the multifaceted nature of children's functioning. Both ICD-9 and DSM-III feature multiple axes. However, we think of the assessment process itself in terms of multiple axes that represent different types and sources of data on children. Tab. 1 illustrates the concept of multiaxial assessment. The five axes here include parent data, teacher data, data on cognitive functioning obtained by standardized tests, biomedical data, and data obtained through direct assessment of the child. The specific assessment procedures would vary with the age of the child, but these are some examples. I will discuss some of the procedures we have developed for obtaining data from parents, teachers, and self-reports.

Tab. 1:   Examples of Multiaxial Assessment (from Achenbach and McConaughy, 1987)

Age Range	Axis I Parent Reports	Axis II Teacher Reports	Axis III Cognitive Assessment	Axis IV Physical Assessment	Axis V Direct Assessment of Child
0-2	Minnesota Child Development Inventory (Ireton & Thwing, 1974) Developmental history Parent interview		Developmental testing e.g., Bayley (1969) Infant Scales	Height, weight Medical exam Neurological exam	Observations during developmental testing
2-5	Child Behavior Checklist (CBCL) Developmental history Parent interview	School records Teacher interview	Intelligence tests, e.g., McCarthy (1972) Scales of Children's Ability Perceptual-motor tests Speech and language tests	Height, weight Medical exam Neurological exam	Observations during play interview (DOF) Direct Observation Form
6-11	CBCL Developmental history Parent interview	Teacher's Report Form (TRF) School records Teacher interview	Intelligence tests e.g., WISC-R (Wechsler, 1974) Achievement tests Perceptual-motor tests Speech and language tests	Height, weight Medical exam Neurological exam	DOF Semistructured Clinical Interview for Children (SCIC) SCIC-Observation Form SCIC-Self Report Form
12-18	CBCL Developmental history Parent interview	TRF School records Teacher interview	Intelligence tests, e.g., WISC-R, WAIS-R (Wechsler, 1981) Achievement tests Speech and language tests	Height, weight Medical exam Neurological exam	Youth Self-Report (YSR) Clinical interview Self-concept measures Personality tests

3. Parents' Reports

We started with parents, because parents' perceptions are typically crucial in determining what will be done about children's problems, and parents' reports must be obtained in the evaluation and treatment of nearly all children referred for mental health services.

Based on a survey of instruments for obtaining data on behavioral and emotional problems and extensive pilot testing in clinical settings, we developed the Child Behavior Checklist, which is designed to obtain parents' reports of their children's problems and competencies in a standardized format.

The checklist and related materials are described in detail by Achenbach and Edelbrock (1983). Briefly, the first two pages of the checklist consist of competence items, including parents' reports of their child's participation in activities and social relationships, plus school performance and problems. Pages 3 and 4 of the checklist consist of 118 specific problem items, plus open-ended items for describing additional problems. The parents score 0 for each item that is not true of their child, 1 for each item that is somewhat or sometimes true, and 2 for each item that is very true or often true.

4. The Child Behavior Profile

In order to score the Checklist in a way that reflects age and sex variations in behavior and that provides a well-differentiated picture of problems and competencies, we have constructed different forms of what we call the Child Behavior Profile. I will describe the profiles derived from the Checklist for 4- to 16-year-olds, but there is also a version of the checklist for 2- to 3-year-olds (Achenbach, Edelbrock, and Howell, 1987). The various forms of the Profile are standardized separately for each sex at ages 4 to 5, 6 to 11, and 12 to 16. These particular age ranges were chosen because they demarcate significant changes in cognitive and emotional functioning, social and educational status, and physical development. The social competence scales are scored in a uniform fashion for all forms of the Profile but are normed separately for each form, so that, for each scale, a child is compared with normal peers of his or her sex and age group. The norms are based on data obtained in a home interview survey of 1,300 randomly selected parents of normal children.

Unlike the social competence scales, the problem scales of the Profile are empirically derived from factor analyses of Checklists filled out by parents of children referred for mental health services. In order to detect syndromes of problems actually occurring for each sex within each age range, we have done separate factor analyses for children grouped by sex and age. For example, problems reported for boys aged 6 to 11 were factor analyzed separately from problems reported for the other groups. Syndromes of problems found to be reliable for a particular age and sex provided the basis for the behavior problem scales for that group. We performed the factor analyses on clinical samples because they afford greater differentiation of behavior problem patterns than would be obtained from normal samples, in which the absence of extremely deviant behavior would preclude detection of clinically significant syndromes. However, once we formulated problem scales reflecting the syndromes of problems for a particular group, we computed norms for these scales on the same nonclinical samples as are used to norm the social competence scales.

To provide a picture of the Profile in concrete form, Fig. 1 shows a computer scored version of the social competence portion of the profile for boys aged 6 through 11. Hand-scored versions are also available. The portion shown in Fig. 1 consists of the social competence scales and a graphic display that enables you to compare the boy's score on each scale with scores obtained by 300 normal 6- to 11-year-old boys. The first social competence scale, entitled Activities, includes the amount and quality of participation in sports and non-sporting hobbies and activities, plus jobs and chores. The second scale, entitled Social, includes participation in organizations, number of friends, frequency of contacts with them, how well the boy gets along with others, and how well he plays and works by himself. The third scale reflects school performance and problems. A score for each of the social competence items on the checklist is entered in the appropriate column, the scores are summed, and the number corresponding to the sum is marked in the graphic display in order to draw a profile. To the left of the graphic display are percentiles that enable you to compare the boy with normal boys of the same age.

The second portion of the Profile, shown in Fig. 2, lists in abbreviated form all the items of the behavior problem scales for 6– through 11–year-old boys, plus items that did not correlate highly with any of the syndromes on which the scales are based. Scores for each behavior problem on a boy's Checklist are entered in the appropriate columns beneath the graphic display. The scores in each column are then summed, and the corresponding score is marked in the graphic display. The graphic display enables you to compare the boy's score on each scale with scores obtained by normal 6– through 11–year-old boys in the same general format as the social competence scales. However, because *low* social competence scores are clinically significant, the *low* ends of the social competence scales are more finely differentiated, whereas the *top* ends of the problem scales are more differentiated.

The Profile provides an overview of competencies and problems reported by a parent, shows whether they are concentrated in particular areas, and compares the child with normal children of the same age in each area. The data thus provided can be used as a take–off point for interviewing the parents and child, as well as a baseline against which to evaluate subsequent changes in behavior.

In each of the sex and age groups for whom we have staldardized profiles for this Checklist, we have found either 8 or 9 factors that were reliable enough to be retained as bases for problem scales. The names of the scales for each group are listed in Tab. 2. These scale names are intended merely as short-hand descriptions of the problems comprising the scales. They are not intended to be diagnostic labels. For example, a high score on the Schizoid scale is not necessarily intended to argue for a diagnosis of schizoid personality or schi-zophrenia. It should be remembered that the Profile is intended to *aid* rather than to *substitute for* a complete evaluation, which should include investigation of organic and cognitive functioning, possible etiological factors, family dynam-ics, and the feasibility of various interventions.

THE CHILD BEHAVIOR PROFILE, REVISED EDITION - PARENT'S REPORT VERSION
PARENT-REPORTED SOCIAL COMPETENCE - BOYS AGED 6-11

T SCORE

I-55
I-FORM FILLED
I- OUT ON: 05/05/86
I-50
I- CASE # F60760
I-45
I- BOY
I- AGE 11
I-40 CARD #01
I-
FILLED OUT BY:
I-35 —→MOTHER
      FATHER
      OTHER
I-30 MISSING
I-
I-25 TOTAL   9.5
I-20 TOTAL T 25
I-
I-15
I-
I-10

%ILE
69 -I
  -I
  -I   8.0   7.5
50 -I
  -I
  -I   7.0   6.0
31 -I
  -I   5.5   5.0
16 -I
  -I   5.0
  -I   3.5   3.5
 7 -I
  -I   4.0
  -I   2.5
 2 -I
  -I   2.5   3.0
  -I
  -I   1.5   2.0
  -I   1.5
  -I
  -I   0.5   0.5
  -I
  -I   0.0   0.0
  -I

ACTIVITIES	SOCIAL	SCHOOL
---------	------	------
2.0 I. # OF SPORTS	0.0 III. # OF ORGANIZATIONS	1.2 VII. MEAN PERFORMANCE.
1.3 MEAN OF PARTICIPATION AND SKILL IN SPORTS	0.0 MEAN OF PARTICIPATION IN ORGANIZATIONS	0.0 SPECIAL CLASS
0.0 II. # OF OTHER ACTIVITIES	0.0 V. # OF FRIENDS	0.0 REPEATED GRADE
0.0 MEAN OF PARTICIPATION AND SKILL IN ACTIVITIES	2.0 FREQUENCY OF CONTACTS WITH FRIENDS	0.0 SCHOOL PROBLEMS
2.0 IV. # OF JOBS	0.0 VI. BEHAVIOR WITH OTHERS	
**** JOB QUALITY	0.0 BEHAVIOR ALONE	
6.5 TOTAL	2.0 TOTAL	1.0 TOTAL
T SCORE = 44	T SCORE = 21	T SCORE = 20

TOTAL SCORE FOR EACH SCALE IS ROUNDED TO NEAREST .5

** INDICATES THE SCORE WAS NOT COMPUTED DUE TO MISSING DATA

Fig. 1: Computer-scored competence scales of the Child Behavior Profile (from McConaughy and Achenbach, 1988)

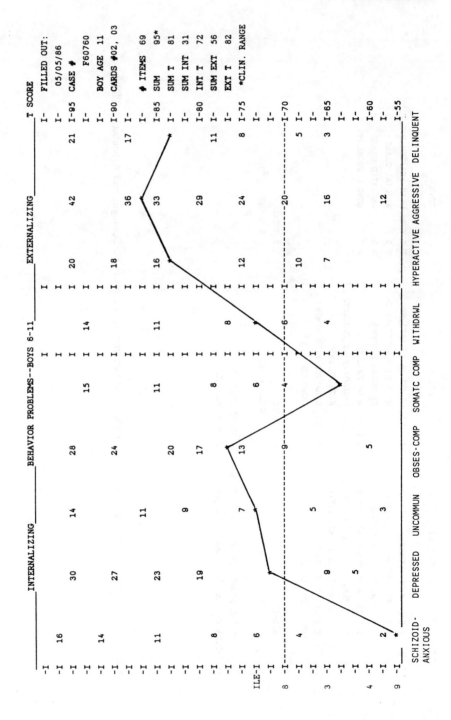

Fig. 2 — Computer-scored problem scales of the Child Behavior Profile

SCHIZOID-ANXIOUS
- 0 11.CLINGS
- 0 29.FEARS
- 1 30.FR SCH
- 0 40.HEARS THINGS
- 0 47.NTMARE
- 1 50.ANXIOS
- - 59.PUBLIC MASTUB
- 0 70.SEES THINGS
- 0 75.SHY

TOTAL= 1
T SCORE= 55
CLINC T=41

DEPRESSED
- 0 12.LONELY
- 2 14.CRIES
- 1 18.SUICID
- 0 31.FR IMP
- 0 32.PERFCT
- 1 33.UNLOVD
- 2 34.FEELS PERSCT
- 1 35.WRTHLS
- 1 45.NERVOS
- 1 50.ANXIOS
- 0 52.GUILTY
- 0 71.SLFCON
- 2 88.SULKS
- 0 89.SUSPCS
- 0 91.TALKS SUICID
- 1 103.SAD
- 0 112.WORRY

TOTAL=13
T SCORE= 71
CLINC T=54

UNCOMMUN
- 1 13.CONFUS
- 0 65.WON'T TALK
- 1 69.SECRTV
- 0 71.SLFCON
- 0 75.SHY
- 1 80.STARES
- 2 86.STUBRN
- 1 103.SAD

TOTAL= 6
T SCORE= 73
CLINC T=51

OBSES-COMP
- 1 9.OBSESS
- 1 13.CONFUS
- 1 17.DAYDRM
- 1 46.TWITCH
- 0 47.NTMARE
- 1 50.ANXIOS
- 0 54.TIRED
- 1 66.COMPLS
- 1 76.SLEEPS LITTLE
- 1 80.STARES
- 2 83.HOARDS
- - 84.STRANG BEHAV
- 1 85.STRANG IDEAS
- 1 92.SLEEP WLKTLK
- 1 93.TALKS
- 1 100.CAN'T SLEEP

TOTAL=14
T SCORE= 77
CLINC T=62

SOMATC COMP
- 0 49.CONSTP
- 0 51.DIZZY
- 0 54.TIRED
- 0 56A.PAINS
- 1 56B.HEAD
- 0 56C.NAUS
- 1 56F.STOMC
- 0 56G.VOMIT
- 0 77.SLEEPS MUCH

TOTAL= 2
T SCORE= 63
CLINC T=50

WITHDRWL
- 2 25.POOR PEER
- 2 34.FEELS PERSCT
- 2 38.TEASED
- 0 42.LIKES ALONE
- 1 48.UNLIKD
- 0 64.PREFER YNG CH
- 0 102.SLOW
- 0 111.WITHD

TOTAL= 7
T SCORE= 73
CLINC T=57

HYPERACTIVE
- 2 1.ACTS YOUNG
- 2 8.CAN'T CONCNT
- 2 10.HYPER
- 1 13.CONFUS
- 1 17.DAYDRM
- 2 20.DS OWN
- 2 41.IMPULS
- 1 61.SCHOOL
- 2 62.CLUMSY
- 0 64.PREFER YNG CH
- 1 79.SPEECH

TOTAL=15
T SCORE= 83
CLINC T=64

AGGRESSIVE
- 2 3.ARGUES
- 2 7.BRAGS
- 2 16.CRUELO
- 1 19.DEM AT
- 2 22.DSOB H
- 2 23.DSOB S
- 2 25.POOR PEER
- 1 27.JEALOS
- 2 37.FIGHTS
- 2 43.LIES
- 1 48.UNLIKD
- 1 57.ATTACK
- 1 68.SCREAM
- 2 74.SHOWOF
- 2 86.STUBRN
- 1 87.MOODY
- 2 88.SULKS
- 1 90.SWEARS
- 1 93.TALKS
- 1 94.TEASES
- 1 95.TEMPER
- 1 97.THREAT
- 1 104.LOUD

TOTAL=34
T SCORE= 86
CLINC T=65

DELINQUENT
- 2 20.DS OWN
- 1 21.DS OTH
- 0 23.DSOB S
- 2 39.BAD FRIEND
- 2 43.LIES
- 0 67.RUNAWY
- 1 72.FIRES
- 1 81.STEALS HOME
- 1 82.STEALS
- 0 90.SWEARS
- 0 101.TRUAN
- 1 106.VANDL

TOTAL=14
T SCORE= 84
CLINC T=71

OTHER PROBS
- 0 2.ALLERGY
- 0 4.ASTHMA
- 0 5.OPP SEX
- 0 6.ENCOPR
- 0 15.CRUELA
- 0 24.NO EAT
- 0 26.NO GLT NNFOOD
- 0 28.EATS
- 2 36.ACCDNT PRONE
- 1 44.NAILBT
- 1 53.OVREAT
- 0 55.OBESE
- 0 56D.EYES
- 0 56E.RASH
- 0 56H.OTHER PHYS
- 1 58.PICKS
- - 60.EXCESS MASTUB
- 2 63.PREFER OLD CH
- 0 73.SEXPRB
- 0 78.SMEARS
- 1 96.SEXPRE
- 0 98.THUMB
- 0 99.NEAT
- 1 105.ALCHL DRUG
- 0 107.WETS
- 0 108.WETBD
- 2 109.WHINE
- 0 110.WISH OP SX
- 0 113.OTHER

PROFILE TYPE:	A.SCHIZ-WITHDRW	B.DEP-WITHDR-AG	C.SCHIZOID	D.SOMATIC COMP	E.HYPERACTIVE	F.DELINQUENT
INTRACLASS CORR:	-0.540	-0.039	-0.783	-0.765	0.380	0.497

Fig. 2: Computer-scored problem scales of the Child Behavior Profile (from McConaughy and Achenbach, 1988)

Tab. 2: Syndromes found through Factor Analysis of the Child Behavior Checklist (from
         Achenbach and Edelbrock, 1983)

Group	Internalizing syndromes[a]	Mixed syndromes	Externalizing syndromes[a]
Boys aged 4–5	Social withdrawal Depressed Immature Somatic complaints	Sex problems	Delinquent Aggressive Schizoid
Boys aged 6–11	Schizoid or anxious Depressed Uncommunicative Obsessive–compulsive Somatic complaints	Social withdrawal	Delinquent Aggressive Hyperactive
Boys aged 12–16	Somatic complaints Schizoid Uncommunicative Immature Obsessive–compulsive	Hostile withdrawal	Hyperactive Aggressive Delinquent
Girls aged 4–5	Somatic complaints Depressed Schizoid or anxious Social withdrawal	Obese	Hyperactive Sex Problems Aggressive
Girls aged 6–11	Depressed Social withdrawal Somatic complaints Schizoid–obsessive		Cruel Aggressive Delinquent Sex problems
Girls aged 12–16	Anxious–obsessive Somatic complaints Schizoid Depressed withdrawal	Immature Hyperactive	Cruel Aggressive Delinquent

a) Syndromes are listed in descending order of their loadings on the second–order Internalizing and Externalizing factors

As Tab. 2 shows, Aggressive and Somatic Complaints syndromes were found for all groups, although the exact composition of these syndromes differed somewhat from group to group. Versions of the Schizoid, Withdrawal, Hyperactive, and Depressed syndromes were also found for most groups, but their composition was more variable, and in some groups they were combined with items that formed a separate syndrome in other groups. The Cruel syndrome was found only for girls, whereas the Uncommunicative syndrome was found only for boys. It should be pointed out, however, that the presence of such syndromes in data from only one sex does not necessarily mean that the *behaviors* are not reported for the other sex. It merely means that the behaviors do not consistently *occur together* in a discriminating fashion for that sex. Thus, *cruel to animals* is reported somewhat more frequently for disturbed boys than disturbed girls, but among girls it occurs more consistently with certain other behaviors to form a distinct syndrome. Combining data from both sexes would have obscured this tendency for behaviors to covary in a particular way for one sex but not the other.

Likewise, syndromes occurring in only one age group would have been obscured by combining data across age groups.

Notice now that the scales are grouped under headings labeled Internalizing, Mixed, and Externalizing. In order to determine whether particular narrow-band behavior problem scales correlate with one another to form broadband groupings of items, we performed second-order factor analyses of the scores obtained by the clinical subjects in each of the sex and age groups on their respective editions of the profile. On all editions of the Profile, the narrow-band problem scales were found to form two broad-band groupings. One of these groupings was similar to a broad-band grouping variously labeled overinhibited, personality disorder, and internalizing in other studies; the second was similar to a broad-band grouping variously label acting out, conduct disorder, and externalizing in other studies.

In order to represent a child's problems in terms of the broad-band groupings as well as the narrow-band scales, all the items on the narrow-band scales of the Internalizing grouping can be summed to provide a score for Internalizing. Likewise, all the items on the narrow-band scales of the Externalizing grouping can be summed to provide a score for Externalizing. To determine how a child's Internalizing and Externalizing scores compare with those of normal children, standard T scores based on our normal samples are provided on the Profile.

4.1 Assessment of Change

The Profile can be viewed as an assessment device designed to provide a standardized description and measure of behavioral problems and competencies. However, the value of assessment depends on how it relates to what happens later, in terms of intervention decisions, the responses of children and their families, predictions of outcome, and long–term adaptation under various conditions. One way of integrating the Profile into the postassessment process is to use it to measure change in reported behavior over time. We have done this over periods of different lengths with different samples (Achenbach and Edelbrock, 1983. As a measure of test–retest reliability, mothers were asked to respond to the Checklist at intervals averaging about one week. The median of the correlations between Time 1 and Time 2 scores on the various scales of the Profile was .89 (total $N = 80$). This indicates satisfactory stability in mothers' reports over periods when their children's behavior is presumably not changing much.

We also conducted a 6–month follow–up of children being seen in outpatient psychiatric clinics. Parents filled out the Checklist at intake and again 6 months later, whether or not their child was still in treatment. The mean of the Pearson correlations between the intake and 6–month follow–up scores on all scales was .65 (total $N = 295$). During this same period, the average scores of most problem scales declined, while scores on the social competence scales remained stable or improved. Thus, while reported problems were generally decreasing and competencies were remaining stable or improving, the correlations indicate significant stability in the rank ordering of clinic–treated children on the scales of the profile over a 6–month period.

As an additional test of changes in Profile scores, children seen in three psychiatric clinics were followed up after they had terminated with the clinics, 1? years after their parents had filled out Checklists at intake. The children and their families had received an average of about 15 clinical interviews. Considering the 1/2-year interval between ratings and the fact that the children had all completed their clinic contacts during that interval, the stability in the rank ordering of ratings was again substantial. The mean of the Pearson correlations between the intake and follow-up problem scales was .62 (total $N = 105$).

At the same time, there was a decrease in nearly all the problem scales for each group, with the decrease in total score for problems being highly significant ($p = .001$) in all groups. According to the parents' ratings, their children thus appear to have generally improved between intake and follow-up. Nevertheless, despite the decreases in problem scores, the mean scores obtained at follow-up were still well above those obtained by normal children of the same age. This underlines the need for judging any set of scores in relation to norms for the child's age.

4.2 Typologies of Profile Patterns

Another way to use the Profile is to determine whether differences in profile patterns can *predict* other important differences among children. To provide a basis for predicting from assessment to outcome, we have sought to identify children who share similar profile patterns and to determine whether typologies based on these patterns relate consistently to outcome under various conditions. In the absence of well-established clinical diagnoses against which to validate profile types, we have opted for an empirical approach to the construction of typologies through cluster analysis. Fig. 3 illustrates the general strategy of cluster analysis. We start with a number of individuals designated here as Subjects 1-10, each of whom has a profile. The clustering program finds individuals who have the most similar profiles and then forms progressively larger clusters of individuals according to the similarity of their profiles, beginning with relatively small clusters of very similar profiles and ending up with a cluster that includes everybody but in which the average similarity among members is low. The most desirable clustering solutions are usually those that fall in the intermediate range in which the sample is broken up into a few groups, each of which is very homogenous.

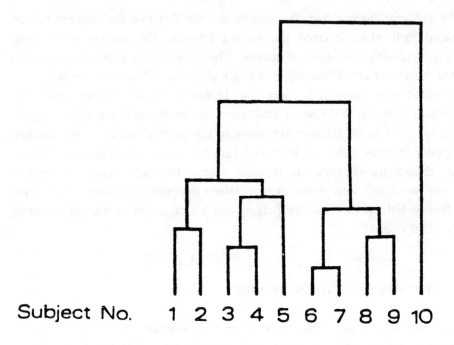

Fig. 3:   Illustration of hierarchical clustering sequence (from Achenbach and Edelbrock,
          1983)

There are many clustering algorithms, but few have been developed specifically
for behavioral data. After trying a variety of approaches, we have found that
centroid cluster analysis appears to be the most effective for behavior profiles
(Edelbrock and Achenbach, 1980). Briefly, centroid cluster analysis starts by
finding the two profiles in a sample that are the most similar to one another.
These are brought together to form the first cluster. The next step is to take the
average of thses two profiles to form a new profile that is an amalgam of the
two. The profile formed by taking the average of the two is called the *centroid*
of the cluster. In effect, the centroid becomes the operational definition of the
cluster. The next step is to determine whether any remaining member of the
sample has a profile more similar to this centroid than to the profile of any
other member of the sample. If such an individual is found, his or her profile
is added to the cluster, and the centroid of the cluster is recomputed as the
average of the first two members' profiles, plus the profile of the new member.

The process is then repeated, with the centroid of a cluster being recomputed each time a new profile is added. Whenever no member of the sample has a profile more similar to the centroid than to some other individual, a new cluster will be started which consists of the two most similar individuals. Their profiles are then averaged to form a centroid which defines their cluster, and the process continues until everyone becomes a member of a cluster.

In order to test the reliability of clusters, we performed cluster analyses of randomly selected samples drawn from large pools of profiles scored from Checklists filled out for clinically referred children. For each sex and age group, profile types that replicated well across two random samples of profiles were considered to be reliable.

We found either six or seven profile types for each of the six age and sex groups whose profiles have been cluster analyzed. These profiles are illustrated in the *Manual for the Child Behavior Checklist and Revised Child Behavior Profile* (Achenbach and Edelbrock, 1983). Fig. 4 shows the centroids of the profiles found for boys aged 6–11. Correlates of the profile types have been reported by Edelbrock and Achenbach (1980) and by McConaughy, Achenbach, and Gent (1988).

To determine the relative distribution of these profile types, the profiles of 1,050 boys seen in a wide variety of outpatient mental health facilities were classified according to their similarity to the six profile types. To do this, the correlations between each boy's profile and the centroids of the replicated profile types were calculated. Each boy was then classified according to the profile type he correlated most highly with. Boys having a total score of less than 25 or more than 100 on the Child Behavior Checklist were excluded, as their profile patterns are unreliable for purposes of classification. The box for each profile type in Fig. 5 indicates the percentage of boys classified by that profile type.

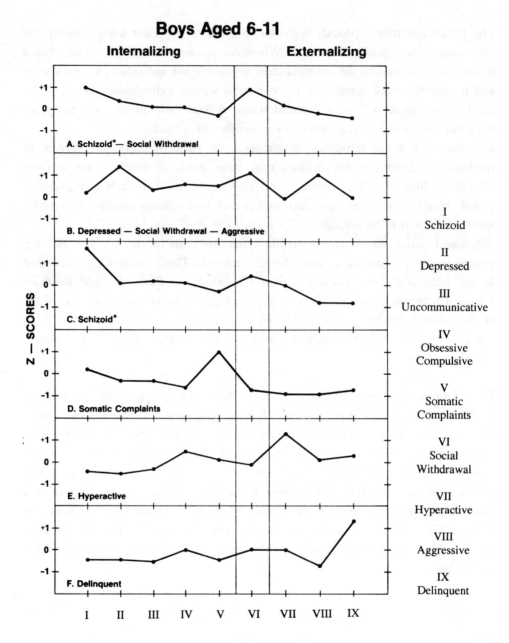

Fig. 4:   Child Behavior Profile types found for boys aged 6–11 (from Achenbach and
          Edelbrock, 1983)
          * Schizoid or Anxious

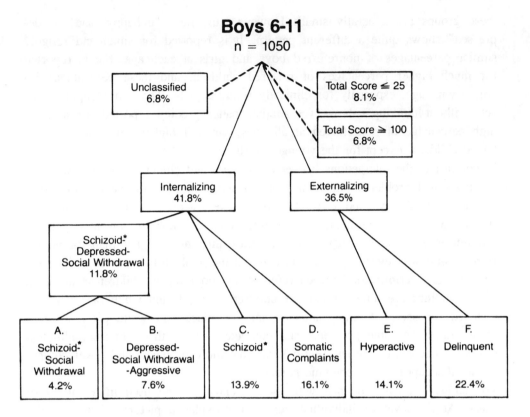

Fig. 5:   Distribution of profile types found for clinically referred boys aged 6–11 (from
          Achenbach and Edelbrock, 1983)
          * Schizoid or Anxious

4.3   Epidemiological Analyses

We have also made quasi–epidemiological analyses of each problem and compe-
tency item on the Checklist, as well as on total scores across items (Achenbach
and Edelbrock, 1981). These analyses provide normative baselines for the
frequency with which each item is reported for children of each age, sex, and
socioeconomic status within referred and nonreferred populations. As an example, we found that specific fears, a problem about which there is considerable
clinical lore, do not in fact discriminate very well between referred and nonreferred children who are matched for age, race, sex, and socioeconomic status.
The percentage of children from whom fears are reported declines steadily with
age for both the referred and nonreferred groups, and the differences between

these groups are generally small. However, the item "unhappy, sad, or depressed" shows quite a different pattern. It is reported for small and roughly similar percentages of nonreferred boys and girls at each age, but is reported for much higher percentages of referred children, and these percentages increase with age, especially for clinically referred girls. The item "impulsive or acts without thinking" shows yet another pattern, being reported for a fairly high percentage of nonreferred at all ages, but still higher percentages of referred children, except for the youngest girls.

In contrast to the interactions between sex, age, and clinical status for some of the individual problems, the total problem score shows remarkable similarities for nonreferred boys and girls. For both sexes, scores decline gradually but steadily with age. Total scores for referred children show somewhat larger sex differences at a couple of ages, but are uniformly much higher than for nonreferred children at every age. We have found the total problem score to be quite an accurate discriminator between referred and nonreferred children at all ages. These findings are quite similar for children of black and white race who are matched for socioeconomic status — that is, black and white parents report pretty much the same problems and competencies for their children, although lower socioeconomic parents report somewhat more problems and fewer competencies than upper socioeconomic parents.

To summarize, data obtained with the Checklist can be used in a variety of ways: At the level of individual items, it provides a picture of the specific problems and competencies reported for a child; at the level of total problem scores, it provides a summary index of deviance from norms for the child's age and sex; at the levels of narrow- and broad-band scales, the Child Behavior Profile reflects the ways in which the child's problems are concentrated in particular areas; and at the level of the profile pattern it offers a taxonomy of behavior disorders. Changes in a child's behavior as a function of time or treatment can also be assessed at any or all of these levels through periodic readministrations of the Checklist.

5. Relations between Empirically Derived Scales and DSM Diagnoses

To briefly address the interface between prevailing nosological approaches and the empirically based approach, Fig. 6 shows relations between scores on our empirically derived syndrome scales and DSM–III diagnoses derived from interviews of parents using the Diagnostic Interview Schedule for Children–Parent Version (DISC–P) in a study by Edelbrock and Costello (1988).

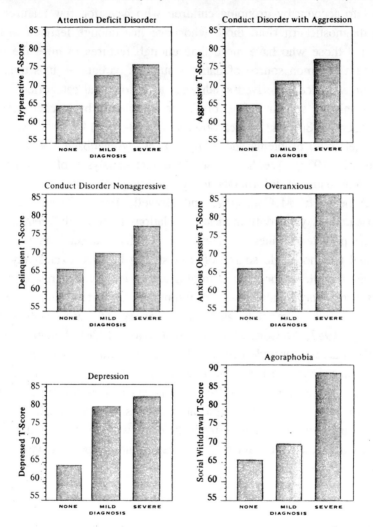

Source: Achenbach (1985) from data reported by Edelbrock & Costello (1988)

Note: A T–score of 70 is the upper limit of the normal range on scales of the Child Behavior Profile

Fig. 6:   Relations between DSM–III Syndrome Scores from the DISC–P and T Scores on Corresponding Scales of the Child Behavior Profile

For those DSM diagnoses that have explicit descriptive features, there is quite a strong relationship, especially when the quantitative aspects of the DSM criteria are taken into account by grouping children who have too few features to meet the DSM diagnostic criterion, those who have just enough features to meet the criterion, and those who have more than enough features to meet the criterion. When using a common source of data — such as parents — it is thus possible to relate our empirically derived syndromes to nosological categories.

We have developed similar rating forms for completion by teachers (Achenbach and Edelbrock, 1986) and direct observers, and for 11- to 18-year-olds to report on their own problems and competencies, (Achenbach, 1986; Achenbach and Edelbrock, 1987). We have also done meta-analyses of correlations between different pairs of informants using a variety of instruments in different samples (Achenbach, McConaughy, and Howell, 1987). Because even highly reliable instruments yield only modest correlations between different informants, and because prevalence rates for particular problems depend on the source of data, we feel that no single source of data should be used exclusively in evaluating individual children or in epidemiological or longitudinal research. Instead, different sources may validly reveal different, but important facets of children's functioning as we have illustrated in a variety of cases (Achenbach and McConaughy, 1987; McConaughy and Achenbach, 1988). Rather than expecting a single source to provide decisive data or expecting all sources to converge on a single diagnostic construct, we must be prepared for the complex realities of differences in functioning in different contexts and with different interaction partners. For most child and adolescent problems, neither diagnosis, nor prevention, nor intervention can be effectively dealt with in the singular, but must be approached through coordination between multiple perspectives and multipronged efforts.

References

Achenbach, T.M. (1985): Assessment and taxonomy of child and adolescent psychopathology. Newbury Park, CA: Sage

Achenbach, T.M., and Edelbrock, C. (1983): Manual for the Child Behavior Checklist and Revised Child Behavior Profile. Burlington, VT: University of Vermont Department of Psychiatry

Achenbach, T.M., and Edelbrock, C. (1986): Manual for the Teacher's Report Form and Teacher Version of the Child Behavior Profile. Burlington, VT: University of Vermont Department of Psychiatry

Achenbach, T.M., and Edelbrock, C. (1987): Manual for the Youth Self-Report and Profile. Burlington, VT: University of Vermont Department of Psychiatry

Achenbach, T.M., and McConaughy, S.H. (1987): Empirically-based assessment of child and adolescent psychopathology: Practical applications. Newbury Park, CA: Sage

Achenbach, T.M., Edelbrock, C., and Howell, C.T. (1987): Empirically-based assessment of the behavioral/emotional problems of 2- to 3-year-old children. Journal of Abnormal Child Psychology, 15, 629-650

Achenbach, T.M., McConaughy, S.H., and Howell, C.T. (1987): Child/ adolescent behavioral and emotional problems: Implications of cross-informant correlations for situational specificity. Psychological Bulletin, 101, 213-232

American Psychiatric Association (1st ed. 1952; 2nd ed. 1968; 3rd ed. 1980; 3rd rev. ed. 1987): Diagnostic and statistical manual of mental disorders. Washington, D.C.: Author

Bayley, N. (1969): Bayley Scales of Infant Development. New York: Psychological Corporation

Edelbrock, C., and Achenbach, T.M. (1980): A typology of Child Behavior Profile patterns: Distribution and correlates for disturbed children aged 6-16. Journal of Abnormal Child Psychology, 8, 441-470

Edelbrock, C., and Costello, A.J. (1988): Convergence between statistically derived behavior problem syndromes and child psychiatric diagnoses. Journal of Abnormal Child Psychology,

Ireton, H., and Thwing, E.J. (1974): Minnesota Child Development Inventory. Minneapolis, MN: Behavior Science Systems

Kraepelin, E. (1st ed. 1883): Psychiatrie. Leipzig: Abel

McCarthy, D. (1972): McCarthy scales of children's abilities. New York: Psychological Corporation

McConaughy. S.H., and Achenbach, T.M. (1988): Practical guide for the Child Behavior Checklist and related materials. Burlington, VT: University of Vermont Department of Psychiatry

McConaughy, S.H., Achenbach, T.M. and Gent, C.L. (1988): Multiaxial empirically based assessment: Parent, teacher, observational, cognitive, and personality correlates of Child Behavior Profiles for 6- to 11-year-old boys. Journal of Abnormal Child Psychology

Wechsler, D. (1974): Wechsler Intelligence Scale for Children − Revised. New York: Psychological Corporation

Wechsler, D. (1981): Wechsler Adult Intelligence Scale − Revised. New York: Psychological Corporation

World Health Organization (1978): Mental disorders: Glossary and guide to their classification in accordance with the Ninth Revision of the International Classification of Diseases. Geneva: Author

The Use of a Standardized Assessment Instrument (the Achenbach Child Behavior Checklist) in Longitudinal Epidemiological Research

Frank C. Verhulst

1. Introduction

To advance our knowledge of psychopathology in children, we need to view children's maladaptive behavior in relation to their developmental course. Developmental psychology has been concerned with variation and stability across time of certain capacities emerging during *normal* development. Likewise, research in developmental psychopathology is concerned with the stability and change of problems of adaptation within a developmental framework. This kind of research is necessary for the following reasons:

1. To assess which problems tend to persist and which do not;
2. To assess which early problem or combination of problems predict later psychopathology;
3. To evaluate the necessity and efficacy of treatment;
4. To judge which behavior is normative and age–appropriate and which is not;
5. To assess the validity of diagnostic constructs in terms of outcome.

To describe development, whether normal or deviant, longitudinal studies have played an important role. A major obstacle to longitudinal research, however, has been the choice of the variables studied. In developmental psychopathology it is especially the lack of standardized assessment procedures and of procedures to define syndromes or diagnostic categories that has severely limited the results across studies and across time periods (Rutter, 1981). To advance our knowledge of abnormal development it is therefore essential to employ standardized assessment procedures, especially ones that potentially provide a basis for constructing groupings of problems that tend to co–occur. Therefore, we used such a procedure in our two–year follow–up of children aged 4–14. At both points the child's functioning was assessed by obtaining standardized parents' reports of behavioral/emotional problems and social competencies using the Achenbach Child Behavior Checklist (CBCL) (Achenbach, 1983).

1.1   The Child Behavior Checklist and Comparisons between Dutch and American Children

The Child Behavior Checklist is designed to obtain parents' ratings of 20 competence items and 118 behavioral/emotional problems. In separate studies using the American and Dutch versions of the CBCL, the instrument was found to discriminate strongly between children referred for mental health services and demographically–matched nonreferred children (Achenbach and Edelbrock, 1983; Verhulst, Akkerhuis, and Althaus, 1985). Children referred to mental health agencies obtained significantly higher scores than nonreferred children on nearly all of the 118 behavioral/emotional problem items, as well as on total problem scores. These results supported the discriminative validity of the instrument. The significant associations of CBCL scores with clinical psychiatric judgment and diagnosis as reported in an earlier study (Verhulst, Berden, and Sanders–Woudstra, 1985) further supported the utility of this instrument. Furthermore, both in the United States and in Holland the CBCL yielded high reliability.

To test the applicability of the CBCL across the United States and Holland, two countries differing in language, traditions, and mental health systems, we compared the prevalence rates of competence items and problem items reported by parents for large samples of randomly selected American and Dutch children (Achenbach, Verhulst, Baron, and Akkerhuis, 1987). We found a remarkably great similarity in mean total–problem scores across the two countries. A nonsignificant difference of only less than half a point on the 240–point scale was found. There were significant but small nationality differences on 52 out of

120 problem items; half showing higher scores for American and half for Dutch children. Competence scores showed significant nationality differences, however, with American parents tending to score their children higher on most items.

Achenbach and Edelbrock (1983) factor-analyzed parents' ratings of large samples of clinically referred children separately for both genders and for each of the age groups 4-5, 6-11, and 12-16 years. For each age- and sex group, factors were identified to represent syndromes of problems that tend to occur together. The degree to which a child manifests problems as reported by the parents is expressed by a score on each scale representing an empirically de-rived syndrome. By providing normative data, the child's score on each scale can be compared with those of same-sexed age-mates. Second-order factor analyses of the syndromes derived from the CBCL revealed two broad-band syndromes called internalizing and externalizing. We separately factor-analyzed CBCL ratings of parents for large samples of Dutch clinically referred boys (Achenbach, Verhulst, Baron, and Althaus, 1987)˙and girls (Verhulst, Achen-bach, Althaus, and Akkerhuis, 1988) aged 6-11 and 12-16. The high correla-tions between most of the American and Dutch syndrome scores strongly support the cross-cultural construct validity of the empirically derived syn-dromes.

We also found great cross-national similarities in the distribution of scores for normative samples. These findings support the use of the same empirically derived syndrome scales by researchers and clinicians in the United States and Holland. Results concerning children's problem behavior assessed with the CBCL in one country are applicable to children in the other country as well. If similar cross-national comparisons are conducted between other European countries and the United States, the generality of findings obtained with this instrument may increase; potentially resulting in an even more solid core of knowledge.

1.2   Aims of the Present Study

Some of the most important questions about child psychopathology concern persistence and change in behavioral/emotional problems and competencies; but existing studies provide only limited answers. In a previous paper we have presented a detailed overview of existing longitudinal studies (Verhulst and Althaus, 1988). Major shortcomings include: the restriction of the sample to a single locality or the use of selected samples; large sample attrition; the use of different assessment instruments at different times; the small number of specific behavioral/emotional problems; or the use of very broad categories of functioning.

The present study was designed to test the persistence and change of behavioral/emotional problems and competencies as reported by parents of children over a two–year period in a representative sample of the general population. The specific aims of the present study were:

1. to test the two–year persistence and change of behavioral/emotional problems reported by parents of a representative sample of children from the general population;
2. to identify differences in persistence–related sex and age.

2. Method

2.1   Data Collection Procedure

As described earlier, the Child Behavior Checklist was used to obtain standardized parents' reports of children's competencies and behavioral/emotional problems. For a more detailed description of the instrument see Achenbach and Edelbrock (1983) and Achenbach's contribution to this volume.

The CBCL was translated into Dutch with the help of a linguist. The translation was kept as close as possible to the description of problems covered by the English version in order to enhance comparability with results obtained in other studies.

2.2   Description of Sample

Sample and procedure at Time 1
As described in detail elsewhere (Verhulst, Akkerhuis, and Althaus, 1985), the original sample of 4- to 16-year-old children was drawn between February and May 1983 from the Dutch province of Zuid-Holland, encompassing over 3,000,000 people living in environments that range from rural to highly urbanized. Using municipal birth registers which list all residents, a random sample was drawn of 100 children of each age and sex with Dutch nationality (N = 2,600).

Parents were visited by interviewers trained in advance. When parents consented to the interview, the interviewer handed over the CBCL and asked each question on the CBCL while recording the answers on a computer optical reader form. The response rate was 85.1%.

The respondents consisted of 89% mothers, 9% fathers and 2% others. Ethnic background of the parents was 9% Caucasean, 2% Surinam, 1% other.

Socio-economic status (SES) was scored on a 6-point scale of occupation as reported by the parent (van Westerlaak, Kropman, and Collaris, 1975). If both parents worked, the higher status occupation was scored. The mean SES of parents was 3.6 and S.D. was 1.6 which is slightly above the midpoint of the scale (3.5).

Sample and data collection procedure at Time 2
In April 1985, we wrote to the parents of 1,774 children belonging to age-groups 4-14 years at Time 1 with a request for their participation in the follow-up study. Enclosed were a CBCL, written scoring instructions, a life-event questionnaire, and a prepaid return envelope. Parents were asked to fill in the questionnaires and return them by mail. If they had questions, parents were to contact members of the research team by telephone. From the end of April through May 1985, parents who had not responded were telephoned by one of three research assistants familiar with the CBCL. In case parents needed help in filling the questionnaires, the interviewers gave assistance by telephone following the same instructions that were given for the Time 1 interview procedure. Parents for whom no telephone number was listed in the telephone directory or

who could not be reached after three attempts were sent a reminder by mail. Parents who did not respond after one telephone request were telephoned again after two to three weeks. The summer holidays made an interruption of the data collection procedure necessary. In September 1985, the remainder of tele-phone calls were made. The second time, parents who could not be reached after three attempts, as well as nonresponding parents for whom no telephone number was known, were sent a reminder with questionnaires enclosed. The life–event questionnaire is part of another study to be reported elsewhere (Ber-den, Althaus, and Verhulst, 1988).

Of the 1,774 CBCL's sent out, 1,412 (79.6%) usable CBCL'S were returned. A number of families had moved during the study's time interval. The new addresses of most of these families were provided by the municipalities. Except for a few cases, it was possible to track the home address of virtually all fami-lies. From the 1,774 children in our sample, 14 were untraceable (5 children had moved abroad and for 9 children the new address was unknown). The response rate corrected for untraceable children is 80.2%.

The mean interval between Time 1 and Time 2 assessment was 2.16 year (S.D. = .14). Although the time interval is slightly larger than two years, we will call it a two–year follow-up for simplicity.

On the 6–point scale of parental occupation, the mean SES was slightly, though significantly, higher at Time 2 than at Time 1 (3.8, S.D. = 1.7 versus 3.6, S.D. = 1.6, T = 3.54, df = 1,390, p < .001). On average, the socio- economic status thus improved for the sample over the two–year period.

Nonresponders

Because information was available on the nonresponders at Time 1, it was possible to trace differences between the responders and nonresponders.

First, we looked at SES in both groups at Time 1. The mean SES at Time 1 for the nonresponders (3.2; S.D. = 1.6; n = 359) was significantly lower than the mean SES (3.6; S.D. = 1.6; n = 1,410) for the responders (T = 4.41; df = 1,767; p < .001).

Next we investigated the total problem scores of the CBCL in both groups. The mean total problem score for the nonresponders (23.2; S.D. = 17.6; n = 360) was slightly, though significantly, higher than the mean total problem score

(21.2; S.D. = 15.9; n = 1,412) for the responders (T = 2.13; df = 1,770; p < .05). In conclusion, nonresponders were parents with somewhat lower socio–economic background who scored their children as somewhat more problematic than parents in the responder group.

3. Results

3.1 Total Problem Score

The total problem score is calculated by summing the scores for each of the 118 problem items (0 if the item is not true of the child, 1 if the item is somewhat or sometimes true, and 2 if it is very true or often true). The higher the total problem score, the higher the level of disturbance of the child.

Tab. 1 presents the mean total problem scores at Time 1 and Time 2 for combined two–year age*– and sex groups for the general population sample (N = 1,412). The mean total problem scores as presented in the Tab. are adjusted for SES. In Fig. 1, the mean total problem scores are graphically portrayed for the combined two–year age groups.

Tab. 1:   Mean Total Problem Scores* Split for Age and Sex at Time 1 and Time 2

Age at	Boys		Girls	
Time 1	Time 1	Time2	Time 1	Time 2
4 – 5	22.7	20.2	21.9	16.6
6 – 7	25.6	20.8	20.0	17.6
8 – 9	23.3	19.8	20.6	16.4
10 – 11	23.1	19.2	18.5	15.1
12 – 13	20.4	13.9	17.5	17.0
14	17.1	15.3	17.4	20.6

* mean scores adjusted for SES

* unless otherwise stated, ages refer to ages at Time 1

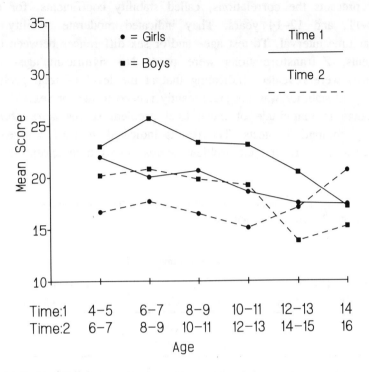

Fig. 1: Total Problem Score

In order to assess the effects of time of assessment, age, and sex on total problem scores, we performed a repeated measures analysis of covariance (ANCOVA) with two between factors (age and sex), one within factor (time), and one covariate (SES) changing over levels of the within factors.

Averaged across both times of assessment, boys obtained higher total problem scores than girls $(F(1,1332)=5.31; p<.05)$, and scores tended to decline with increasing age $(F(5,1332)=2.55; p<.05)$. SES had a significant $(F(1,1332)=19.67; p<.001)$ effect on total problem scores, with higher scores obtained by lower SES children.

Total problem scores at Time 2 were significantly lower than scores at Time 1 across ages and both sexes $(F(1,1332)=68.81; p<.001)$.

The difference between Time 1 and Time 2 SES scores did not contribute to differences between Time 1 and Time 2 total problem scores.

To assess the stability in rank order of scores, product–moment correlation coefficients were computed between Time 1 and Time 2 total problem scores.

Tab. 2 presents the correlations, called stability coefficients, for age-groups 4-5, 6-11, and 12-14 years. They indicated moderate stability across the two-year time interval. To test age- and/or sex differences between the stability coefficients, Z-transformations were used. No significant age- and/or sex differences were revealed, indicating that at the level of total problem scores the two-year stability was not significantly related to age or sex.

The change in magnitude of mean total problem scores across time was assessed by computing t-tests. The results indicated in Tab. 2 revealed significant decreases in mean total problem scores across time except for girls aged 12-14.

Tab. 2:   Stability Coefficients (r) and t-Tests Between Total Problem Scores at Time 1 and Time 2 Split for Age and Sex

	Age at Time 1					
	4 − 5		6 − 11		12 − 14	
	r	change	r	change	r	change
Boys	.67	D*	.71	D***	.66	D***
Girls	.62	D***	.67	D***	.66	n.s.

D = significant decrease in mean scores across the 2-year time interval
n.s.   = non-significant difference between mean scores
* p < .05; ** p < .01; *** p < .001
Note: All stability coefficients are significant at the p < .001 level

3.2   Syndromes

Achenbach and Edelbrock (1983) have factor-analyzed parents' ratings of large samples of children referred to mental health agencies. Analyses were performed for both sexes and age groups 4-5, 6-11, and 12-16. For each age/sex-group, the authors computed several narrow-band factors and two broad-band factors named "internalizing" and "externalizing". The names of the narrow-band factors summarize the items comprising each scale. The broad-band syndrome called internalizing comprises items that mainly involve internal conflicts and stress, whereas externalizing problems reflect conflicts with other people and their expectations of the child.

For each of the empirically derived syndromes, the stability was assessed by computing product–moment correlations and t–tests between syndrome scores at Time 1 and Time 2 for both sexes and the three age groups.

Tab. 3 presents the stability coefficients and the results of the t–tests by age group and sex. Note that not all syndromes appeared in the factor analyses of each age– and sex group. Stability coefficients and differences in mean scores indicated in the Tab. were significant at the p < .01 level of significance. The last column presents the stability coefficients averaged across age– and sex groups. Z–transformations were used to compute average stability coefficients.

Tab. 3: Stability Coefficients (r) and Results of t–Tests Between Syndrom Scores at Time 1 and Time 2

Age group	Boys			Girls			Total
	4 – 5	6 – 11	12 – 14	4 – 5	6 – 11	12 – 14	
Syndrome	r change	r change	r change	r change	r change	r change	average r
Agressive	.65 D**	.70 D***	.66 D***	.59 D***	.70 D***	.68	.66
Cruel					.50 D**	.60	.56
Delinquent	.47	.55 D*	.57		.41	.51 I**	.51
Depressed°	.66	.62 D*		.45	.54 D***	.58	.57
Hostile withdrawal		.71 D***					.71
Hyperactive		.65 D*	.60 D***	.53 D***	.59 D*		.60
Immature	.51		.57 D***			.64 D*	.58
Obsessive		.59 D***	.46 D***	.35 D***		.60	.51
Sex problems	.38			.30	.50 D***		.40
Schizoid	.28	.49 D***	.38	.52 D***	.44	.48	.44
Somatic complaints	.32	.46	.50	.46 D***	.48	.40 I*	.44
Social withdrawal	.51	.66 D*		.68 D***	.58 D*		.59
Uncommunic.		.60	.57 D*				.59
Average r	.48	.60	.56	.51	.53	.58	.56
Internaliz.	.51 D**	.64 D*	.53 D***	.43	.58 D*	.56	.54
Externaliz.	.61 D*	.66 D***	.64 D***	.47 D*	.69 D***	.64	.62

o   for girls 12–14 stability coefficient for the depressed–withdrawal syndrome is presented
D = decrease in mean scores; I = increase in mean scores
* p < .05; ** p < .01; *** p < .001
Note: All stability coefficients are significant at p < .01 level

Because stability may be related to types of problems, we tested the differences of stability coefficients between Time 1 and Time 2 scores for the internalizing and externalizing syndromes. Significance levels were computed for differences between two stability coefficients for correlations based on the same sample.

For the total sample (N=1,412), stability coefficients between Time 1 and Time 2 were significantly higher for the externalizing syndrome than for the internalizing syndrome (t=4.59; df=1,409; p<.001).

Total competence scores

Total competence scores were calculated in the same way as outlined by Achenbach and Edelbrock (1983). The higher the total competence score, the more adaptive the behavior of the child.

Tab. 4 presents the mean total competence scores at Time 1 and Time 2 for combined two–year age groups and both sexes. The mean scores were adjusted for SES. During the first period of data collection, the two items requesting parents to list the child's jobs or chores were erroneously interpreted to mean only remunerated work. We therefore omitted this item from the analyses. The mean total competence scores are graphically portrayed in Fig. 2.

Tab. 4:   Mean Total Social Competence Scores* at Time 1 and Time 2 Split for Age and Sex

Age at	Boys		Girls	
Time 1	Time 1	Time2	Time 1	Time 2
4– 5**	8.7	9.7	10.0	11.2
6– 7	14.7	15.5	16.5	16.9
8– 9	15.5	15.1	16.3	15.9
10–11	15.4	14.0	16.8	15.0
12–13	15.0	13.9	15.3	14.4
14	14.8	13.1	15.1	13.9

*   mean scores adjusted for SES and exclude items on number of jobs and job performance
** scores for 4–5-year-olds do not include school scale

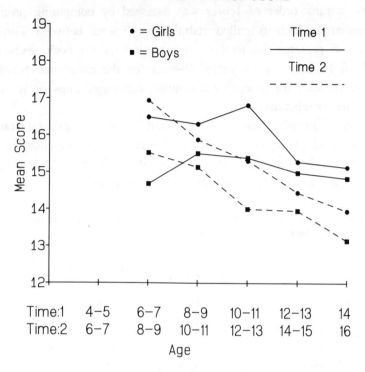

Fig. 2: Total Social Competence Score

Repeated measures analysis of covariance (ANCOVA) was used to assess the effects of time of assessment, age and sex on total competence scores. Because no data on school functioning were available for the 4–5-year-olds, they were omitted from the analyses of total competence and school scale scores.

Averaged across both Time 1 and Time 2 assessments, girls obtained higher total competence scores than boys $(F(1,927)=25.19; p<.001)$. Age also revealed a significant effect $(F(4,927)=10.43; p<.001)$. It can be seen from Tab. 4 and Fig. 2 that older children scored somewhat lower than younger children except for boys at Time 1. SES also revealed a highly significant effect with lower scores for lower SES children $(F(1,927)=50.15; p<.001)$.

Total competence scores were found to decrease somewhat between Time 1 and Time 2, except for age group 6–7 for which a slight increase could be noted.

The difference between Time 1 and Time 2 SES did not contribute to differences between Time 1 and Time 2 competence scores $(F(1,927)=0.37$; ns).

The stability in rank order of scores was assessed by computing product–moment correlation coefficients called stability coefficients between Time 1 and Time 2. Tab. 5 presents the total competence scores for both sexes and age groups 4–5, 6–11, and 12–14 years. Z-tests for the difference between two correlation coefficients for independent samples significant age- or sex differences between the correlations.

The change in magnitude between Time 1 and Time 2 mean total competence scores was assessed by computing t-tests. The results are presented in Tab. 5. They show a significant increase in scores for 4- to 5-year-olds and a significant decrease for other children, except 6- to 11-year-old boys.

Tab. 5:   Stability Coefficients (r) and t-Tests Between Total Social Competence Scores at Time 1 and Time 2 Split for Age and Sex

| | Age at Time 1 | | | | | |
| | 4 – 5 | | 6 – 11 | | 12 – 14 | |
	r	change	r	change	r	change
Boys	.45	I***	.55	n.s.	.43	D***
Girls	.36	I***	.51	D**	.39	D**

D = significant decrease in mean scores across the 2–year time interval
I = significant increase in mean scores across the 2–year time interval
n.s. = non–significant difference between mean scores
** p < .01; *** p < .001
Note: all stability coefficients are significant at the p < .001 level

3.3   Movement Between the Two Times of Assessment

Another way of assessing the persistence of behavioral/emotional problems across the two–year interval is to ask what happened at a later age to the children who could be regarded as disturbed at an earlier age. We chose the 90th percentile of the cumulative frequency distributions of total problem scores as the cut–off point. Children scoring at or above this cut–off point were considered to score in the clinical range (Verhulst, Akkerhuis, and Althaus, 1985). Next we looked at the distribution at Time 2 of children who were in the top 10% category at Time 1. We also looked at the distribution at Time 2 of those children who were in the bottom 50% category at Time 1. We took the lowest 50% of the children to represent the normal or nondisturbed group. This cut-off is rather arbitrary although it seems reasonable to contrast this group of children with those in the disturbed group.

Tab. 6 shows the cumulative frequency distributions of total behavior problem scores for the above–mentioned groups in the total sample.

Tab. 6:   Change in Total Problem Scores Between Time 1 and Time 2

% bands	percentage of children above each Time 2 band who, at Time 1, were in the:	
at Time 2	bottom 50 %	top 10 %
100	100 (n = 741)	100 (n = 140)
90	87	100
80	69	99
70	54	97
60	41	96
50	31	95
40	19	92
30	10	81
20	7	69
10	2 (n = 14)	54 (n = 76)

From the Tab. we can see, for example (third column), that 54% (n = 76) of the children who scored at or above the 90th percentile (top 10%) of the cumulative frequency distribution at Time 1 were still in the top 10% (first column) at Time 2. In other words, 54% of the children defined as disturbed at Time 1 could still be regarded as such two years later. This also means that about 46% of the children in the disturbed group at the earlier age moved out of this category. However, this does not mean that they necessarily moved into the group designated as normal. On the contrary, it can be inferred from Tab. 11

that 95% of the children in the disturbed group at Time 1 (third column) scored above the 50% band. In other words, only 5% of the children scoring in the deviant range at the earlier age moved into the normal group, scoring in the bottom 50% at a later age. Movements in the reverse direction, that is, from the normal into the disturbed group, can also be demonstrated from Tab. 7. For example, only 2% (n=14) of the children scoring in the normal, bottom 50%, range at Time 1 (second column) moved into the top 10%, or disturbed category, two years later.

Results for samples divided according to sex and age
The previous results refer to the total sample of boys and girls aged 4–14. To get a clearer picture of the movements between the two times of assessment we must take account of age- and sex differences in the scorings. Therefore, children were divided according to their sex- and age groups 4–5, 6–11, and 12–16 years. Cumulative frequency distributions were computed for the six groups, and for each of them the number of children was determined who, at Time 1, scored at or above the 90th percentile (D=deviant) as well as the number of children who, at Time 1, scored at or below the 50th percentile (L=low). Next we looked at the proportion of children that belonged to the following "change categories":

1. LL = Low on both occasions;
2. DL = Deviant at Time 1 and low at Time 2;
3. DD = Deviant on both occasions;
4. LD = Low at Time 1 and deviant at Time 2;
5. R   = Remainder of children.

Tab. 7 and 8 present the proportion of boys and girls respectively in each change category for the three age groups.
As can be seen, the proportion in each of the change categories was not very much affected by age and sex.

Tab. 7: Proportion of Boys in Each Change Category by Age Group

Time 1

Age Group	LL %(n)	DL %(n)	LD %(n)	DD %(n)	R %(n)	Total %(n)
4 – 5	34.6(45)	0.8(1)	-(-)	5.4(7)	59.2(77)	100(130)
6 – 11	32.4(122)	0.3(1)	0.8(3)	5.0(19)	61.5(232)	100(377)
12 – 14	35.3(61)	1.2(2)	1.7(3)	5.2(9)	56.6(98)	100(173)

Tab. 8: Proportion of Girls in Each Change Category by Age Group

Time 1

Age Group	LL %(n)	DL %(n)	LD %(n)	DD %(n)	R %(n)	Total %(n)
4 – 5	35.3(47)	1.5(2)	2.3(3)	3.0(4)	57.9(77)	100(133)
6 – 11	34.0(137)	0.5(2)	1.0(4)	5.7(23)	58.8(237)	100(403)
12 – 14	40.3(74)	0.5(1)	0.5(1)	5.4(10)	53.5(99)	100(185)

The persistence in each category was determined by computing the percentage of children in each Time 1 category that belonged to the same category two years later. Tab. 9 and 10 present the percentages by age group and sex respectively.

Tab. 9: Percentage of Children in Each Time 1 Category Belonging to the Time 2 Category for Both Sexes Combined (Number of Children in the Time 1 1 Category in Brackets)

Age Group	LL	DL	LD	DD
4 – 5	68(136)	13(24)	2(136)	46(29)
6 – 11	63(409)	4(76)	2(409)	55(76)
12 – 14	73(186)	9(34)	2(186)	56(34)

Tab. 10: Percentage of Children in Each Time 1 Category Belonging to the Time 2 Category for Both Sexes Combined (Number of Children in the Time 1 Category in Brackets)

Age Group	LL	DL	LD	DD
4 — 5	68(136)	13(24)	2(136)	46(29)
6 — 11	63(409)	4(76)	2(409)	55(76)
12 — 14	73(186)	9(34)	2(186)	56(34)

For example, it can be seen from Tab. 9 that 55% of the 76 6- to 11–year-old children who, at Time 1, scored in the deviant range could still be regarded as deviant two years later. Also, it is shown that only 2% of the children who could be considered as low scorers at Time 1 moved into the disturbed group at Time 2.

SES influence

The distribution of SES across the different change categories was examined. For the DD group, mean SES was 3.3 (sd=1.45); for the LL group, mean SES was 3.8 (sd=1.54); for the LD group mean SES was 3.6 (sd=1.60); and for the DL group mean SES was 3.6 (sd=1.13). T-tests for the differences between means were calculated. The only significant difference between SES was found between the DD and LL groups (T=2.64, df= 617; $p < .01$). Deviant children who remained deviant over time were from a lower socio–economic background than children who were stable and non deviant.

4. Discussion

Information on the stability and change of behavioral/emotional problems is fundamental to the study of child psychopathology. The present study assessed the 2-year course of problems and competencies in a general population sample of children as reported by their parents on the Child Behavior Checklist (Achenbach and Edelbrock, 1983).

Although the recovery rate of 80% of the original sample seems satisfactory, the nonresponders included an overrepresentation of children from lower SES and those with relatively high problem scores on the CBCL. Hence, we lack information on a group with a higher probability of being deviant than those in the responder group. However, we do not know to what extent the lack of information on the 20% nonresponders affected our results.

For the 1,412 children on whom information on both times of assessment was available we found a small, though significant, increase in parents' occupational scores across the follow–up period. A possible explanation for this increase is that parents of children in the age range of our sample were advancing in their careers. Although this finding is worth noting, we could not demonstrate that the increase in SES contributed to the changes in total problem scores or to the changes in total competence scores.

4.1   Total Problem Scores

Averaged across the two times of assessment, older children obtained slightly lower total problem scores than younger children. As discussed in our earlier study (Verhulst, Akkerhuis, and Althaus, 1985), this decrease in the absolute number of problems as children mature probably reflects the greater diffusiveness of behavioral problems in earlier developmental stages, rather than a decrease with age in the prevalence of psychiatric disorders. However, the significant decrease in mean total problem scores across the follow–up period cannot be attributed to the effect of age only. Over the two–year time period, there was a significant decrease in problem scores. Although possible, it is unlikely that the mental health of the children in our sample increased dramatically. Other explanations for the decrease in problem scores must therefore be considered. First, there is the possibility that a retest effect is responsible for the difference in total problem scores. Another factor possibility influencing parental scores is the fact that at follow–up the parents were sent a questionnaire by mail, whereas the first assessment was carried out by interviews. Although the interviewers were instructed not to give examples or interpretations of behavior or to judge parental answers, the fact that someone is in the home posing questions and recording answers may exert a significant influence, by which parents are inclined to score their children as more problematic. It is not clear, however, which mechanisms are involved in this effect.

Another explanation may be that parents of children who, on average, had improved somewhat in their behavior during the time interval were somewhat more inclined to participate the second time than parents of children whose behavior had deteriorated.

Robins (1980) extensively discussed the results of a study comparing lay interview results using the DIS (Diagnostic Interview Schedule) to obtain lifetime diagnoses with results achieved by psychiatrists repeating the DIS some six weeks later. During the second interview, respondents reported fewer symptoms than in the first interview. This resulted in a shrinkage of the number of lifetime cases over time, rather than an increase as could be expected, since more of the respondents' lifetime had already been lived. Robins points out that certain explanations for the decline between first and follow-up interviews in clinical samples do not explain the decline in the reporting of lifetime symptoms in a general population sample. In clinical samples it may be that (1) the initial interview itself is therapeutic; (2) the first interview occurrs at a time when subjects are referred, usually at the height of their illness, while the second interview takes place at a time selected by the interviewer that is random with respect to the severity of symptoms; and (3) focusing only on the disturbed end of the distribution of symptoms causes regression to the mean across time. However, these explanations cannot explain the decline in scores in general population samples such as the ones described by Robins, as well as ours. Robins accentuates the fact that in their study the first interview was carried out by a lay interviewer, whereas the second interview was performed by a psychiatrist. Robins points out the possibility that this may account for finding some disorders less frequently in the psychiatric interview. It is not clear, however, why respondents should claim less symptoms during the interview with the psychiatrist than with the lay interviewer. The reverse seems to be even more plausible, namely, that psychiatrists are likely to elicit more symptoms than lay interviewers. In summary, it is unclear what methodological or developmental factors affect the magnitude of group scores over time. However, stability coefficients can tell us whether individual children tend to preserve their rank orders irrespective of changes in the magnitude of group scores.

The stability coefficients between Time 1 and Time 2 total problem scores ranged from .62 (girls, aged 4–5) to .71 (boys, aged 6–11). These coefficients indicate moderate stability of problem behavior across a two–year period.

4.2   Age and Sex Differences

We found no significant differences between stability coefficients for different age groups. This indicates that: (1) the variability of problem behavior across time in preschool children is not greater than that in older children, despite the fact that cognitive and social development show rapid changes in the preschool years, and (2) that adolescence is not characterized by rapid changes in the level of problems that adolescents manifest. Our findings agree with those of Richman, Stevenson, and Graham (1982) who found considerable stability in preschool behavioral problems and Rutter, Graham, and Chadwick (1976) who concluded that adolescents do not grow out of their problems to a greater extent than younger children. However, our study is the only one, as far as we know, to present follow–up data separately for ages covering the preschool period to adolescence, making it possible to compare stabilities in the occurrence of behavioral/emotional problems across various developmental levels. Sex was not significantly associated with stability of total problem scores.

4.3   Syndromes

We investigated stability and change for the dimensions or syndromes derived from the CBCL by Achenbach and Edelbrock (1983). Stability coefficients indicating two–year stability were significant for every syndrome and for each age– and sex group, ranging from r = .28 for Schizoid in 4– to 5–year–old boys to r = .71 for Hostile–withdrawal in 12– to 14–year–old boys. Averaged across both sexes and the three age groups, the lowest stability coefficient was for the syndrome called Sex problems (= .40), while the highest was Hostile withdrawal (r = .71). However, the Hostile withdrawal syndrome was present only in one age–sex group, namely boys aged 12–14. The syndrome present for all age– and sex groups that showed the greatest stability was the Aggressive syndrome (average r = .66).

In reviewing 16 studies, Olweus (15) also found substantial stability in aggressive behavior, although his data pertained only to boys. Our data, however, show similar stability for the Aggressive syndrome in boys (average $r = .67$) and girls (average $r = .66$). Another feature of the Aggressive syndrome was that the stability coefficients were in the same high range for both sexes at all ages. This means that many children showing aggressive behavior at one age are likely to show it two years later.

Most other syndromes showed moderate stability. Only the syndromes called Sex problems, Schizoid, and Somatic complaints showed relatively low stability coefficients, especially for boys aged 4–5.

Although stability coefficients for various syndromes are informative with respect to the stability of symptom groupings, low stability coefficients do not necessarily imply low validity of the syndromes. Low stability coefficients do indicate, however, that problems at one time do not strongly predict the same constellation of problems two years later. Nevertheless, problems that show little persistence may cause considerable concern during the time they are present. Furthermore, we do not know to what extent these problems may be indicative for other problems of adaption at a later age.

4.4   Competence Scores

Averaged across both times of assessment, there was a slight decline in total competence scores with increasing age, and girls obtained higher competence scores than boys in ANCOVA.

Stability expressed as correlation coefficients between competence scores at both times of assessment was generally weaker than that found for problem scores. Stability coefficients for total competence scores ranged from $r = .36$ (girls aged 4–5) to $r = .55$ (boys aged 6–11). This difference across both age and sex between the two stability coefficients was significant at the $p < .05$ level ($Z = 2.27$). Although stability coefficients were somewhat higher for boys than for girls and highest for the 6- to 11-year-olds, these age- and sex differences were not significant.

4.5   Stability at a Categorical Level

We found that 54% of the children from the total sample who were initially classified as disturbed still scored in the disturbed range two years later. The remaining 46% moved out of the deviant category. However, only 5% improved to a degree that placed them in the "normal" category (i.e., < percentile). At Time 2, 69% of the disturbed children scored in the top 20% range. We also presented the proportions of children changing from one category to another across time separately for both sexes and for three age groups. We found that the proportions of children remaining in the deviant category across time were not very much influenced by sex. The percentage of children remaining in the deviant category was only for the 4- to 5-year-olds somewhat smaller, whereas the percentage of children moving out of the deviant category into the normal or low-scoring category was greater than that found for the other age groups.

For the whole sample, between 3 (girls aged 4–5) and nearly 6% (girls aged 6–11) of all children could be regarded as remaining disturbed across a two-year time-span.

In conclusion, moderate stability was found for child psychopathology as reported by parents on the CBCL. Somewhat more than half of the children regarded as disturbed at the first assessment were still deviant two years later. It was rare for children in the disturbed category to move into the low-scoring or normal category (5%). Even more exceptional was a change from the normal into the disturbed group (2%). Although extreme changes were the exception more than the rule, considerable change did occur in the level of behavioral/emotional disturbance across a rather short time interval.

5. Conclusion

Our findings underscore the notion that behavioral/emotional problems should not be regarded as static. The study of child psychopathology should take account of the many variations in the types and level of pathological manifestations across time. It is therefore important that changes in behavioral/emotional problems be viewed against a background of normative data obtained by standardized assessment such as we have presented.

References

Achenbach, T.M., and Edelbrock, C.S. (1983): Manual for the child behavior checklist and revised child behavior profiles. Burlington: University of Vermont, Department of Psychiatry

Achenbach, T.M., Verhulst, F.C., Baron, G.D., and Akkerhuis, G.W. (1987): Epidemologic comparisons of American and Dutch children: (I) Behavioral/emotional problems and competencies reported by parents for ages 4 to 16. Journal of American Academic Child and Adolescent Psychiatry, 26, 317–325

Achenbach, T.M., Verhulst, F.C., Baron, G.D., and Althaus, M. (1987): A comparison of syndromes derived from the child Behavior Checklist for American and Dutch boys aged 6–11 and 12–16. Journal of Child Psychology and Psychiatry, 28, 437–453

Berden, G.F.M.G., Althaus, M., and Verhulst, F.C. (submitted 1988): Do major life events contribute to changes in the behavioral functioning of children?

Richman, N., Stevenson, J., and Graham, P.J. (1982): Preschool to school: a behavioral study. London: Academic Press

Robins, L.N. (1980): Longitudinal methods in the study of normal and pathological development. In Earls, F. (ed.): Studies of children. New York: Prodist, 34–84

Rutter, M., Graham, P., Chadwick, O.F.D., and Yule, W. (1976): Adolescent turmoil: fact or fiction? Journal of Child Psychology and Psychiatry, 17, 35–56

Rutter, M. (1981): Longitudinal studies: a psychiatric perspective. In Mednick, S.A., and Baert, A.E. (eds.): Prospective longitudinal research: an empirical basis for the primary prevention of psychosocial disorders. Oxford: Oxford University Press, 326–336

Verhulst, F.C., Akkerhuis, G.W., and Althaus, M. (1985): Mental health in Dutch children: (I) a cross–cultural comparison. Acta Psychiatrica Scandinavica, 72, Suppl. No. 323

Verhulst, F.C., Berden, G.F.M.G., and Sanders–Woudstra, J.A.R. (1985): Mental health in Dutch children: (II) The prevalence of psychiatric disorder and relationship between measures. Acta Psychiatrica Scandinavica, 72, Suppl. No. 324

Verhulst, F.C., Achenbach, T.M., Althaus, M., and Akkerhuis, G.W. (1988): A comparison of syndromes derived from the Child Behavior Checklist for American and Dutch girls aged 6–11 and 12–16. Journal of Child Psychology and Psychiatry, 29, 879–895

Verhulst, F.C., and Althaus, M. (1988 in press): Persistence and change in behavioral/emotional problems reported by parents of children aged 4–14: an epidemiological study. Acta Psychiatrica Scandinavica, 77, Suppl. No. 339

Van Westerlaak, J.M., Kropman, J.A., and Collaris, J.W.M. (1975): Beroepenklapper. 2 delen. Nijmegen: Instituut voor Toegepaste Sociologie

Developmental Diagnosis with Pre-School Children

Ursula Kastner-Koller, and Pia Deimann

A large number of studies in the field of developmental psychology deal with childhood disorders. Scientists attempt to give detailed descriptions and accurate classifications of psychic disorders. In doing so, they often neglect normal development.

However, to be able to identify deviations — that is, to state outstanding abilities on the one hand and lack of talent or behavioral problems on the other — it is absolutely necessary to provide means for diagnosing what can be called "normal development". As a matter of fact, there are various tests to measure intelligence, abilities, and personality characteristics beyond the age of 6. However, as far as younger children are concerned, there is an obvious lack of proper diagnostic tools — let alone that younger children rarely have the ability to express their problems.

With the exception of physiological examination during the first years of life, patterns of normal childhood development are usually concluded from behavioral observations and comparison with other children.

As early as during the first half of our century, there were attempts to underpin empirically this intuitive understanding of normality. Gesell (1925, 1928) elaborated a schedule to observe infants. This schedule formed the basis for a number of developmental tests, for example, Bühler–Hetzer–Kleinkinder–Test (Bühler and Hetzer, 1932), Echelle de Développement (Brunet and Lézine, 1951), Sprachfreie Entwicklungstestreihen (Baar, 1957).

There are some useful and reliable tests for children up to the age of 3, such as the Bayley Scales of Infant Development (Bayley, 1969) and the Münchener Funktionelle Entwicklungsdiagnostik (Hellbrügge, Lajosi, Menara, Schamberger, and Rautenstrauch, 1978; Köhler and Engelkraut, 1984).

As far as children between 3 and 6 years of age are concerned, many tests for specific aspects of childhood development are in use (see Tab. 1); however, only the Bühler–Hetzer–Kleinkinder–Test (Bühler and Hetzer, 1932) and the Denver Developmental Screening Test (Frankenburg and Dodds, 1967) attempt to cover the entire range of development.

Tab. 1: Survey of General and Specific Developmental Tests (Rennen-Allhoff and Rennen 1987, p.XIIf.)

Test	Aspects of new-born behavior	General	Motor	Perceptual	Cognitive	Language	Social-Emotional	Age range
Aktiver Wortschatztest für 3 − bis 6jährige Kinder						×		3 – 6 and above
Altersinventarium der aktiven mimischen Psychomotorik								
Bayley Scales of Infant Development					(×)			
Bender Gestalt Test for Young Children				×			×	
Beobachtungsbogen für Kinder im Vorschulalter							(×) ×	
Brazelton Neonatau Behavioral Assessment Scale	×							0 – 6
Bühler − Hetzer − Kleinkindertest		×	(×)		(×)		(×) (×)	
Burks Behavior Rating Scales. Preschool and Kindergarten							(×) ×	
Cattell − Infant Intelligence Scale		×			(×)			
Chalop − Atwell Scale of Motor Coordination								
Columbia Mental Maturity Scale					×			
Denver − Entwicklungsskalen		×		×		×		
Developmental Test of Visual − Motor Integration		× ×						
Duisburger Vorschul − und Einschulungstest		×	(×)	×	(×)	(×)	× (×) ×	
Echelle de Développement		×	× (×)		× (×) (×)		× (×) ×	
Educational Evaluation		×						
Entwicklungsgitter								
Entwicklungskontrolle für Krippenkinder				×				
Fragebogen zur Erfassung praktischer und sozialer Selbständigkeit								
French − Bilder − Intelligenz − Test	×			×		×		
Frostigs Entwicklungstest der visuellen Wahrnehmung		×	(×)	(×)	(×)	(×)	(×)	
Gesell Developmental Scales	×	×	(×)		(×)	×	× (×) ×	
Graham − Rosenblith Behavior Test for Neonates					×		×	
Griffith Entwicklungsskalen		×	(×)		(×) (×)	(×)	(×) (×)	
Grundintelligenztest Skala 1					× ×			
Hannover − Wechsler − Intelligenztest für das Vorschulalter					×			
Heidelberger Sprachentwicklungstest						×		
Infant Psychological Development Scales					×			

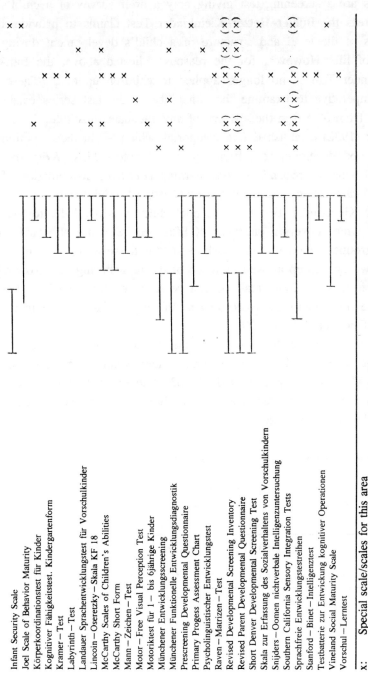

Infant Security Scale
Joel Scale of Behavior Maturity
Körperkoordinationstest für Kinder
Kognitiver Fähigkeitstest. Kindergartenform
Kramer – Test
Labyrinth – Test
Landauer Sprachentwicklungstest für Vorschulkinder
Lincoln – Oseretzky – Skala KF 18
McCarthy Scales of Children's Abilities
McCarthy Short Form
Mann – Zeichen – Test
Motor – Free Visual Perception Test
Motoriktest für 1 – bis 6jährige Kinder
Münchener Entwicklungsscreening
Münchener Funktionelle Entwicklungsdiagnostik
Prescreening Developmental Questionnaire
Primary Progess Assessment Chart
Psycholinguistischer Entwicklungstest
Raven – Matrizen – Test
Revised Developmental Screening Inventory
Revised Parent Developmental Questionnaire
Short Denver Developmental Screening Test
Skala zur Erfassung des Sozialverhaltens von Vorschulkindern
Snijders – Oomen nichtverbale Intelligenzuntersuchung
Southern California Sensory Integration Tests
Sprachfreie Entwicklungstestreihen
Stanford – Binet – Intelligenztest
Testbatterie zur Entwickung kognitiver Operationen
Vineland Social Maturity Scale
Vorschul – Lerntest

x: Special scale/scales for this area
(x):   Although a special scale/scales intended for this field, its interpretability is questionable
(When there are several versions of a test, the age guidelines refer to either the German or the most recent version)

The Denver Scales are a screening test giving only a brief survey of a child's development, whereas the Bühler–Hetzer–Kleinkinder–Test claims to provide a profound diagnosis of the level and structure of a child's development during the first 6 years of life. However, for the reasons indicated above, the Bühler–Hetzer–Kleinkinder–Test is no longer applied to children up to 3. Therefore, it appears imperative to examine the suitability of the test series established for children from 3 to 6 in the absence of any adequate substitute.

Bühler and Hetzer (1932) established five categories which − in their opinion − describe childhood development sufficiently, viz., motor skills (*Körperbeherrschung*), social behavior (*Soziale Reife*), learning (*Lernen*), manipulation of materials (*Materialbearbeitung*), and intelligence (*Geistige Produktivität*).

The Bühler–Hetzer–Kleinkinder–Test for preschool children is divided into four test series each of which covering one year of life. Ten items are allocated to each of the age groups. The children's task is to try to solve the ten items relevant to their own age group as well as those of the neighboring age groups. As a result of the test, a developmental age can be retrieved for the whole test and for each of the five categories. According to Bühler and Hetzer, the median Developmental Quotient (DQ) is 100.

In the present study, a total of 409 Viennese middle–class children between 3 and 6 years of age were tested with the Bühler–Hetzer–Kleinkinder–Test over the last 12 years. The test group consisted of 183 children from 3 to 4, 174 children from 4 to 5 and 52 children from 5 to 6. Boys and girls were equally distributed within the age groups (see Tab. 2).

Tab. 2: Distribution of Boys and Girls Within the Age-Groups

	Age in Years							
	3 − 4		4 − 5		5 − 6		Total	
	n	%	n	%	n	%	n	%
Boys	88	48.1	93	53.4	29	55.8	210	51.3
Girls	95	51.9	81	46.6	23	44.2	199	48.7
Total	183	44.7	174	42.5	52	12.7	409	100.0

Chi–Square: 1.49
df: 2
p: 0.47

The test results were submitted to a complete test analysis (Kastner–Koller and Deimann, 1987). This test analysis showed, inter alia, that the value of the item statistics and the reliability coefficients were rather poor. Moreover, the median DQ had increased significantly (see Tab. 3).

Tab. 3:   Developmental Quotient: Minimum, Maximum, Mean, and Standard Deviation

	Age in Years			
	3 – 4	4 – 5	5 – 6	Total
Minimum	80	75	84	75
Maximum	152	133	114	152
Mean	117.3	111.1	102.0	112.7
SD	13.4	9.9	6.9	12.3

The distributions of DQs for the total group and for each of the age groups are presented graphically in Fig. 1 (a–d).

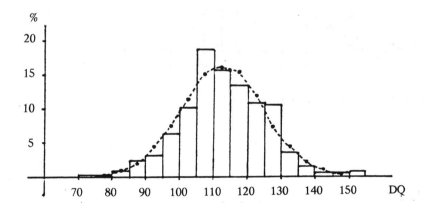

Fig. 1a: Distribution of DQ for the total group

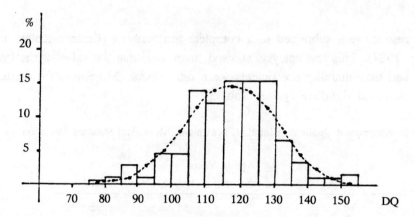

Fig. 1b: Distribution of DQ for the Age Group 3–4

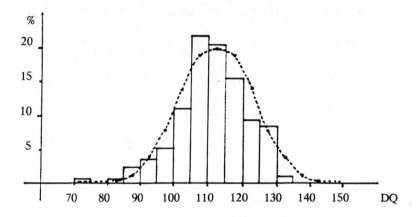

Fig. 1c: Distribution of DQ for the Age Group 4–5

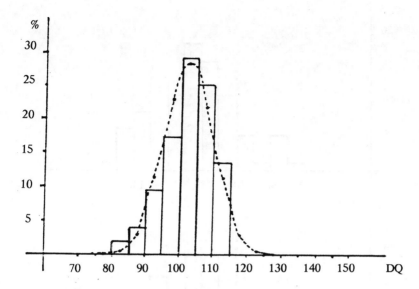

Fig. 1d: Distribution of DQ for the Age Group 5-6

A normal curve was superimposed on the histogram, and it can be noted that the experimental distributions of DQs for the total group and for the age groups 3–4 and 4–5 approximated the normal distribution rather closely. Due to the ceiling effect, the experimental distribution for the age group 5–6 was unilateral: In the absence of any test series for children beyond the age of 6, it was impossible for children between 5 and 6 years of age to achieve a DQ higher than 120. For this reason, the age group 5–6 was excluded from further considerations.

As shown in Tab. 3 above, the DQs for the total group as well as for the age groups 3–4 and 4–5 were significantly above the median of 100. This means that the results of the application of the Bühler–Hetzer–Kleinkinder–Test today are biased in so far as a DQ of 100 can no longer be considered to be normal.

Furthermore, a trend analysis of the DQ development over the past 12 years (i.e., the reference time span) was of certain interest. For that purpose the sample — that is 357 children between 3 and 5 years of age — was divided into three subgroups: 81 children tested in the years 1975 to 1979, 101 children tested during 1980 to 1982 and 175 children tested during 1983 and 1987. Chart 2 shows the distribution of DQs. In spite of a major increase from the second to the third period — a fact which cannot be interpreted satisfactorily — the result was that there is no general trend.

P. Deimann, and U. Kastner–Koller

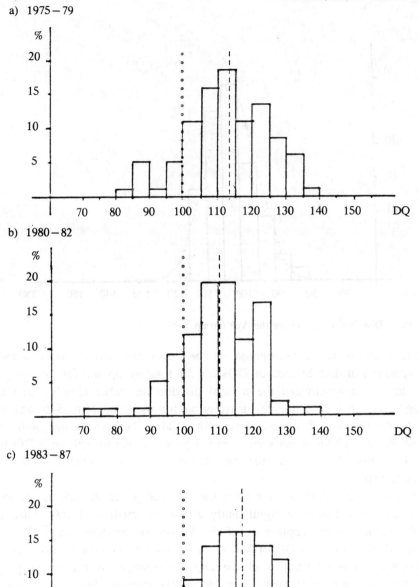

a) 1975–79

b) 1980–82

c) 1983–87

∘ ∘ ∘ median DQ assumed by Bühler and Hetzer
– – – experimental median DQ

Fig. 2:   Distribution of DQs (1975–79, 1980–82, 1983–87)

Item analysis pointed out that a large number of items have become too easy (Kastner–Koller and Deimann, 1987), so that the alleged difficulty level of 66% (Bühler and Hetzer, 1932) could not be confirmed. Some items showed a significant decrease of difficulty even within the last 12 years. The children of the third period (1983 to 1987) were much more skilled on items in the motor, manipulating, and learning categories. Compared to the prior periods, they succeeded more often in solving the following items: *Wassergefäß tragen* (carrying a bowl of water), *Soziales Rollenspiel* (social role playing), *Wetteifer* (pretended rivalry), *Nachahmendes Bauen* (imitative brickbuilding), *Nachzeichnen eines Kreises* (sketching a circle), *Schematische Darstellung* (sketching a house, a tree, etc.), *Zeichnung benennen* (defining a self–made drawing), *Kaufmannsladen 4 von 5* (a memory item) and *Ding vom Haken holen* (hook–and–eye principle). The frequencies and Chisquare statistics are presented in Tab. 4.

Tab. 4: Frequencies and Chi–Square Statistics of Items With Decreasing Difficulty in at Least One Age Group

Item	Sketching a circle (Kreis Nachzeichnen)							
Age group	3 – 4				4 – 5			
Period	75 – 79	80 – 82	83 – 87	total	75 – 79	80 – 82	83 – 87	total
0	15	17	14	46	9	11	2	22
1	21	26	90	137	36	47	69	152
Total	36	43	104	183	45	58	71	174
Chi–Square:		17.49				10.51		
df:		2				2		
p:		0.0002				0.0052		

Item	Imitative brickbuilding (Nachahmendes Bauen)							
Age group		3 – 4				4 – 5		
Period	75 – 79	80 – 82	83 – 87	total	75 – 79	80 – 82	83 – 87	total
0	7	15	10	32	2	2	1	5
1	29	23	94	151	43	56	70	169
Total	36	43	104	183	45	58	71	174

Chi–Square:	13.58	Gart's 2I:	0.83
df:	2 2		
p:	0.0011		0.66

Item	Carrying a bowl of water (Wassergefäß tragen)							
Age group		3 – 4				4 – 5		
Period	75 – 79	80 – 82	83 – 87	total	75 – 79	80 – 82	83 – 87	total
0	17	22	17	56	11	20	3	34
1	19	21	87	127	34	38	68	140
Total	36	43	104	183	45	58	71	174

Chi–Square:	23.19	19.52
df:	2	2
p:	0.0000	0.0001

Item	Social role playing (Soziales Rollenspiel)							
Age group		3 – 4				4 – 5		
Period	75 – 79	80 – 82	83 – 87	total	75 – 79	80 – 82	83 – 87	total
0	8	10	5	23	2	1	1	4
1	28	33	99	160	43	57	70	170
Total	36	43	104	183	45	58	71	174

Kullback's 2I:	13.50	Gart's 2I:	0.818
df:	2		2
p:	0.0012		0.66

Item	Pretended rivalry (Wetteifer)							
Age group		3 − 4				4 − 5		
Period	75 − 79	80 − 82	83 − 87	total	75 − 79	80 − 82	83 − 87	total
0	12	15	62	89	4	14	6	24
1	24	28	42	94	41	44	65	150
Total	36	43	104	183	45	58	71	174
Chi − Square:		11.64				7.83		
df:		2				2		
p:		0.0030				0.02		

Item	Memory (Kaufmannsladen 4 von 5)							
Age group		3 − 4				4 − 5		
Period	75 − 79	80 − 82	83 − 87	total	75 − 79	80 − 82	83 − 87	total
0	19	28	36	83	6	12	12	30
1	17	15	68	100	39	46	59	144
Total	36	43	104	183	45	58	71	174
Chi − Square:		12.42				0.97		
df:		2				2		
p:		0.002				0.62		

Item	Defining a self−made drawing (Zeichnung benennen)							
Age group		3 − 4				4 − 5		
Period	75 − 79	80 − 82	83 − 87	total	75 − 79	80 − 82	83 − 87	total
0	21	26	60	107	14	18	9	41
1	15	17	44	76	31	40	62	133
Total	36	43	104	183	45	58	71	174
Chi − Square:		0.097				7.89		
df:		2				2		
p:		0.953				0.019		

Item	Hook–and–eye principle (Ding vom Haken holen)							
Age group		3 – 4				4 – 5		
Period	75–79	80–82	83–87	total	75–79	80–82	83–87	total
0	15	13	25	53	10	8	4	22
1	21	30	79	130	35	50	67	152
Total	36	43	104	183	45	58	71	174
Chi–Square:		4.08				6.97		
df:		2				2		
p:		0.1298				0.031		

The increasing percentage of children attending kindergarten and generally using more highly sophisticated toys may explain these results.

Another problem is the structure of the Bühler–Hetzer–Kleinkinder–Test. The five categories assumed by Bühler and Hetzer could not be reproduced by factor analysis. In the present study the extracted factors were not valid for the entire sample, but differed from age group to age group. Although it is true that the factors could be interpreted meaningfully within each age group, they did not cover the entire range of childhood development. In Tab. 5 the age-specific factors and the corresponding items are presented.

Tab. 5:   Age-Specific Factors and Corresponding Items

Age group 3–4

Factor 1:   Motor coordination
             Sorting I (Blättchen Sortieren I)
             Sorting II (Blättchen Sortieren II)
             Carrying a bowl of water (Wassergefäß tragen)
             Sketching a circle (Nachzeichnen eines Kreises)
             Imitative brickbuilding (Nachahmendes Bauen)

Factor 2:   Achievement motivation
             Following the rules of a game (Spielregel)
             Pretended rivalry (Wetteifer)
             Puzzle I (Geduldspiel I)

Continued

Factor 3:   Performance intelligence
              Solving a problem by using tools (Matador)
              Recognizing the pulley-block principle (Baustein herunterlassen)
              Hook-and-eye principle (Ding vom Haken holen)
              Memory 3 out of 4 (Kaufmannsladen 3 von 4)
              Memory 4 out of 5 (Kaufmannsladen 4 von 5)

Factor 4:   Verbal intelligence (visual stimuli)
              Realizing impossible details in a picture (Fehlerbild)
              Telling a picture story (Kausale Folge)

Factor 5:   Verbal intelligence (acoustic stimuli)
              Repeating a sentence of 8 syllables (8 Silben)
              Repeating a sentence of 4 syllables (4 Silben)
              Verbal comprehension (Pläne formulieren)

Age group 4-5

Factor 1:   Verbal factor
              Repeating a sentence of 8 syllables (8 Silben)
              Repeating a sentence of 12 syllables (12 Silben)
              Defining a self-made drawing (Zeichnung benennen)
              Assigning commodities to pertinent shops (Laden und Waren)

Factor 2:   Fine motor coordination and perseverance
              Puzzle I (Geduldspiel I)
              Puzzle II (Geduldspiel II)

Factor 3:   Structuring ability
              Sketching a house, a tree, etc. (Schematische Darstellung)
              Realizing impossible details in a picture (Fehlerbild)
              Copying a complex brickbuilding (Kompliziertes Bauwerk)
              Following 3 instructions (3 Aufträge)

Factor 4:   Comprehension of coherencies
              Comprehension of complex rules (Eisenbahnspiel)
              Telling a picture story (Kausale Folge)
              Recognizing the pulley-block principle (Baustein herunterlassen)

Factor 5:   Specific factor
              Memory 4 out of 5 (Kaufmannsladen 4 von 5)

Continued

Age group 5-6

Factor 1:   Fine motor coordination and perseverance
             Puzzle I (Geduldspiel I)
             Puzzle II (Geduldspiel II)
             Margin embellishing with a given pattern (Randverzierung)

Factor 2:   Structuring ability
             Margin embellishing with a given pattern (Randverzierung)
             Sketching a house, a tree, etc. (Schematische Darstellung)
             Copying a complex brickbuilding (Kompliziertes Bauwerk)
             Drawing a man (Abbildendes Merkmal)

Factor 3:   Repeating a sentence with 12 syllables (12 Silben)
             Repeating a sentence with 16 syllables (16 Silben)
             Recognizing the pulley-block principle (Baustein herunterlassen)

In the age group 3-4 the first two factors *Motor Coordination* and *Achievement Motivation* describe two aspects essential for the development of children of this age; whereas Factors 3 to 5 include different aspects of intelligence. These five factors are certainly not a sufficient description of developmental tasks in the 4th year.

According to the present analysis, the Bühler-Hetzer-Kleinkinder-Test shows substantial deficiencies. Due to the improved environmental conditions after World War II, the test no longer appears to be a reliable instrument for estimating the development of preschool children. Children of the 1980s are more likely to pass an item of a test series above their age group than was the case in the 1930s. Moreover, there is reason to question the presumption that the Bühler-Hetzer-Kleinkinder-Test covers the whole range of childhood development. With a view to diagnosing childhood development reliably and more comprehensively, it is necessary to observe a wider stream of behavior than is actually done by the Bühler-Hetzer-Kleinkinder-Test.

Substituting by specific developmental tests cannot be a satisfactory solution as far as the diagnosis of general development is concerned. The only possible substitute, the Denver-Scales, show similar deficiencies as described for the Bühler-Hetzer-Kleinkinder-Test (Nawrat, 1987).

The deficiencies after some 50 years of existence of the Bühler-Hetzer-Kleinkinder-Test revealed by the analysis are of a size and nature that a remedy cannot be expected from sheer restandardizing. Therefore, the development of an entirely new test appears to be the only solution.

References

Bayley, N. (1969): Manual for the Bayley Scales of Infant Development. New York: The Psychological Corporation

Baar, E. (1957): Psychologische Untersuchung von tauben, schwerhörigen und sprachlich speziell gestörten Kleinkindern. I. Sprachfreie Teste in verschiedenen Ländern. II. Sprachfreie Durchführung der regulären Entwicklungsteste von Bühler und Hetzer sowie Schenk-Danzinger für das Alter von 1-7 Jahren. Basel: Karger

Brunet, O., and Lézine, I. (1951): Le développment psychologique de la première enfance. Paris: Presses Universitaires de France

Bühler, C., and Hetzer, H. (1932): Kleinkindertests. Entwicklungstests vom 1. bis 6. Lebensjahr. Leipzig: Barth

Frankenburg, W.K., and Dodds, J.B. (1967): The Denver Developmental Screening Tests. The Journal of Pediatrics, 71, 181-191

Gesell, A. (1925): The mental growth of the preschool child. New York: Macmillan

Gesell, A. (1928): Infancy and human growth. New York: Macmillan

Hofstätter, P.R. (1939): Was besagen Testergebnisse? Ein Beitrag zum Dimensionsproblem der Entwicklungstests. Zeitschrift für Kinderforschung, 47, 72-96

Kastner-Koller, U., and Deimann, P. (1987): Ein Klassiker auf dem Prüfstand. Ergebnisse einer testtheoretischen Analyse des Bühler-Hetzer-Kleinkindertests. Vortrag, 8. Tagung Entwicklungspsychologie. Bern

Nawrat, S. (1987): Kognitive Komplexität dargestellt am Beispiel des Traumes. Unpublished master's thesis, Grund- und Integrativwissenschaftliche Fakultät der Universität Wien, Wien

Rennen-Allhoff, B., and Allhoff, P. (1987): Entwicklungstests für das Säuglings-, Kleinkind- und Vorschulalter. Berlin, Heidelberg: Springer

Labeling Versus Support Diagnosis in Special Education: The Concept of an Intervention–Oriented Diagnostic Strategy for Children With Learning Disabilities

Dietrich Eggert

1. Introduction

Classification of individuals sometimes has enormous practical consequences, particularly in the field of education. Any suggested scientific classification poses serious problems if it is consequently administered to label and categorize individuals. If special institutions are built up on the basis of such classifications, and diagnostic procedures have been established as routine rituals of selection for these institutions, the assumptions underlying the classification are crucial. If they are criticized or become doubtful, a lot of organizational and practical consequences are to be expected. The following article tries to consider these consequences from a (special) educational point of view. Special education of mentally retarded and learning disabled children in Germany has been based on the belief in a classification of students into different types of schools or institutions. Now it seems evident that the basis of this classification has become doubtful. Let us start the discussion with a historical, but not unimportant remark.

Everything started with Alfred Binet. At the turn of the century he made his ingenious suggestions for the identification and education of intellectually subnormal children in France (Binet et al., 1907; Binet et al., 1911). He developed a complex, combined strategy for identification, classification, and education, comprising a psychological, an educational, and a medical examination of the child and a technological device for the measurement of intelligence: the intelligence test.

All three records together should lead to a classification and the subsequent placement in a special school or institution. He also suggested a curriculum for the organization of learning (orthopedie mentale) in such institutions (Wolff, 1961–1969, see Matarazzo, 1982).

Binet's successors in the following decades of our century — who were probably more simple minded than he was — gradually reduced the complex identification and intervention procedure he had suggested to a simple administration of an intelligence test and the placement of a child with an IQ below 80 or 85 in a special school for mentally retarded or learning handicapped children. (The German term "Lernbehinderte" includes "Learning disability" and "Moderate mental retardation" of the WHO classification). Several vital elements of Binet's complex strategy were omitted, and even his advice to control the validity of the technological device — the intelligence test — at least yearly was neglected. From this point of view, it seems almost ridiculous that from 1956 to 1983 in Germany a test like the German adaptation of the WISC (Wechsler Intelligence Scale for Children; German version: Hamburg Wechsler Intelligenztest für Kinder, HAWIK, Bondy, 1956) was mainly used for the identification of children with learning handicaps — for nearly 30 years without any revision or significant alterations.

Many further aspects support the conclusion that a huge amount of pedagogical and psychological energy is wasted every year in an almost illogical routine ritual: the so-called 'testweek', when children with learning problems are tested — mostly by special education teachers — labeled, and afterwards sent to special schools solely on the basis of the administration of an intelligence test (90%) and school achievement tests (60% in 1980, as Schuck and Eggert reported in 1982). In some West German states the use of intelligence tests is still compulsory by an order of the school administration.

The resulting dilemma for the teacher working as a diagnostic agent may best be illustrated by the confusion which arose when the revision of the WISC-R by Tewes (HAWIK-R) in 1983 showed a remarkable difference between the "old" and the "new" IQ's. New IQ's tended to be much lower then the older ones (mean difference 15–20 IQ points, when both tests were compared in the same sample). An application of the old classification rule (learning handicap = IQ lower then 85) placed almost 50% of the tested children with learning problems in the group of Lernbehinderte (Schuck and Ahrbeck, 1986).

After about 10 years of critical discussion (Kornmann, 1976; Kornmann, Meister, and Schlee 1983; Kretschmann 1985; Eggert 1986), there is a growing discomfort and uneasiness and dissatisfaction among teachers and psychologists with such a "special school selection procedure" (SAV as it is legally called in the state of North Rhine Westfalia), particularly with the procedure of labeling children.

This uneasiness led to the development of various concepts for alternative diagnostic strategies. Nowadays the criticism is also applied to the institution "special school" itself. Following the discussion of the usefulness of the "normalization principle" (Kugel and Wolfensberger, 1974) for the integration of handicapped children in general, there is a growing uneasiness with the very differentiated system of special schools in Germany. Integrative kindergartens and experiments with integrative school classes have shown that there is a wide range of possibilities for successfully educating children within the framework and mainstream of the regular schools, and that for some children many special schools are sometimes handicaps to their social integration into everyday life, because of the social stigmatization associated with being a "handicapped" child.

This article aims to specify some of the characteristics of the so-called "labeling or selection diagnosis" as opposed to concepts of alternative strategies called "support or intervention-oriented" diagnosis. Furthermore, I want to demonstrate some of the consequences for the construction and administration of alternative diagnostical devices — the diagnostic inventories or surveys. The problem of a valid diagnostic strategy for children with learning problems is most important when there is a special institution or school that must be filled with children labeled "learning disabled".

But I think that it is worth considering whether these problems also apply to any attempt to classify or label children as belonging to "clinical groups" with certain assumped features or trait profiles such as, for instance, "dyslectic", "minimal brain damage", or "hyperkinetic syndrome". When educational, psychotherapeutic, or medical help for children is based on a labeling proce-dure, including the administration of psychometric tests, the same questions might easily be posed.

2. Labeling and Selection Diagnosis Versus Support- or Interven-tion-Oriented Diagnosis

Let us now try to sketch some of the arguments in the debate about the two different forms of diagnostic strategies in special education.

1. The main argument of the advocates of any kind of labeling or selective

diagnosis is the belief in a "typical" syndrome of "learning disability" with specific trait constellations, measurable with standardized psychometric tests or similar instruments. In Germany this belief — based on the assumption of intellectual subnormality as the key trait — has led to the establishment of a special school for this group: the school for learning handicapped children ("Schule für Lernbehinderte"). This special school has the largest population of special pupils in Germany (about 4% of each yearly school intake attend a school for learning handicapped children). Since the 1973 definition by the German Education Council (Dt. Bildungsrat, 1973) of "learning disability" as "enduring, global, and serious learning handicap, associated with an IQ more than 1 1/2 standard deviations lower than the mean and correlated with problems of behavior and social integration" many schools have been set up for these children, and approximately 5,000 children (minimum) have been tested with psychometric and educational tests every year.

The poor prognostic validity of cognitive tests for school achievement school and the poor psychometric criteria in general for most of the German tests in the field of (special) education has led to the above-mentioned uneasiness and dissatisfaction on the side of the user of psychometric tests for school selection — focusing on the criticism of the IQ.

The lack of reasonable investments in tests due to an extreme cutback in budgets for education in general and educational research in particular during the last 10 years has made the situation even more serious. At the moment there are only a couple of tests with satisfactory test criteria available; many of the others are poorly standardized or completely invalid and out of date.

The concept of a support- or intervention-oriented diagnostic strategy tries to avoid any labeling of a child as deviant in general or "learning handicapped" in particular. Classifications are only useful for statistical purposes; they do not contribute to a real assessment or prognosis of the development of an individual child, as Mercer (1973), Spreen (1978), and Zigler and Balla (1982) have noted for mentally retarded children. Support diagnosis is the attempt to structurize a description of the individual competences of a child as a basis of an optimal intervention strategy to help the child develop its potentials. Competences are defined as the product of abilities and motivational factors, that is, how the child really acts and performs and not what potentials it has.

2. When placement in a special school is the aim of labeling and selection diagnosis and the argument that such a syndrome exists is accepted, the assessment of an IQ is understood to be a sufficient base for further treatment of a child in the school system (it is also believed that there is a vindication for a selective school system). Or in short: A measured IQ below 80 or 85 is accepted as a valid indicator of further development. The absurdity of such an argumentation can easily be demonstrated by a contradiction that arises from the application of this classification formula. If only 4–5% of a yearly school intake are "learning handicapped" and attend a special school, there seems to be a remarkable logical error to use an IQ of 85 for labeling and selection: Because of the properties of the normal distribution, 15.6% of the population fall into this range. How can the criterion be valid, if 5% are in these schools when 15.6% require identification? From the perspective of support diagnosis, a quantitative measure is only a report about the product of a learning process and the outcome of some aspects of development and does not provide any information about the process of the individual development. Test scores do not give information about special social conditions in relation to lower social status or about a child's deprived learning situations or previous learning experiences. A test score does not tell us why a child cannot solve a certain problem, nor what experiences the child has made or not made.
Support diagnosis tries to describe the process of the individual development in its specific life environment (Individuum–Umwelt–Einheit: Oerter, 1982) as a whole as far as this is necessary to understand its influence on the learning process of the child in school and to compensate for the different learning preconditions of the child.

3. The third argument concentrates on the basic philosophy of the procedures; whether the basis of the theories are found in psychology or education. Labeling or selection diagnosis is psychological in the sense that it makes use of the trait concept of differential psychology and has a conception of a deviant personality pattern as a sufficient basis for educational treatment.

The psychological type is emphasized. There is only an indirect connection between diagnostic categories and educational setting and intervention categories.

Support diagnosis tries to describe the needs for support and intervention in the school as a result of a report about the individual development compared with its potential for the acquisition of the structure of the subjects reading, writing, and mathematics, including a concept of the 'critical crossroads' and typical faults of students in acquiring this structure. Here – with regard to the contents – the educational dimension is emphasized: Diagnosis is part of the educational process and is categorized in didactic terms. Didactics is the master of diagnosis and prepares the theoretical framework; diagnosis and didactics should be based on theories of development and change.

4. Another argument in the comparison of selective and supportive strategies is concerned with the result of the procedure. Labeling diagnosis searches for the "special type of child" for an existing special school, fitting the child into the school; whereas supportive strategies search for the optimal educational intervention strategy for the individual child in a regular school (as long as this is possible).

    The search for an early labeling of deviant children in a highly selective school system in Germany and the establishment of a widespread and very differentiated system of special schools clearly shows a trend to segregate as early as possible.

    Supportive diagnostic strategies are associated with the concept of "de–institutionalization" (Bruininks et al., 1981): the integration of handicapped children either by mainstreaming or total integration of most deviant children into regular schools.

    These concepts are the subject of a highly controversial debate among scientists and practitioners in the field of special education in Germany. Selection is an important feature of the German school system and of rehabilitation measures for handicapped persons.

5. Labeling, selection, and the following placement are based on the assumption that it is possible to determine a "deviant" or "defective" development

in comparison to a "normal" development of a child, combined with the idea of measuring the amount of deviance in quantitative terms, that is, with psychometric tests. An intelligence, motor proficiency, or social adjustment quotient or similar score is believed to allow a successful classification of a child in terms of its prospective development. The clinical group dominates all features of the individual.

Therefore it is only necessary to identify the correct rationale for the identification of a person as a member of a specific group (the person's type) to have a complete picture of his or her personality. Traits are normally distributed in the population: a constant deviation from the mean of a group of normal individuals is a certain indicator of subnormality.

The point of reference for the individual assessment in support diagnosis is not the group or the normal distribution of test scores in a reference group. Only intra individual differences are the rationale for the evulation of changes. Instead of a quantitative description (which is in case of deviance mostly a negative difference) observational methods and inventaries are trying to give a more qualitative description of the individual development in terms of the process of academic achievement and learning. Closely connected with these arguments is the notion, that psychodiagnosis in general has to reconsider some basic assumptions. The development of more sophisticated developmental theories and the criticism against the trait theory as a basis of the classical test theory in general has shown, that for instance the concept of a 'true score' could be questionned. Furthermore, the concept of 'objectivity', i.e. the measurement of abilities in standardised 'laboratory' situations under strictly experimental conditions is too doubtful –particularly in the field of education 'open' situations, including aspects of the everyday life of the child at school and at home, seem to be more useful for the educational support of the child.

6. One of the most important questions posed by the intervention–oriented position is concerned with the compatibility of diagnostic and intervention categories. Diagnosis as an orienting procedure before the start of education and in the process of education and intervention itself should emphasize the complex character of the educational process as a whole, particularly in the field of learning handicaps. The compatibility of diagnostic and intervention

categories in the field of education is possible when there is a structural theory of the subject matter, that is, about the process of the acquisition of reading, writing, and mathematics in children based on a structural content analysis and a developmental theory. Brügelmann's concept (1983) of the "didactic map" as a structural, but not hierarchical model of the acquisition of reading and writing has led to a remarkable theoretical framework for teaching, diagnosis, and support. The Regenbogen Lesekiste (Ballhorn, Brügelmann, Kretschmann, and Scheerer–Neumann, 1987) (rainbow reading box) provides useful material for a support diagnosis as a substite for psychological tests as well as for instruction. There are other concepts for mathematics (Kutzer, 1983) including a structural and hierarchical theory of the subject matter and materials for instruction, diagnosis, and intervention with learning handicapped children. They have demonstrated that the basic assumptions of a supportive diagnosis can effectively be administered to school problems.

Any teacher or psychologist trying to administer support diagnosis must know that the concept in itself is neither a metaformula for the solution of every problem with children with learning problems nor is it applicable without the teacher possessing a reasonable, basic instructional knowledge. The primacy of didactic content means that a teacher should possess knowledge about the first steps in learning and the typical problems of a child — the teacher should really be a master of the learning process.

3. Some Characteristics of Diagnostic Inventories

In this section, we will demonstrate some practical aspects of alternative diagnostic instruments following some of above mentioned principles of support diagnosis. The list contains some characteristics that led to the construction of the diagnostic inventory of basic motor competences (DMB: Eggert, 1987) and the diagnostic inventory of auditory situations (DIAS: Eggert, 1988) as part of a program for the diagnosis and therapy of basic motor factors as motivational and physical prerequirements for social, verbal, and cognitive learning at school. The program is a further development of well–known perceptual–motor programs. The structured theory of the development of these competencies in the child is the framework for diagnosis and intervention.

Competence is defined as the ability to interact effectively with the surrounding world. It implies the construction of a conception of the self and the mastering and organizing of personal skills to perform specific activities. The use of these skills depends on the individual's own assessment of competence. This influences the person's choice of activities, the situations in which these activities will be carried out, and the amount of effort the person would be prepared to invest if difficulties arise. The above–mentioned diagnostic inventories try to measure these competencies. We will not describe these inventories in detail; a description of the basic assumptions underlying the construction of the inventories shall merely demonstrate the elements of a support diagnostic device.

A diagnostic inventory should at first contain a broad spectrum of heterogeneous actions and operations instead of homogeneous test items covering only a small range of objective situations.

Second, it should offer "open diagnostic situations" instead of standardized test items. Open situations mean that there should be a wide range of instructional help during the observation to obtain an idea of the child's process of problem–solving and its capacity to interact efficiently with the instructor in the situation. A feature of these diagnostic situations is that the process of solving is more important than the result. (This requires the inclusion of a detailed observation).

In the third place, these situations should include as much information as possible from the everyday life of the child in school or in its natural environment, even when this poses problems in the appraisal of the situation and means more subjectivity in measurement and interpretation.

Since the aim is the measurement of change instead of a result of a development, the appraisal of the individual result in terms of a difference to a reference group (standardization sample) seems only of a minor importance.

Multiple interrelated phases of diagnostic and interventional steps should further realize the concept of an integration of the diagnostic and therapeutic process. The first step could be the administration of a short version of the inventory (perhaps with formalized instructions and some reference group results using the 90th percentile line) for a screening to plan the first steps of instruction or intervention. In the DMB these items are called "focus items". Additional items for a more specific observation and a tryout of different intervention situations form the second step of intervention. These items take the form of more "open situations". The control of the effectiveness of the intervention could follow (in the form of a reconsideration of the effects of the planned intervention), constantly alternating diagnostic and interventional steps. Such a process could include different combined steps in the forming of diagnostic hypotheses; steps of planned intervention and control of effectiveness of intervention. The process itself is a never-ending story, that is, the combined phases of diagnosis and intervention do not stop until the end of the educational process.

IQ's and similar scores are not very important for such a process. They could possibly play a role in the posthoc evaluation, but not in the actual process of education or intervention.

Any observation should take place in natural groups, that is, in the classroom and not in a test room in the classic dyadic situation of examiner and examinee, because the learning problems of the child are generated in the classroom environment.

Teamwork of two observers on the basis of team teaching in observation and intervention is necessary, if possible.

The diagnostic situations should be compatible with categories of the teaching and should be rooted in the structure of the subject matter, so that diagnostic observations and intervention suggestions are closely linked together. A manual of possible situations should suggest a wide variability of different situations according to different intervention steps, that means, that the theory should be so differentiated that a large variety of possible interventions could be included. It is questionable whether the concept of classical test theory (insofar as the trait concept, the axiom of a true score, an orientation toward the criteria of the experiment, and the classification of individuals in units of the normal distribution are concerned) is still useful for such a diagnostic procedure. A methodological framework could possibly be seen in statistical models on a more simple base than the assumption of interval scales and the normal distribution curve. Path analysis and similar techniques have shown satisfying results with the diagnostic inventory of basis psychomotor competences (DMB: Ratschinski, 1987).

The administration of such an inventory is not only a possible way of orienting the diagnosis and intervention more closely to the individual needs of the student, but also of training professionals in new methods of observation, instruction, and didactics. It is crucial for the implementation of support oriented strategies that not only the everyday child, but also the teacher is willing and able to cooperate. Whether or not this cooperation will occur could be the touchstone of the realization of the strategy.

4. Summary

At the present time, there is no satisfactory theoretical basis for classifying children with deviant learning competences and placing them in special schools. The uneasiness of practitioners and scientists in the field of special education in Germany with diagnostic strategies that mainly use psychometric tests as a device for the identification of children with learning handicaps in a highly selective school system with many schools for handicapped children has led to the development of the concept of support- or intervention-oriented diagnosis.

The basic philosophy of this support diagnosis or "Förderdiagnostik" is to put off any labeling of these children as long as possible. Diagnosis as an orienting educational operation should, like all kinds of intervention, be rooted in a structural and developmental theory of learning: reading, writing, mathematics, and their basic prerequirements.

It is questionable whether the technological framework of the trait concept and psychometric tests is still useful for this purpose. At the moment it seems that tests are more helpful for labeling and selectional purposes and not for the concept of integrating handicapped children. New methods, emphasizing observational procedures and the measurement of intraindividual changes seem to be more appropriate.

The task of developing a satisfying rationale for the measurement and a technology for the concept of support diagnosis is very complex. It includes saying good-bye to a couple of basic psychological technologies and assumptions in education and teaching.

But it seems more challenging to work at solutions for a new point of view in coping with the problem of learning handicapped children as individuals in the school, including the concepts of integration, normalization, and trying to make school more satisfying for students and teachers. I think that in the small area of diagnostic teacher activity, support diagnosis could provide a path to such solutions.

References

Binet, A., and Simon, T. (1907): Les enfants anormaux — Guide pour l'admission des enfants anormaux dans les classes de perfectionnement. Paris: Colin

Binet, A., and Simon, T. (1911): La mesure du developpement de l'intelligence chez les jeunes enfants. Paris: Ed. Bourrelier

Ballhorn, Brügelmann, Kretschmann, and Scheerer-Neumann (1987): Die Regenbogen Lesekiste. Verlag für Pädagogische Medien: Hamburg

Bondy, C. (Ed.) (1956): Hamburg Wechsler Intelligenztest für Kinder (HAWIK). Bern-Stuttgart: Huber

Brügelmann, H. (1983): Kinder auf dem Weg zur Schrift. Konstanz: Faude

Bruininks, R.H., Meyers, C.E., Sigford, B.B., and Lakin, K.C. (Ed.) (1981): De-institutionalization and community adjustment of mentally retarded people. American Association on Mental Deficiency

Deutscher Bildungsrat (1972): Gutachten und Studien der Bildungskommission, Sonderpädagogik 3: Geistig Behinderte, Lernbehinderungen, Verfahren der Aufnahme. Stuttgart: Klett

Eggert, D. (1986): Von der Umschulungsdiagnostik zur lernentwicklungsorientierten Förderdiagnostiksonderschule in Niedersachsen: Zur Problematik der Anwendung psychologischer Testverfahren in der sonderpädagogischen Praxis Sonderschule in Niedersachsen, 1, 9-23

Eggert, D. et al. (1987): Diagnostisches Inventar psychomotorischer Basiskompetenzen. Weinheim: Beltz

Eggert, D., and Peter, T. (1988): Diagnostisches Inventar auditiver Alltagshandlungen von Kindern. Weinheim: Beltz

Kornmann, R. (Ed.) (1976): Diagnostik bei Lernbehinderten. Rheinstetten: Schindele

Kornmann. R., Schlee, J., and Meister, H. (Ed.) (1983): Förderdiagnostik. Heidelberg: Schindele

Kretschmann, R. (1985): Aufgaben und Grenzen der Förderdiagnostik. Zeitschrift für Heilpädagogik 12, 901-904

Kugel, and Wolfensberger (1974): Geistig Behinderte — Eingliederung oder Bewahrung? Stuttgart: Thieme

Matarazzo, J.D. (1982): Die Messung und Bewertung der Intelligenz Erwachsener. Bern-Stuttgart: Huber

Mercer, J.R. (1973): Labelling the mentally retarded –Clinical and social system perspectives on mental retardation. Berkeley: University of California Press

Oerter, R., and Montada, L. (Eds.) (1982): Entwicklungspsychologie. München: Urban & Schwarzenberg

Ratschinski, G. (1987): Grunddimensionen motorischen Verhaltens im Grundschulalter — multivariate Analysen motorischer Basisfaktoren. Universität Hannover, FB Erz.Wiss.I, Diss.

Schuck, K.D., and Eggert, D. (1982): Anspruch, Realität und Alternativen der diagnostischen Tätigkeit der Sonderschullehrer. In Ingenkamp, Horn, and Jäger (Eds.): Tests und Trends 1982. Weinheim: Beltz

Schuck, K.D., and Ahrbeck, B. (1986): Eine empirische Untersuchung zur meßtechnischen Güte und diagnostischen Bedeutung des HAWIK-R in der Sonderschule für Lernbehinderte

Spreen, O. (1986): Geistige Behinderung. Heidelberg − New York: Springer

Tewes, U. (Ed.) (1983): Hamburg Wechsler Intelligenztest für Kinder (HAWIK-R). Bern-Stuttgart

Zigler, E., and Balla, D.A. (1982): Mental retardation. The developmental-difference controversy. Hillsdale, N.J.: Erlbaum

The Reading Development of Normal and Poor Readers in the First Grade: How Helpful is the Concept of Developmental Stages for the Understanding of Reading Acquisition in German–Speaking Children?*

Christian Klicpera

1. Introduction

Reading development can be understood as the gradual development of information processing routines, or simply put, as the development of component skills (Barron, 1981; Perfetti, 1985). According to this view, the acquisition of written language requires different component skills, some of which are learned early and become automatic through continual practice. These might include letter recognition and the development of schemata for the relevant features of individual characters. Other skills are acquired later, however, like the knowledge of the origin of certain words as foreign or loan words.

In an alphabetic writing system, one particularly important component skill for the initial development of reading is the knowledge of grapheme–phoneme correspondences. The application of this knowledge in the form of phonological recoding allows for the reading of new words. In information processing models, phonological recoding is viewed as an indirect access route to word meaning. The notion is that the recognition of a written word is made possible by its first being transformed into its spoken form. Thus, the development of grapheme–phoneme conversion abilities is especially important for learning to

---

*) This research was conducted in conjunction with the Department of Child Psychiatry of the Max Planck Institute for Psychiatry in Munich. It was partially supported by the Hochschul–Jubiläumsfond of the city of Vienna. I wish to thank Dr. E. Hütter for help in analyzing the data.

read, in that instead of being dependent on outside help, it allows for independent reading (Jorm and Share, 1983).

On the other hand, the development of reading ability requires the building up
of word–specific and orthographic knowledge. This is accumulated through
increasing familiarity with the written form of repeatedly read words. This
word–specific knowledge can facilitate the reading of words by beginners who
do not know the alphabet and cannot yet read, but perhaps know from others
what the word is. They then can recognize a word on the basis of a few
features. It is also the case that word–specific knowledge is used by fluent
readers, in that they identify and read frequent words more rapidly than in-
frequent ones (Henderson, 1982). The word–specific knowledge of fluent readers is more differentiated than that of beginning readers. This is due to the fact
that fluent readers have stored in an abstract form the entire sequence of letters,
or, at least, the important parts of the letter sequence from which the word is
built. Thus, a word is stored not as concrete visual features, but abstracted
from the particulars of its outward shape such as type or font into an abstract
alphabetic code. This internal representation results in a particular type of
lexicon, a written, or orthographic lexicon (Henderson, 1982). Once a word is
identified, this lexicon makes accessible how the word should be pronounced.
Thus phonological recoding during reading is no longer necessary. In information processing models, because of this word–specific orthographic knowledge,
reading allows direct access between the written word and the lexicon.

Skilled reading depends on the development of accurate word reading abilities.
These are supplemented and supported by the contextual expectation of the
child, his understanding of the reading situation as a form of linguistic communication. The contextual expectation of the child permits him to employ
previous knowledge and already developed linguistic abilities in the decoding
and recognition of the words. Although the use of context can supplement those
abilities necessary for word recognition, the main task for the beginning reader
is the development of word–specific reading ability and the mastery of phonological recoding.

The view of reading development as a process in which different component
skills, processing routines, or strategies are acquired leaves open how this
process develops. It can be seen as a gradual, more or less continuous learning
process. The other possibility is to view the process as one that progresses in

stages or steps (Chall, 1983; Frith, 1985). This view has already been hinted at in pointing out that different component skills are developed at different times.

Is this approach also appropriate for early reading development? Which stages can be differentiated in learning to read? We want to speak of stages when the development between two points in time distinctly diverge from one another. Ideally, this difference should not only be quantitative, but also qualitative. That is, the transition from one stage to another should not only lead to a change in reading performance, but also a change in reading behavior. An improvement in one feature of the reading process should bring with it a deterioration in another feature. The influence of the features of written language on reading behavior should change qualitatively, in that as one feature increases its influence, another should decrease. When we have evidence that between two points in time a new reading skill or strategy has developed, then we can say that a transition has occurred from one stage of reading development to another.

We have briefly sketched the general hypotheses of information processing theory with respect to the reading process and reading development. What stages can be derived from these general assumptions? In the past few years, many stage models of reading development have been proposed based on information processing theory, all of which are quite similar in their main features (Frith, 1985; Marsh et al., 1977; Seymour and MacGregor, 1984; Jorm and Share, 1983). A brief description of these stages will focus on the commonalities among the various conceptions, abstracting away from the differences in specific characteristics. The names we will use for the stages are identical with those used by Frith (1985) and Seymour and MacGregor (1984).

Logographic Stage: In an initial phase, reading is based predominantly on the familiarity of specific features of individual words. Children identify words only on the basis of characteristic, often global features. The features used at this stage are visual and do not lead to, or only partially lead to, the identification of the letters that make up the word. In addition, the order of the letters receives only very limited attention. According to Marsh et al. (1977), further reading development in this stage is relatively limited. On the other hand, Frith (1985) maintains that the features utilized for reading can be further differentiated, and in this way it is possible to see noteworthy reading development in the logographic stage.

Alphabetic Stage: In this stage, the recognition of letter and phoneme identity and the knowledge of the systematic correspondence between them is applied to the reading of words. This is also the stage of letter–by–letter reading. A word is no longer directly recognized on the basis of a few features associated with it. Instead, words are recognized by virtue of the fact that they can be reconstructed through the pronunciation of the phonemes that correspond to individual graphemes. In other words, the identification of words results from the phonological recoding of the letter sequence.

Orthographic Stage: In this stage, words are once again directly recognized without phonological recoding. However, for this recognition, information about the sequence of letters is utilized. Based on this information, the appropriate entries in the orthographic lexicon are activated, and in this way the word is identified. To facilitate the process, it is most likely the case that the words are segmented into morphemes, and eventually into syllables, or other smaller, frequently occurring letter sequences at the subword level. In this way, certain complex features of print can be taken into consideration, such as the knowledge of the origin of words based on shared written features of certain word groups. At issue during this stage is word specific reading, but of a different sort from that of the logographic stage.

The description of these stages has been developed for English, and the question remains as to how applicable they are for the learning of other alphabetic systems. The German writing system differs from the English in the considerably greater regularity of the grapheme–phoneme correspondence. It is possible that the greater transparency of the grapheme–phoneme correspondence facilitates the learning of this type of alphabetic principles. It is further possible, then, that one might not find a fully developed, definable logographic stage, at least for the reading acquisition process in the context of school instruction.

2. An Investigation of the Development of Reading Ability in the First Grade

In order to be able to differentiate between word–specific logographic reading skills and phonological recoding, we investigated the reading performance of first graders on familiar and new words, and nonsense, pronounceable letter sequences, so–called pseudowords. Word–specific knowledge and familiarity with the written form of words plays a roll primarily in the reading of familiar words, that is, words that have already been read repeatedly. The reading of new words, those that are not yet familiar to the children in their written form, on the other hand, is much more strongly dependent on the knowledge of the letter–sound relationships. To be sure, even with these words, other factors enter into reading performance. When it is a question of words that the child is familiar with from everyday spoken language, it may be possible, due to a certain familiarity with written language, to identify these words based on a few features, without really reading through the whole word. A complete consideration of the graphic information is really only required for pseudowords. In order to correctly read these sequences of letters, each letter must be identified in its proper position, and the pronunciation must be based on knowledge of grapheme–phoneme correspondences. (This is at least true for beginning readers. Later it may also be possible to base the reading of these words on analogies made to real words and on the mastery of smaller units, such as frequently occurring syllables, obviating the necessity for a letter–by–letter recoding.)

A comparison of the reading performance for these three types of words should make it possible to describe the development of both types of strategies of word recognition and to differentiate between different phases of reading development.

The quality of the reading errors and the reading behavior give a further indication of the transition from the logographic to the alphabetic stage. Studies of English by Weber (1970), Biemiller (1970), Cohen (1975), and Francis (1977, 1984), have demonstrated differences in the quality of reading errors for the various stages in the process of reading acquisition. At first, there is very little similarity between the errors and the actual words the children are supposed to read. Instead these early errors consist of other words that the children already know how to read. When the children are not able to spontaneously read the word correctly, their errors display only limited graphic similarity to the target word, usually sharing only the first letter. Later, around the second half of the 1st–grade year, the incorrectly read words look much more similar to their targets. A greater number of features of the target word are taken into consideration, not just the first letter, but the other letters as well. As mentioned above, at first the reading errors were made up exclusively of real, meaningful words, generally words previously familiar to the children. Now, however, the errors are frequently nonsense words, that do bear a high similarity to the target word, albeit not the correct word. The transition between these two reading approaches has been described as discontinuous. During the transition one often finds a phase when children will simply refuse to even try to read the word out loud.

This yields the following questions and hypotheses for investigation:

1. If it is the case that the beginning of reading development consists largely of word–specific reading, then children should be able to read words already familiar to them, but new words to a much lesser extent. They should not be able to read pseudowords at all. Moreover, the increase of newly introduced words during the course of reading instruction should, after only a short time, lead to greater uncertainty and a decrease in reading accuracy even for familiar words.

   With more progress in reading development, however, one should see phonological recoding abilities develop. Then, not only should the reading accuracy for familiar words improve, but the difference between familiar words, new words, and pseudowords should become smaller.

2. By looking at the quality of reading errors, can one identify a stage of reading that looks like as if it were based on a few global features? This stage can be characterized by only a minimal graphic similarity between the reading error and the target word. In addition, instead of the word to be read, the child frequently says another word that is familiar to him or her from the course of reading instruction.

3. We expect that the greater regularity of the grapheme–phoneme correspondence in written German and the earlier systematic introduction of these correspondences in instruction should lead to a relatively frequent sounding out of new words. As sounding out is an indication of letter–by–letter phonological recoding, this behavior should not be observed in the first phase of reading acquisition, but instead should increase in frequency over the last course of reading development.

2.1   Method

Subjects. 120 German–speaking first graders from five Viennese elementary schools, who went to day care in the afternoons, participated in the research. For this longitudinal study, however, there are 82 children (35 girls and 47 boys) who participated in all testing sessions. The remaining children could not be tested on one of the test times.

In school they used a reading course that largely followed the principles of analytic–synthetic reading instruction (*Das Lesehaus, Frohes Lernen*).

Procedure. During the course of the first grade each child's reading performance level was individually tested five times. Testing started at the beginning of November, after they had been in school for about 9 weeks. Further testing followed in intervals of 5 to 6 weeks. For each test time the children received the following texts to read:

1. Lists of familiar words: A word was considered familiar if the child had read it already in the basal reader. These words consisted only of the letters that had already been introduced during reading instruction.

2. Lists of new words, not yet familiar from the basal readers: The new words were taken from the core vocabulary and the narrow vocabulary from Plickat (1983) and were as frequent as the familiar words. They were similarly made up of only those letters that had been introduced during reading instruction prior to the time of testing.

3. Lists of pseudowords: The pseudowords were constructed from words already familiar to the children, by reordering the letters or exchanging individual letters. Care was taken that the pseudowords be made up of letter sequences that are frequent in written German and exhibit a high orthographic regularity.

For all tasks reading errors and reading times were recorded. We will only report the reading errors here. For each task, the number of errors was converted into a percentage of the total number of words on that list.

Qualitative analysis of reading behavior. For each task the response of the child during reading was recorded. The following measures were taken for the three types of words:

1. Graphic similarity of the reading errror to the target word: Applying Soederbergh's formula (1977) we differentiated among low, middle, and high similarity and calculated the percentage of errors that fell into each of these groups. We will examine more closely only those errors that fell into the high similarity group.

2. Naming an incorrect, familiar word: We recorded how often the children named a word which they already knew from the reading book, instead of the actual word to be read. It was then determined what proportion of the total number of errors these errors made up.

3. Sounding out: We recorded the percentage of words in which the children employed the technique of letter–by–letter, distinctly audible sounding out. It was also noted even when this only occurred for part of the word.

Statistical evaluation. The results of the five test times were condensed into three research periods, with mean values calculated where appropriate: Beginning (first testing), Middle (second and third testings), and End of the school-year (fourth and fifth testings). In order to address the research questions, a multivariate analysis of variance was performed. We investigated the effect of test time and task, that is, type of list (as a repeated measure) on reading errors, on the categories from the error analysis, and on reading behavior. Through the application of contrasts in the MANOVA, the factors List Type and Test Time were classified in such a way that each testing time could be compared with the following one, comparing familiar words with new words, and new words with pseudowords.

2.2   Results and Discussion

At the beginning of reading instruction, there was a distinct difference between the ability to read familiar words and the ability to read new words. There were virtually no errors in the reading of familiar words, in contrast to new words and pseudowords which, in comparison, were both read relatively inaccurately. Although there is a large difference between the accuracy with which familiar words as opposed to new and pseudowords were read, it is important to emphasize that new and pseudowords are read quite competently right from the beginning. A few weeks after the beginning of reading instruction, two–thirds of the new and pseudowords were read correctly.

The growth of reading performance was not equally distributed over the course of the first year of school. The changes that occured in the first few months of reading instruction were particularly striking when you take into consideration that in the beginning, the children have learned the grapheme–phoneme correspondences for only a few letters, and the remaining letters are only gradually introduced over the course of the first half of the year. At first, the children were limited in their ability to apply their knowledge of grapheme–phoneme correspondences to the reading of new words and pseudowords. The difference between familiar and new words then decreased relatively quickly. Within a few months, in fact, within a few weeks (the greatest change took place within the first and second testing times, meaning within 6 weeks), the reading of new words was managed much more successfully. One can see this as a qualitative change in reading behavior or reading strategies.

What argues for a qualitative change in reading behavior is that the progress in reading new words is accompanied by a temporary decrease in the accuracy with which familiar words are read. This is obviously related to the fact that the number of new words introduced in the course of reading instruction has greatly increased, so that logographic reading is no longer maintained.

The development of reading ability for familiar, new, and pseudowords is indicative of a qualitative change in reading strategy during the course of the first year of school. This development, however, does not show the kind of radical change one would have expected from the stage theory of reading development.

During the course of the first year of school there are also marked changes in reading behavior and in the type of reading errors. These changes are particularly striking in the first months. This is characterized by a sharp increase in the graphic similarity of the reading errors made on words that were already familiar from reading instruction. In the beginning, as one would expect for logographic reading, the errors scarcely resembled the target word. This, however, changed after only a few weeks. This change in reading development is closely correlated with another characteristic of reading behavior, that is, the naming of another familiar word from the reading instruction instead of the target word. This was observed almost exclusively during the reading of familiar words, and decreased markedly from the beginning to the middle of the school year.

This change in the quality of reading errors was limited to those made for familiar words. Errors on new and pseudowords, from the outset, show a high graphic similarity to the intended letter sequence and only rarely was another already read word named instead. From the beginning of reading instruction, one frequently observed a slow sounding out of the word. This kind of sounding out is employed much less often for familiar words. Those words that had been read during reading instruction were read quickly, without any perceptible delay.

The development of reading behavior confirms the assertion that familiar words, primarily at the beginning of learning to read, are read differently from new words and pseudowords. Whereas for familiar words, all the features of reading behavior attributable to the logographic stage can be observed, this is not the case for the new words and the pseudowords. Early on, one observes letter–by–letter reading for these words, at a time that still should be characterized by the use of a logographic route. The early use of the sounding out of words fits into the picture yielded by the analysis of the development of reading accuracy. There again, it appears that from the beginning the children can read a portion of the new and pseudowords without error. Instruction with a synthetic reading method results in a certain amount of phonological recoding right from the start.

The development of reading behavior clearly shows that the view of reading development as one divided into stages has only limited validity for German.

3. Reading Development in Poor Readers

Does the reading development of children who later exhibit reading difficulty follow the same, albeit temporally delayed, course as that of children who read without any problems? Or, can one identify, at least for some children, a qualitative deviation in the course of development?

This question becomes more concrete when one refers to the concept of component skills in reading: Is it the case that certain component skills are acquired by these children only with great effort, or not at all? This would mean that reading, to the extent that it is learned, would have to be supported by the overdependence on certain component skills, and that these children would not be able to perform certain tasks.

This question can be further expanded with a view to the concept of reading stages: Do poor readers fail to make the transition between certain stages of reading development? Are they not able to achieve the appropriate transition, or perhaps only partially? Or is it the case that they pass through all the stages, but that the problem is that the process is slowed down?

For English, the prevalent opinion is that it is primarily the acquisition of phonological recoding abilities that causes problems for poor readers (Barron, 1981; Jorm, 1984). Poor readers are therefore stuck in the stage of logographic reading (Frith, 1985), and the progress they are able to make in learning to read is reduced primarily to the expansion of a sight–word vocabulary. This would mean that the first stage of reading development is unimpaired and only after a period of time should one see a lagging behind.

Up to this point there has been little research on German. The prevalent opinion is that by the end of grade school all normally endowed children acquire sufficient reading accuracy, if not fluency (Schenk–Danzinger, 1968). An example of this is the paucity of relevant studies on dyslexia. There appears to be a greater interest in children's writing difficulties than their reading problems. It could be that the regularity of the German writing system does allow all, or almost all normally endowed children the achievement of sufficient reading accuracy.

On the other hand, the difficulties of learning to read in an alphabetic writing system can be attributed not only to a lack of regularity in grapheme–phoneme correspondences, but also to difficulties in understanding the internal structure of the language and to an inability to reflect on the organization of language into abstract phoneme units. These difficulties should be found when learning any alphabetic writing system, no matter how regular it is in its grapheme–phoneme correspondences. Based on this assumption, we would expect persistent reading difficulties for German, also.

This yields the following hypotheses for investigation: Poor readers differ from good readers primarily in the reading of words that require phonological recoding. They should have little difficulty with familiar words, particularly at the beginning of reading development when the number of familiar words is small. On the other hand, they should show great difficulty in the reading of new and pseudowords, and these difficulties should remain throughout the course of the school year.

A further question is whether this course of reading development is characteristic of all children who later have reading problems. Might there be children who at first have reading problems, but later catch up and achieve a normal level of reading development? Or, alternatively, might there be children who at first have no difficulties, but later develop problems? In the past few years, repeated reference has been made to the heterogeneity within the group of poor readers. Different divisions have been proposed: children with reading and spelling difficulties versus children with only spelling difficulties (Frith, 1985); division according to the type of reading and writing errors (Boder, 1973); or according to the relationship between reading speed and reading accuracy (Lovett, 1984). The value of these divisions is still being discussed. But even if these divisions into subgroups of reading and writing difficulties represent only the extreme forms of the heterogeneity found in normal reading and writing development (Bryant and Impey, 1986; Seymour, 1986), they can help us understand the specific, individual difficulties of many children. It therefore seems sensible to look for different types of reading development.

We chose to use the method of cluster analysis in order to construct subgroups that showed similar processes. It appeared too complicated to take into account all of the various views as to the relevant criteria, and too arbitrary to choose among criteria.

The reading errors that the children made at the beginning, the middle, and the end of the first grade on lists of familiar, new, and pseudowords were used as a basis for the division into groups. The cluster analysis was performed following Ward's method. The division of the entire group ($N = 82$) into three subgroups was accepted as the most sensible solution.

Of the three groups, the largest ($N = 49$; 59.8%), had no problems in learning to read. A second group ($N = 26$; 31.7%), had certain problems at the beginning, but by the end of the year learned to read quite well. Only the third group (N = 7; 8.5%) had great difficulty in learning to read and persistent problems throughout the school year. There was no homogeneous group that had no difficulties in the beginning, but developed problems later, during the course of the school year. This is not to say that no such children exist, only that their process of development was too heterogeneous to be identified as a single group.

As a follow–up to the cluster analysis, we used an analysis of variance to examine the influence of these three groups on the reading of word lists.

3.1   The Influence of Type of Word and Test Time on Reading Ability in the First Grade

What characterizes the *initially poor readers* is that in the beginning they have great difficulty with new words and pseudowords (Fig. 1). This group clearly differentiates itself at the beginning of reading development from those children who exhibit a problem–free course. These differences are evident during the entire first year of school (F (1,79) = 160.9; p = < .001), with a decrease in the difference from the beginning to the middle of the school year (F (1,79) = 9.9; p < .005), and then an even more considerable decrease from the middle to the end of the school year (F (1,79) = 39.7; p < .001). In addition, it is characteristic for this group, as opposed to the good readers, that they have problems reading new words, but no difficulty reading familiar words (F (1,79) = 91.2; p < .001). Also, for these children the number of errors increases from the beginning to the middle of the school year, which is not the case for the good readers. At the same time, the initially poor readers show a sharp decrease in the number of errors when reading new words (F (1,79) = 20.3; p < .001). This is related to the fact that during the course of the first half of the school year the number of words introduced during reading instruction increases, and thus already by the middle of the school year, the familiar words can no longer be recognized on the basis of a few features. It is the difficulty with reading new words that noticeably decreases over the course of the school year, especially in the second half (F (1,79) = 22.0; p < .001). Consequently, by the end of the course of instruction in the first grade the difficulties with these words have almost completely disappeared.

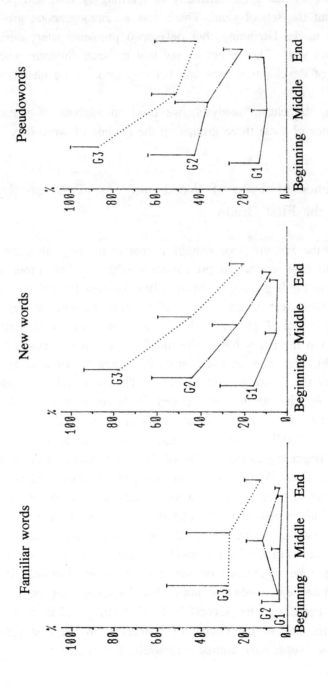

Fig. 1: The development of reading accuracy in the reading of familiar, new, and pseudowords by first graders with different courses of reading development (G_1: good readers; G_2: initially poor readers; G_3: persistently poor readers).

The difficulties initially poor readers have in reading pseudowords are similarly defined. These difficulties throughout the entire process are even more striking than those for new words (F (1,79) = 8.3; p < .01). The tendency for these difficulties to subside corresponds to that for new words. To be sure, these problems remain in the second half of the school year.

The *persistently poor readers* clearly exhibit a lower level of performance than either of the other two groups, especially in comparison to the initially poor group (F (1,79) = 124.6; p < .001). The persistently poor readers differ from the other two groups primarily in that from the outset they make many more errors. From its very high level, the number of errors decreases more sharply in the first half of the year for this group than for the initially poor readers (F (1,79) = 15.1; p < .001), but it still remains very high. In the second half of the year they might make as much progress as any child, but they never catch up. The level of reading performance at the end of the school year is low.

These children make relatively frequent errors on familiar words, and even more errors on new words. Thus the difference in the error percentage between familiar words and new words is even larger for these children than for the initially poor readers (F (1,79) = 9.1; p < .01).

A third difference has to do with the type of improvement in the second half of the year. For these children it is only a marked improvement for new words, whereas for pseudowords it is very small, much smaller than that for the initially poor readers (F (1,79) = 11.7; p = <.001).

In sum, one can say that the results of the analysis of variance clearly show differentiated courses of reading development for the three groups. How are these differences relevant to the processes of interest in reading development, particularly to the notion that reading development is a process carried out in stages?

All children, except those in the problem-free learning group, have marked problems in learning grapheme–phoneme relations. For the initially poor readers this is clearly the main reason why they remain behind in their reading development during the first half of the school year. They have problems only with those words in which the grapheme–phoneme relationship is crucial for reading, namely, in the reading of new words and pseudowords. The reading of new words and pseudowords also caused marked problems for the persistently poor readers. What differs from the initially poor readers is that these difficulties remain through the end of the school year. At that point they can still barely read half the pseudowords.

What is this difference in the persistence of these difficulties dependent upon? We assume that for the persistently poor readers, in addition to a severe impairment in phonological recoding abilities, another factor plays a role. As we have seen, at the beginning of the school year, there is a very striking difference betwen the two groups in their ability to read familiar words. The mastery of a sight–word vocabulary that has been gradually developed, helps the initially poor readers to learn the grapheme–phoneme correspondences during the school year. The existence of a sight–word vocabulary enables the children to test the correspondence between the spoken and the written form with enough examples so that it supplements the formal instruction. The persistently poor readers do not have this possibility to the same degree, and this could contribute to the fact that up to the end of the year the persistently poor readers have not really mastered phonological recoding.

Alternatively, one might suppose that the persistently poor readers, during most of the first grade year, have completely deficient phonological recoding abilities, and this makes the development of a sight–word vocabulary impossible. Whichever of these suggestions one prefers, they both make clear the early interaction between direct reading and phonological recoding.

The profile of the reading ability of the initially poor readers for the three types of words corresponds most closely to the description of reading development as formulated in a stage model. At the beginning they have no trouble with familiar words, but marked difficulties with new words and pseudowords. The reading skills which they acquire first appear to be based largely upon direct, logographic reading. Is this impression confirmed when one analyses the reading behavior of these children and the types of errors they make?

3.2   Reading Behavior

Graphic similarity. The errors of the initially poor readers show a smaller graphic similarity to the target word than those of the problem–free readers. This is true both for the first half of the year (F (1,24) = 4.2; p = .05), and for the second half of the year (F (1,50) = 6.5; p = .01). The graphic simi-larity of the error is particularly low at the beginning of the school year, and then increases until the middle of the school year, so that there is a closer approximation in this feature (F (1,24) = 8.2; p < .01). It is also noteworthy, that at the beginning of the year, the initially poor readers produce errors with low graphic similarity only for familiar words. For new words and pseudo-words the graphic similarity of the errors is higher. In contrast, this occurs with the good readers from the outset not only for new words and pseudo-words, but also for familiar words. (This interaction was not statistically relia-ble.) This tendency, however, means that initially poor readers, who make almost no errors on familiar words, must read them differently from new words.

The errors of the persistently poor readers in both the first and second halves of the year, are less similar to the target than those of the initially poor readers (F (1,24) = 2.1; p = .16; F (1,50) = 3.1; p = .08, respectively). At the beginning of the school year, their errors on familiar, new, and pseudowords all bear little graphic similarity to their targets. The similarity to the word to be read increases more sharply from the beginning to the middle of the year for the persistently poor readers than for the initially poor readers (F (1,24) = 3.4; p = .08), although the value remains lower.

Incorrect, familiar words. In the first half of the year, in contrast to the good readers, the initially poor readers frequently make errors in which they say another previously read word instead of the target (F (1,25) = 4.2; p = .05). This occurred primarily during the first testing and for the reading of familiar words (F (1,25) = 5.9; p < .05).

The persistently poor readers made this type of error less often than the init-ially poor readers (F (1,25) = 1.8; p = .18; F (1,51) = 1.8; p = .18, respectively).

Sounding out. At all test times, the initially poor readers used sounding out to read words as often as the problem–free readers (Fig. 2).

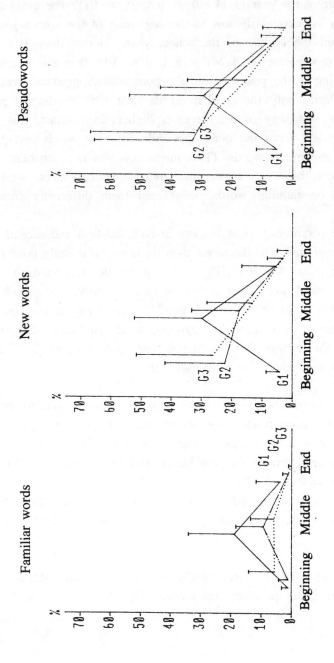

Fig. 2: The frequency of sounding out in the reading of familiar, new, and pseudowords by first graders with different courses of reading development (G_1: persistently poor readers; G_2: initially poor readers; G_3: good readers).

In contrast, the persistently poor readers at the beginning almost never sounded a word out. However, in the middle of the school year they sounded words out more often than the other two groups (F (1,78) = 8.2; $p <$ .01). In contrast to the other children, during the first testing the persistently poor readers did not sound out familiar, new, or pseudowords, although the sounding out of new and pseudowords was frequently observed in the other two groups. In the middle of the school year, sounding out was frequently used by the persistently poor readers for all types of words, even for familiar words, which the other children did not do (F (1,78) = 5.8; $p <$ .05).

To summarize, we can say that the three groups clearly differentiate themselves from one another both in their reading behavior and in the types of reading errors. Since these variables were not entered into the cluster analysis, this provides an outside validation of the formulation of the groups.

The results draw a more detailed picture of the reading difficulties of the three groups than would be possible from error frequencies alone. It is now clear that the initially poor readers, although they can identify familiar words via a direct, logographic route, have a lot of trouble with the reading of new words and pseudowords, because in these cases the logographic route is not very successful. This is why we find the high graphic similarity to the target word in the errors they make when reading new words and pseudowords, and the relatively frequent use of sounding out. Their behavior when reading these words is very similar to that of the good readers right from the beginning, except that they are not very successful in their efforts. Characteristic for this group of initially poor readers is the simultaneous existence of two different reading strategies. These children use a strategy of logographic reading for familiar words, and phonological recoding for new and pseudowords.

Despite the commonalities, the differences between the initially poor readers and the good readers should be emphasized. The good readers from the beginning of their reading instruction rarely appear to be reading logographically. Even for familiar words, their errors are graphically similar to the target, and they seldom name another previously read word instead of the target.

The persistently poor readers exhibit reading behavior that is very different from the other two groups. At the beginning of reading instruction there is almost no indication of phonological recoding. Their errors for all types of words are less similar to the target, and they do not sound words out. At this point, they are completely in a logographic stage. However, even for them the progress of reading development leads to a change, and this change is even more marked than that of the other children.

It is also noteworthy that the persistently poor readers are less inclined to replace the target word with a previously read word. Here, according to our view, there are once again problems in the acquisition of word–specific knowledge. The poor readers are in less of a position to learn the previously read words and therefore develop only an insufficient knowledge of their written form.

The analysis of reading behavior has shown that in the learning of the German writing system the identification of a logographic stage is in fact helpful. It helps us to understand the beginning of reading acquisition in a portion of children. It is, however, misleading to suggest that for German–speaking children, poor readers are stuck at the logographic stage. Our results show that the difficulties of poor readers most probably are due to their being less in the position to master phonological recoding. Other difficulties then follow as a result of this.

4. Further Development of Reading and Writing in Grade School

In labeling the groups as "initially poor" and "persistently poor" we have made certain assumptions about the further reading and writing development of these groups. We assume that the trend toward the gradual improvement of the reading difficulties of the initially poor readers will continue, but that the persistently poor readers will continue to have reading problems in the future.

The children were tested at the end of first, second, and third grades on a standardized oral reading test. At the same time the children were given a school achievement test, that among other things tested their spelling performance level.

The development of the oral reading ability in the subsequent years in grade school showed that the difficulties for the initially poor readers were in fact only transient. By the end of the third grade this group had caught up with the good readers both as far as reading accuracy and reading rate is concerned. On the other hand, the children who were persistently poor readers in the first grade, despite the fact that they do attain some reading accuracy and have reduced the number of errors they make on simple texts, do not catch up. With respect to reading rate, poor readers increasingly lag behind the performance level of other children.

As a supplement, we would like to report the spelling development of these children. Based on the literature on the difference between children who are poor readers and spellers with spelling problems exclusively, we suggested that the initially poor readers might be those children who no longer have trouble reading, but do have spelling problems. The results did not support this hypothesis.

5. Summary and Conclusions

The concept of developmental stages in reading helped us gain a better understanding of reading development, and turned out to be useful in the description of groups with different courses of reading acquisition. For reading development in German, that is, learning to read a writing system with regular grapheme–phoneme correspondences, one must acknowledge that there is overlapping among the stages, and thus the dissociation of different reading strategies can occur on differing tasks. Children can at the same time read familiar words logographically and read unfamiliar sequences letter by letter.

The suggestion that poor readers get stuck at the logographic stage, and in their later development or at least for a long time do not show any signs of the alphabetic stage, is not supported for German–speaking children. In fact, there was a group of poor readers who at the beginning showed no evidence of phonological recoding, and yet even these children, who at the end of the year were the poorest readers, after only 8 weeks exhibited a change in their reading behavior and in their reading strategies.

The relative regularity of the German writing system gave all the children in the research groups the possibility of the early use of phonological recoding. Despite this, the poor readers had trouble learning this skill and their reading performance remained at a very low level, even after several years. Even in the acquisition of the German writing system, there turn out to be great difficulties in the beginning stages of learning to read, problems which may persist at least until the end of elementary school.

References

Barron, R.W. (1981): Development of visual word recognition: A review. In MacKinnon, G.E., and Waller, T.G. (Eds.): Reading research. Advances in theory and practice, Vol. 3. New York: Academic Press

Biemiller, A. (1970): The development of the use of graphic and contextual information as children learn to read. Reading Research Quarterly, 6, 75–96

Boder, E. (1973): Developmental dyslexia: A diagnostic approach based on three atypical reading–spelling patterns. Developmental Medicine and Child Neurology, 15, 663–687

Bryant, P., and Impey, L. (1986): The similarities between normal readers and developmental and acquired dyslexics. Cognition, 24, 121–137

Chall, J.S. (1983): Stages of reading development. New York: McGraw–Hill

Cohen, A.S. (1975): Oral reading errors of first grade children taught by a code–emphasis approach. Reading Research Quarterly, 10, 616–650

Francis, H. (1977): Children's strategies in learning to read. British Journal of Educational Psychology, 47, 117–125

Francis, H. (1984): Children's knowledge of orthography in learning to read. British Journal of Educational Psychology, 54, 8–23

Frith, U. (1983): The similarities and differences between reading and spelling problems. In Rutter, M. (Ed.): Developmental neuropsychiatry. New York: Guilford Press

Frith, U. (1985): Beneath the surface of developmental dyslexia. In Patterson, K.E., Marshall, J.C., and Coltheart, M. (Eds.): Surface dyslexia: Neuropsychological and cognitive studies of phonological reading. London: Erlbaum

Henderson, L. (1982): Orthography and word recognition in reading. London: Academic Press

Jorm, A.F. (1984): The psychology of reading and spelling disabilities. London: Routledge and Kegan Paul

Jorm, A.F., and Share, D.L. (1983): Phonological recoding and reading acquisition. Applied Psycholinguistics 4, 103–147

Lovett, M.W. (1984): A developmental perspective on reading dysfunction: Accuracy and rate criteria in the subtyping of dyslexic children. Brain and Language 22, 67–91

Marsh, G., Desberg, P., and Cooper, J. (1977): Developmental changes in reading strategies. Journal of Reading Behavior, 9, 391–394

Perfetti, C.A. (1985): Reading ability. New York: Oxford University Press

Plickat, H. (1983): Der deutsche Grundwortschatz. Weinheim: Beltz–Verlag Schenk–Danzinger, L. (1968): Handbuch der Legasthenie im Kindesalter. Weinheim: Beltz–Verlag

Seymour, P.H.K. (1986): Cognitive analysis of dyslexia. London: Routledge and Kegan Paul

Seymour, P.H.K., and MacGregor, C.J. (1984): Developmental dyslexia: A cognitive experimental analysis of phonological, morphemic and visual impairments. Cognitive Neuropsychology, 1, 43–82

Soderbergh, R. (1971): Reading in early childhood: A linguistic study of a preschool child's gradual acquisition of reading ability. Stockholm: Almquist and Wiksell

Weber, R.M. (1970): A linguistic analysis of first–grade reading errors. Reading Research Quarterly, 5, 427–451.

Issues in Assessment and Intervention with Blind Infants and Children

David H. Warren

1. Introduction

The prospectus for the conference on "Prevention and Intervention in Childhood and Youth: Conceptual and Methodological Issues" mentions that the goals will be to explore the conceptual, empirical, and methodological problems in prevention and intervention research and practice with handicapped children, and specifically, today, with visually impaired children. I propose to touch on each of these areas, and I will do so in the context of two different topics. I will begin with the issue of assessment, which I consider to be perhaps the most important conceptual issue in our field. I will then move to the specific issue of spatial–cognitive development, where some of my own research is directed.

2. Assessment

The topic of assessment falls squarely within the scope of the conference, in that it is closely related to intervention, indeed should form the basis for intervention.

Let me begin by asking a very obvious question which turns out not to have a very obvious answer: What should the *goal* of intervention be?

There are many answers, but they fall into two major categories:

One category of answer is that the goal of intervention with visually impaired infants and children should be to have their developmental progression match the developmental norms that have been identified for sighted children.

The other category of answer rejects this goal of sighted equivalence, and says instead that the goal of intervention should be something *other than* sighted norms. The distinguishing feature of this category is the rejection of sighted developmental norms as the goal for visually impaired children.

I will say at the outset that I am an advocate of a form of the second position. I am sure that not all of you will agree with my choice of the second category, let alone with my own particular version of it, but I will state my own views firmly, and give the reasons that I hold this position: Then we can discuss the matter later.

My view is that we should *not* expect visually impaired children to match the developmental norms of sighted children. Furthermore, I suggest that we reject even the quest for developmental norms for visually impaired children as a population. Instead, we should define the goal as follows: Each visually impaired child should be encouraged and aided to reach his or her own optimal level of developmental progress and eventual attainment, without reference to any other child or set of norms.

This is a very important choice for us to make, because our choice will define the goals of intervention, and the goals in turn will direct our strategies for intervention. I want to explain in some detail the reasoning that leads me to this conclusion.

Let me first discuss the rejection of sighted norms: I will return later to the separate question of norms for visually impaired children.

First we should look at intervention itself and its purpose. The situation that calls for intervention is one that contains risk — some circumstance places the child "at risk", and seeing this, we intervene. Why do we intervene? We intervene with the purpose of reducing or eliminating the risk. We want to rearrange the circumstances so that the risk, which is only a *potential* adversity, does not become an *actual* adversity.

In the case of the visually impaired child without additional handicaps, the absence or dysfunction of vision creates a risk circumstance. Why is this a risk? It is a risk because vision is so fundamentally involved in so much of what human beings do. We all know of cases of visually impaired children who have made virtually no adjustment to this circumstance, who essentially vegetate, dependent on others for all of their needs. This is what can happen without effective intervention. We also all know of children who have very little restriction due to the lack of vision — they are bright, active, independent, and they will be successful people. In one case, the potential adversity has become actual; in the other, it has been avoided. How? By intervention. I do not mean to restrict my use of the term "intervention" to formal programs — I use the term to refer broadly to anything constructive that anyone, including the family member as well as the professional, does differently because of the visual circumstance than would be done if there were no visual impairment. Intervention involves actively rearranging the child's environment, rather than leaving it to happenstance.

Now, if we are going to be actively rearranging or manipulating the child's environment, we should certainly have a goal in mind: What do we want to accomplish by doing this manipulation? This is where the question of norms assumes importance. If our goal is to have the visually impaired child meet sighted developmental norms, then our intervention would take one form; if our goal is to minimize the potential adverse effects of the visual risk circumstance, then it might take quite a different form. So we need to have that goal defined. It is here that I wish to suggest that we adopt the goal of minimizing the adverse effects of the visual loss, rather than emulating the development of the sighted child.

I want to offer three examples that will help to illustrate the advantages and disadvantages of comparisons with sighted children.

The first example is the evaluation of intelligence. Whether for blind or for sighted children, intelligence has to do with how well the child will do in educational or other settings in which adaptation depends somehow on how well the child understands the physical world and can think and reason.

It has been recognized for a long time now that we have to use different instruments to evaluate this potential for adaptation in visually impaired children. It is clearly misleading to evaluate the visually impaired child using a test that has items that require vision for their administration, or that require specific knowledge that can only be obtained visually. This recognition has led in two directions. In one, a test such as the Wechsler Intelligence Scale for Children is used, but the parts that require vision are omitted, and individual items are selectively modified or omitted. This, it is generally agreed, produces an evaluation of the visually impaired child that is incomplete and therefore not comparable to the evaluation of the sighted child. Most significantly, it omits

the performance scales. Most will agree that to get a full picture of the visually impaired child's intelligence, it is important to evaluate these spatial abilities as well as verbal abilities. This problem has led to the other approach. This
involves the drastic modification, revision, and supplementation of material
from standardized tests, such as that resulting in the Perkins–Binet test, or even
the design of tests specifically for the visually impaired child, such as the Blind
Learning Aptitude Test of Newland.

But in attempting to evaluate the intelligence of visually impaired children in
this appropriate way, we have created a situation in which it is impossible to
make any legitimate comparison of the intelligence of visually impaired and
sighted children. We cannot use the tests developed for sighted children because
they are inappropriate for the visually impaired. And we should not test sighted
children with the tests that have been developed specifically for visually impaired children, because these tests would similarly misrepresent *their* intelligence or capacity for adaptation.

In my view, this is not a bad situation − I think that it is not only *impossible*
to make this comparison, but that it is also *improper*. Recall the purpose of
doing the evaluation in the first place: It is to assess and predict how well the
individual will do in adaptive situations. That is an individualized question, and
the question of the comparison of sighted and visually impaired populations is
entirely beside the point − it is a question that need not even be asked, because there is no important consequence of its answer. The question should not
be how much like the sighted child we can make the visually impaired child
appear, but how well the visually impaired child can be led to adapt to the life
situations which he or she will encounter.

A second example illustrates the logical, though in my view not sensible,
extreme of the notion of using sighted norms as the benchmark for visually
impaired children. Stephens and Simpkins (1974) studied a wide range of
Piaget–type cognitive abilities in blind and sighted children, over the age range
6 to 18 years. The sighted children performed with vision available, and the
blind children performed the tasks tactually. Severe deficits were found for the
blind children in many tasks. For the sighted children, there was a clear
progression from the 6–to 10–year old group to the 10– to 14–year group, and
again to the 14–to 18–year group. The blind 10–to 14–year–old group showed

little advancement over the 6–to 10–year–old group, and in fact there were few differences in level of performance between the sighted 6–to 10–year–olds and the blind 14–to 18–year–olds. (I should point out that this is a far bleaker picture than has been reported by other researchers using similar tests, for example Tobin (1972), Gottesman (1973), and Cromer (1973)).

Stephens (Stephens and Grube, 1982) went on to design an experiential intervention program whose goal was to bring the performance of the blind children up to that of their sighted age–mates. During the 17–month intervention period, the blind children received an extensive individualized program which averaged about 95 hours per child. Generally, the training was apparently successful: The blind children progressed to the point where they were equivalent on most conservation and classification measures, although there were still some differences in tests of spatial and mental imagery.

Apparently then, the intervention program was a success. But I have serious questions about it, and about the whole basis for conducting it at all. First, most of the research that finds developmental lags in visually impaired children tests the sighted with vision and the blind of course tactually, or haptically. This is not a meaningful comparison. (Nor, of course, is it meaningful to compare the blind performing haptically with a group of blindfolded sighted children performing haptically.) Haptic perception simply plays a different role in the perceptual ecology of the blind child from that which vision plays for the sighted child, and I do not think that they can possibly serve as equivalent indicators of the achievement of cognitive level. So I maintain that the premise on which the intervention was based is faulty.

Second, what about the goal of the intervention, which was to eradicate these apparent differences? This goal is no sounder than the premise on which it rests. Why should we want to make these two different kinds of performance, the haptic for the blind and the visual for the sighted, equivalent? The kinds of performance are different, and making them *appear* the same does not make the underlying cognitive capabilities the same. If we take a pear and an apple, we can see that they are not equivalent: Their shapes are different, and the apple is red while the pear is yellow. What would we accomplish by carving the pear to have the shape of the apple, and coloring its skin red? We would not make it into an apple — it is still a pear, though no longer one with any self–respect.

I do not question the premise that cognitive development is an area in which there is risk for the visually impaired child, and in fact I believe that this is a critically important area for intervention. But the intervention should have as its goal not the achievement of apparent equivalence to sighted children; rather, the goal should be to bring each visually impaired child to the level of having the soundest concepts possible about the nature of the physical world.

A more suitable approach is illustrated in a study by Lopata and Pasnak (1976). Based on a pretest of intelligence and of cognitive skills, the children, who were legally blind, were divided into two matched groups. One group was given individualized training in Piaget–type cognitive skills over a period of some weeks − in this respect, the plan was quite similar to that of Stephens and Grube. The other group received other intervention, but not involving cognitive skill training. At the end, both groups were again given a cognitive skills test and the IQ test. The trained group showed a significant improvement on both tests compared to the untrained group.

Why is this a better study? It is better in two important ways. First, the improvement of the training group of visually impaired children was compared to that of an untrained group, also of visually impaired children: The goal was not to see how much like sighted children they could be made to perform, but rather to see how much they could improve compared to untrained visually impaired children. Second, evaluation was made not just of improvement on the cognitive skills that were involved in the training, but also in performance on an intelligence test, in this case the Slossen test. This step is important because it allows evaluation of whether any improvement was limited to the trained skills, or was more general, of a kind that would show up in a broader, non-specific test.

I would be even more satisfied with such a study if, in addition to maintaining the basic orientation to visually impaired children and their improvement, it would also assess the generalization of performance to adaptive learning situations that are thought to require cognitive skills.

Let me take a final example; one that illustrates an exceedingly difficult problem in considering the desirability and the nature of intervention.

Many people have noticed that blind infants are slow to crawl and then to walk. Fraiberg (1968) reported this, and noted that this slowness occurred in spite of other motor indications that these 1–year–old infants were strong enough to crawl and had been observed resting on their hands and knees for several months prior to the actual onset of crawling. She reported further that crawling did begin very quickly after the infants began to reach outward for sound-producing objects. Apparently the action of reaching outward to sound enabled the similar reach, which consitutes the first action of crawling, to emerge. So Fraiberg's notion is that the developmental delay in crawling is not a result of lags in motor capabilities, but is rather because of a delay in the reach to sound.

Fraiberg's group then devoted considerable effort to getting infants to reach to sounds earlier, on the assumption that this would allow earlier crawling and then walking. This was thought to be important because "failure to achieve locomotion within a critical period of time may be one of the factors that bring about developmental arrest in deviant children" (Fraiberg and Freedman, 1964, p. 163). Although their efforts were not generally successful, the issue is an important one in its own right and a good illustration of the difficult issues of assessment and intervention.

In fact, compared to sighted infants, Fraiberg's blind infants were *not* delayed in reaching to sounds. Although sighted infants do typically reach to visually perceived objects by about 5 months of age, they do not reach to objects purely based on sound cues until late in the first year, just as blind infants do (Freedman, Fox–Kolenda, Margileth, and Miller, 1969). If the reaching–crawling link is a valid one, then it is presumably the earlier reach to objects based on *visual* cues, not *sound* cues, that triggers crawling midway through the first year for sighted infants.

So what should we do? There are good arguments in favor of intervention, to try to stimulate earlier reaching and presumably earlier crawling. At the same time, there are reservations that should be expressed.

In favor of intervention are the following points. First, early locomotor development, and presumably later activities that depend on it, would be facilitated. I do not think that the timing of locomotor development by itself is sufficient justification: I see no reason why crawling at six months of age or walking at a year is desirable simply for its own sake. But second, what if the infant's *cognitive* development is somehow being restricted by the same factors that impede earlier crawling? This is not impossible: Reaching out for objects in the environment may be as important to the development of cognitive skills, such as understanding the critical distinction between the self and the external world, as it is to crawling. If the early stages of cognitive development are being retarded by the failure to reach, then subsequent stages will also be slowed down. We might view this as a more serious kind of delay.

Why should a delay in either locomotor development or cognitive development be a concern, if developmental equity with the sighted infant is not necessarily desirable?

There is one very good reason to be concerned. We usually think of the development of conceptual abilities as an interactive process, in which appropriate experiences encounter a nervous system which is maturationally prepared for them. This combination of neural readiness and appropriate experience produces cognitive development. If there is a serious mismatch, in which for some reason the necessary experience does not occur during the time of neural readiness, then might there be lasting cognitive results? To make the general point more specific, perhaps there is a time of neural readiness in the middle of the first year when the infant is prepared to encounter the kind of information that results from reaching out for objects in the external world. Perhaps the blind infant's failure to reach outward during that time produces a situation in which the period of neural readiness passes by without the infant's having encountered the appropriate experiences. This might produce a cognitive deficit that would be very difficult to overcome.

Of course, there are individuals who are congenitally blind and who have no apparent cognitive deficits whatsoever — do they not disprove this kind of reasoning? Not automatically: It may be that they were provided with some particular kinds of experiences that led to an early reaching outward, with associated progress in locomotion and conceptual development; or it may be that they showed the early lags and yet overcame them later on. This is not a trivial question, either theoretically or practically — certainly wise and effective intervention practice depends on its answer.

One possible solution to this whole problem is to suggest that we should, simply as a matter of routine, intervene to elicit reaching and the other activities earlier. What danger could there be in this?

In fact there *are* some dangers, and I want to mention two. First, children often regress in an aspect of development if they are pushed too hard; further, this regression may often generalize to other areas of performance. If we try to get blind infants to reach outward to sounds before they are ready for this experience, then we may be creating the situation for just this sort of generalized regression. Second, during the first year the blind infant has a vast array of learning tasks before him, and it may be better to let him concentrate his developmental energy in those areas in which he can make spontaneous progress, rather than pushing abilities which are not ready to occur.

In any case, this is a critical area in which we need to get some definite answers; answers based on empirical research. In designing any research, we need to have a motivating goal in mind. I think that the goal in this case should be to provide the blind infant with experiences that are appropriate to that infant's level of neural readiness. This is a very different goal than trying to match sighted developmental norms, and it would require quite a different program of empirical research.

Let me return now to the main conceptual issue that led to these examples: This is the issue of norms, and specifically whether the developmental progress of visually impaired children should be evaluated against the benchmark of sighted norms. I hope that I have made a persuasive case against the use of such norms.

Now, though, I want to push it a step farther and suggest that we abandon the use of *any* norms for visually impaired children, including even those norms that are generated from the visually impaired population itself.

Essentially, my argument is that the population of visually impaired children is so heterogeneous that the very concept of norms is inappropriate. The term *norm* is short for *normal*, or average. The average, the norm, is a way of characterizing a population. We can calculate an average of just about anything, but the fact that it can be calculated does not make it meaningful. The greater the range of values of a variable is in a population, the less meaningful is any descriptive number such as an average or a norm for that population.

This immense variation in the population of visually impaired children is a consequence of the fact that these children differ from one another along a number of important dimensions. They differ in how much residual visual function they may have. They differ in the cause of the visual impairment. They differ in when the impairment began, and whether it was gradual or sudden. And perhaps most important of all, they differ in the presence or absence of additional handicaps, and in the degree of severity of these.

In order to establish a norm for such a diverse population, say of visually impaired 8-year-olds, we would have to be sure that in every important respect, the sample that we select to measure reflects the distribution of these variables in the population. This is probably impossible from a practical point of view. But even if it *were* possible, the result would be largely useless. We know that it does not make any sense to compare two 8-year-olds, one who has been totally blind virtually from birth as a result of Retinopathy of Prematurity with an accompanying hearing loss, with a child who became blind by accident at age 6. So what sense would it make to evaluate either of them with reference to population norms that are based on a sample with even greater heterogeneity? Not much, I suggest.

In order to make any kind of norming approach meaningful, we would have to take all of those six or eight important variables, combine them every possible way in a matrix, and generate a separate set of norms for every resulting subpopulation. I do not think that the result would be worth the effort.

Instead, I think that we should approach the intervention question in an entirely individualized manner. We should generate expectations, and create interventions designed to meet them, for each visually impaired child separately from every other child. I do not have a detailed solution to offer, and I recognize that this is a shortcoming in my treatment. Perhaps there is an analogy that we could pursue: In the educational setting, we attempt to do this with the IEP, the individualized education plan, and I think that we might consider an extension of this concept to the blind child's entire developmental progression.

In short, I suggest that developmental norms for the visually impaired population are theoretically meaningless as well as unhelpful to the goals of intervention. Now, I have no doubt that however much you may have agreed with what I said earlier, some of you will disagree with this conclusion! In any case, I hope you *will* agree that this is one of the major conceptual problems that we face in the field of childhood visual impairment today.

3. Spatial Perception and Cognition

I want to move now to an area of research with which I have been concerned for some time. This is the ability of the visually impaired child to understand the spatial environment, both perceptually and conceptually. I do not want to restrict this concept very much — I mean it to include everything from very minor and practical things like knowing where and how to find one's tooth-brush, to very major and practical things like effective mobility in the spatial environment, to purely conceptual things like understanding what one's current position is in relation to the rest of the room, the building, the local geography, or even the Atlantic Ocean.

That is obviously a vast topic, and I will have to restrict it for today. I will do so by discussing a theme that I think underlies success in every one of these examples. It is the development of the ability to understand the nature of spatial structure. I want to suggest a way of thinking about this area of development that is somewhat different from the way we usually think about it, a way that fits in with the view of intervention that I have presented.

Most people proceed, over years of development and experience, from the neonate's virtual lack of any spatial concept, through a series of intermediate levels, to a set of mature concepts that allow us, for example, to imagine, describe, and follow routes through *known* environments; to learn routes and layouts in *new* environments; to imagine, as we sit in a familiar place, what is behind the wall, below the floor, and above the ceiling; to estimate distances and travel times; to use maps; and so on. All of these tasks require some basic understanding of the nature of spatial structure. And of course some of us are better or worse than others at any given task. Nonetheless, all of us are considerably better at them than a human neonate is.

The developmental question is this: What is necessary to cause the infant or child to progress from one of these levels of spatial understanding to another? I suggest that we may consider the infant to suffer from a limitation: The limitation is a set of inadequate spatial concepts. If he is to progress to a better set of more effective concepts, he has to break out of the restrictions that characterize his present concepts. We can think of developmental progress as a series of phases of breaking out of or escaping from concepts that are too limited, that are insufficient to the individual's current needs. This does not happen all at once: The neonate who lacks virtually any spatial concepts first acquires a set of concepts that suffices for a time, perhaps to guide activities of reaching to visible objects; but this set of limited concepts will in turn prove insufficient for his needs when he begins to locomote in the spatial environment.

Generally, older infants and young children can be characterized as having *egocentric* spatial concepts, in which external locations are interpreted with respect to the child's own orientation and location. This egocentrism gradually gives way to external concepts; using these, the child can relate items in the spatial field to other items in that field, rather than only to himself. Gradually *allocentric* concepts are acquired, with which the young child can deal with relationships among objects in the external space entirely without reference to his own location or orientation.

After this major qualitative change, further change is more quantitative — children acquire spatial understanding of larger-scale environments and spatial relationships, and of course they come to be able to use those concepts to direct their own behavior not only in the immediately accessible space but in larger spatial areas such as neighborhoods and cities.

If we take this idea that spatial concepts are limited at any given developmental level, with restrictions that need to be overcome in order to move on to the next level, then the question becomes: What must happen in order for the infant or child to escape these limitations and to progress to the next level?

This is a good place to direct the issue back to the visually impaired child. We are safe in assuming that the blind neonate has the same limitation of spatial concepts that the sighted neonate has. There is no evidence that blind neonates generally have any trouble finding their mouths with their thumbs; this suggests that they quickly develop at least a rudimentary functional concept of the topology of parts of their bodies. However, the evidence presented by Fraiberg and others tells us that blind infants in the latter half of the first year do not reach out for objects in the external environment. They are apparently working within a conceptual restriction, in which they fail to realize the independent existence of external objects. Piaget, describing pre-object-concept, sighted infants, suggests that for them an object in effect ceases to exist when it is not in perceptual range. Without functional vision, that range is more limited for the blind infant; somehow, the concept of object permanence has to develop despite this greater perceptual limitation. We can think of this as a risk situation of the sort that I discussed earlier, one that may call for intervention in order to bring the infant safely by.

From this point on there is a considerable gap in our knowledge about the spatial-conceptual development of visually impaired children, until we come to the research that falls under the *spatial cognition* rubric. In the past decade, there has been considerable work that shows that visually impaired children have difficulties conceptualizing even moderately familiar environments. I refer here, for example, to a study by Casey (1978), who found most of his visually impaired sample to have serious difficulties in constructing a model of the grounds of the school which they had been attending for at least a year.

Furthermore, visually impaired children generally have difficulty learning the spatial relationships among a set of objects arranged in novel settings. An example is the study by Fletcher (1980), who found visually impaired children to have great difficulty with what she called "map" questions, which require them to learn the objective spatial relationships among objects in an unfamiliar room. They were much better at "route" questions, which required learning which object followed or preceded another in relation to the child's own path through the room. When the locations of objects could be referenced to the child's own route through the room, performance was reasonable. These *route* questions can be answered on the basis of an *egocentric* concept. When objects in the room had to be referenced to one another, performance was very poor. Successful answers to such *map* questions require an *allocentric* concept. The limitation to an egocentric spatial concept, and the related failure to proceed to an allocentric concept, constitutes a serious cognitive problem. There is another risk situation here, and the consequent question of intervention. What kinds of experience can be provided to facilitate the progression from egocentric to allocentric spatial concepts?

I have recently been directing a research project that is designed to explore the nature of this progression from egocentric to allocentric spatial concepts. I want to acknowledge, with thanks, the support of the March of Dimes Birth Defects Foundation that has made this project possible. We are working with visually impaired children of elementary school age. Our first hypothesis is that visually impaired children *do* use some allocentric spatial concepts, and that we would be most likely to find evidence of such allocentric concepts if we test them in environments with which they are highly familiar. This is borne out: Most of our subjects demonstrate a very good spatial understanding of their own living room, and the ability to deal with object–object spatial relations in this setting.

Then we create an artificial spatial setting, in which we can arrange the locations of objects at will. As we expected, after a brief exposure to such a novel setting, the children's responding is not allocentric: It is either egocentric, with responding governed by reference to their momentary location, or less frequently, it is entirely chaotic. Then, we are interested in whether they will gradually acquire allocentric understanding of this novel setting as a result of increased experience in it. We explore this under different conditions.

The reference condition is one in which they simply get repeated exposure to the locations of the items in the setting, by walking to each item from a standard starting point and back to the starting point. In another condition, after pretraining, they use the Sonicguide, an electronic sensory aid. In yet another condition, there is no Sonicguide, but we install an auditory landmark in a fixed location off to the side of the setting: It is a repetitive beeping sound. Presumably, the child might be able to use this stable auditory landmark as an external reference, and to learn the locations of the objects in the setting in relation to that external reference rather than in relation to his or her own locomotor paths.

The research is not completed, but several results are emerging of which I am fairly confident. First, at least some children can acquire an allocentric concept of such a novel space, based on several half-hour sessions of practice. The transition from egocentric to allocentric concepts does not happen all at once; it emerges, when it does, over several test sessions. Second, at least under these limited conditions, the Sonicguide does not generally facilitate the child's acquisition of an allocentric concept of the spatial setting. Third, the auditory reference landmark seems to provide the best condition for allocentric concept acquisition.

What can explain these results? Taking the last point first, the auditory reference landmark apparently can serve as a stable point of reference, one which is consistently perceptually available to the child. He can relate the direction that he is moving to get to a particular object to the sound, and he can hear the difference in the sound's position when he is at one location as opposed to another location.

Why is the Sonicguide not of similar benefit? The Sonicguide is an electronic device which produces an audible signal that denotes the direction and distance of objects. My thinking at this time is that this device is, in effect, simply serving as a longer pair of arms for the child. That is, as the child approaches an object, the Sonicguide gives perceptual evidence of the location of the object before the child can contact that object with his hands. But since the device is mounted on the child's head, it moves around the environment with him, and therefore it does not give him the kind of stable, external reference that the auditory landmark does. It provides an additional source of *perceptual* information, but it does not, under these conditions, facilitate the *conceptual* organization of that information.

These are preliminary results, but they suggest that the acquisition of spatial concepts, particularly mature allocentric concepts of novel environments, can indeed be facilitated by the provision of external perceptible landmarks. We are not taking a very structured approach to this facilitation in the current research, but I am proposing to follow up this work with a project in which we will work specifically with two kinds of strategies for learning spatial relationships. These are *landmark referencing* and *spatial updating*.

Landmark referencing refers to the process of learning the linkages among objects in a space, first in small sets of two and three, then gradually linking additional objects so that the child learns where each new object is in relation to the structured relationship among previously learned objects. Such knowledge is independent of the child's own momentary location.

Spatial updating refers to the child's own movement within the space, to keeping track of his or her continuously changing location in relation to the fixed locations of known objects. Effective updating depends on a good understanding of the stable structure of the spatial environment — the child has to know what is in the space, and where, in order to keep track of his changing relationship to it. And of course, effective mobility depends on updating.

I think that by beginning with these strategies in relatively well-known spaces, we can teach children to apply them in novel spatial settings as well as in larger spaces, and that by this process we will be able to produce not only better concepts of the immediate spaces in which the child exists, but also a good set of spatial conceptualization and learning strategies that the child will be able to use in encountering entirely novel spatial settings.

4. Infancy

I want to return briefly to the other major transition period in the development of spatial concepts, that is the transition from the 6-month-old infant's failure to understand that there are objects whose existence is independent of his own perceptual experience of them, to the stage of object constancy in which the existence of objects is independent of the 18–month–old's immediate perceptual experience of them.

I have already talked about what the positive and negative consequences of intervention might be. But we need to understand more about this developmental era and the particular spatial conceptual restrictions that must be overcome in it. This era is just as important for us to understand as the early childhood transition from egocentric to allocentric concepts, perhaps even more so, since it may involve critical periods which may affect locomotor as well as cognitive development. We need to know whether there is indeed a critical neural period, such that a mismatch between maturation and experience may be created. We need to know what the consequences of such a mismatch are, and whether such consequences are transitory or long–lasting. We need to know what the positive and negative effects of intervention might be. We need to know what kinds of experience might lead to an earlier recognition of the independent existence of objects. We need to know, in particular, what the role of auditory perception is, and how it works. Can auditory spatial experience substitute for visual spatial experience? Might a combination of auditory and tactual experience be effective? Can auditory information be sufficiently spatially structured to substitute for the spatial–organizational role that vision serves in the sighted infant?

These are critical questions for our understanding of the perceptual and cognitive development of the visually impaired infant, and we need much research on them in order to have the basis to design effective intervention programs for visually impaired infants. That we need such intervention programs I do not question. I *am* convinced that we do not at present have enough information on which to base optimally effective interventions.

5. Conclusion

My minor goal has been to provoke your interest in issues of spatial concepts and the circumstances for their development, and to offer a way of looking at these issues within a model for intervention that identifies risk circumstances and seeks to intervene to minimize or eliminate the consequences of the risk.

My more major concern has been with the critical issue of assessment, and with its implications for intervention questions. Here, I have argued that we should not only reject the idea of comparing the developmental progress of visually impaired children to that of sighted children, but that we should also reject the notion that there are useful norms to be developed for the population of visually impaired children. Rather than evaluating any visually impaired child's progress in relation to any norm, we should evaluate that progress in relation to his or her own presumed optimal level of functioning. I do not in any way see this as acceding to a lower level of attainment for the visually impaired child. I see it not as settling for less than is possible, but rather as avoiding the setting of artificial goals for the visually impaired child. Difficult as it may be to attain, our goal should be to intervene to create in every visually impaired child his or her own optimal level of accomplishment, in personal, educational, and vocational goals.

References

Casey, S.M. (1978): Cognitive mapping by the blind. Journal of Visual Impairment and Blindness, 72, 297–301

Cromer, R.F. (1973): Conservation by the congenitally blind. British Journal of Psychology, 64, 241–250

Fletcher, J.F. (1980): Spatial representation in blind children. 1: Development compared to sighted children. Journal of Visual Impairment and Blindness, 74, 381–385

Fraiberg, S. (1968): Parallel and divergent patterns of blind and sighted infants. Psychoanalytic Study of the Child, 23, 264–300

Fraiberg, S., and Freedman, D.A. (1964): Studies in the ego development of the congenitally blind child. Psychoanalytic Study of the Child, 19, 113–169

Freedman, D.A., Fox–Kolenda, B.J., Margileth, D.A., and Miller, D.H. (1969): The development of the use of sound as a guide to affective and cognitive behavior – A two–phase process. Child Development, 40, 1099–1105

Gottesman, M. (1973): Conservation development in blind children. Child Development, 44, 824–827

Lopata, D.J., and Pasnak, R. (1976): Accelerated conservation acquisition and IQ gains by blind children. Genetic Psychology Monographs, 93, 3–25

Stephens, B., and Grube, C. (1982): Development of Piagetian reasoning in congenitally blind children. Journal of Visual Impairment and Blindness, 76, 133–143

Stephens, B., and Simpkins, K. (1974): The reasoning, moral judgement, and moral conduct of the congenitally blind (Report No. H23–3197). Office of Education, Bureau of Education for the Handicapped.

Tobin, M.J. (1972): Conservation of substance in the blind and partially sighted. British Journal of Educational Psychology, 42, 192–197

Methodological and Conceptual Issues in the Construction of a Developmental Test for Blind Infants and Preschoolers

Michael Brambring

1. Introduction

Our knowledge of the development of blind and partially sighted children during infancy and preschool age is still fragmentary, a fact which is also pointed out in the reviews of Vander Kolk (1981), Warren (1984), Ferrell (1986), and Lewis (1987). The reasons for this can be seen, among others, in the small number of children examined and the heterogeneity of the characteristics and conditions investigated. The heterogeneity refers to the variety of visual impairment (i.e., onset, degree, and cause), to the different physical and so-cial–environmental conditions of the individual children, and to the low comparability of the assessment procedures used.

It is expecially serious that, with the exception of the investigations of Norris, Spaulding, and Brodie (1957) and Fraiberg (1977), no longitudinal studies exist in which the individual developmental progress of blind and partially sighted infants has been observed over a long period.

The lack of empirical developmental data restricts the systematic introduction of early prevention strategies, as such strategies could only be planned with sufficiently precise knowledge of the "normal" development of visually impaired children. Also, intervention strategies based on diagnosed developmental retardations presume that the observed developmental retardations indicate significant developmental delays in the individual child. Such a statement, however, is only possible if the developmental data of the individual child can be compared with the developmental data of other visually impaired children of comparable status. It seems that this goal can only be achieved with difficulty because of the above–mentioned heterogeneity of the individual biographies of visually–impaired children. However, these difficulties should not be a reason for abandoning the construction of appropriate assessment procedures, but should lead to more precise formulations of the conditions under which an adequate developmental diagnosis is also possible for visually impaired infants.

Comprehensive developmental assessment means the reliable testing of the developmental characteristics of the child in all relevant developmental areas as well as the assessment of the conditions of the social and family environment in which the child grows up. The last-named aspect in the development of handicapped children requires particular attention.

In the present article only the first-mentioned aspect − the assessment of development in early childhood − will be discussed in detail, with the emphasis on the presentation of the methodological and conceptual difficulties which arise when constructing a developmental test for visually impaired infants. Finally, our own procedures in drawing up the "Bielefeld Developmental Test for Blind Infants and Preschoolers" will be described.

2. Previous Developmental Tests for Visually Impaired Infants

The goal of a developmental test is to obtain, in a relatively short period of time, comparable data about the developmental level of children. The quality of a developmental test − like any other diagnostic procedures such as observation or questionnaires − emerges when inter- and intraindividual developmental differences are reliably detected, and further developmental progress is accurately predicted. Up to now, there are only a few procedures for the assessment of the developmental stage of blind and partially sighted children. This statement applies to observation and questionnaires as well as to test procedures.

Worldwide, there are only three procedures which claim to assess the developmental stage of visually impaired preschool children comprehensively: Oregon Project for Visually Impaired and Blind Preschool Children (Brown et al., 1979, Reynell−Zinkin Scales (Reynell, 1979), Würzburger Testinstrument (Blindeninstitutsstiftung Würzburg, 1980).

The Oregon project consists of a diagnostic section ("Skills Inventory") and a section with instructions for early intervention ("Teaching Activities") which is based on the diagnostic section.

The skills inventory comprises approximately 700 items which are assigned to six developmental areas − cognition, language, self-help, socialization, fine motor, and gross motor. The items were taken from other developmental tests by selecting those items which were most important for the assessment of the developmental level of visually impaired children. The items contain specific codings for totally blind children. In addition to assessing the developmental level, the items should suggest whether the child needs Braille or orientation/ mobility training.

The age range extends from birth up to the age of six, with the items being listed hierarchically within each of the six age groups. The raw data per age group can be converted into relative data.

The skills inventory attempts to fulfill the following objectives:

1. to assess the stage of development in the six developmental domains;
2. to select suitable developmental interventions; and
3. to record the developmental progress of the children.

The skills inventory should assess the developmental level of the children. However, it should not be used in the sense of a normative developmental test because the age data which serve as comparative data are based on normative data from sighted children.

The selection of intervention measures depends on the recorded intraindividual developmental retardations in the six developmental domains.

An empirical examination was carried out with 53 children aged between several months and 8 years; these data, however, have yet to be taken into account in the test instructions.

The Reynell–Zinkin Scales are based on the concept of the Bayley Scales, but the Reynell–Zinkin Scales have only published a "Mental Scale" and as yet no "Motor Scale." The developmental test consists of five subscales with a total of 114 items. The test covers the age groups from birth to the age of five for blind and partially sighted children. The five subscales comprise:

1. Social Adaptation, that is, the social reaction of the children to other persons as well as the adoption of independent routines like eating, drinking, and so forth.
2. Sensorimotor Understanding, that is, the understanding of real objects and the relations between them.
3. Exploration of Environment, that is, the orientation of the child in the room and the appropriate use of large objects like pieces of furniture, doors, and so forth.

4. Verbal Comprehension, that is, the localization of sounds, voices, and so forth; the recognition of words and the following of verbal instructions

5. Expressive Language, that is, the development of language structure such as word utterances and sentence constructions, as well as the language content, that is, the naming of objects and the telling of a story containing a sequence of simple events.

The scale was tested on 109 visually impaired children with no additional severe handicaps. Through multiple testing, 203 data sets were collected which served as an empirical basis for the calculation of the age distribution. The age calculations were made separately for blind and partially sighted children at 3-month intervals. These should serve as reference points — not as norms — for the assessment of the developmental stage of the child.

The test was deliberately not subjected to a test-theoretical examination (reliability and predictive validity) because of the small number of children in each age group and the heterogeneity of the samples involved.

According to the age tables, the developmental differences between blind and partially sighted children on the one hand and a sighted comparative group on the other, reach their highest level at the age of 3 and 4 and amount to approximately two years for the scales "Social Adaptation" and "Sensorimotor Understanding", and to approximately one year for the "Language Scales."

The Würzburger Testinstrument for multiply handicapped visually impaired children is designed to assess the developmental stage and the developmental progress of children who are both mentally-handicapped and visually impaired. The items are mostly taken from the "Munich Functional Developmental Test" (Hellbrügge et al., 1978; Coulin et al., 1977) and the "Kiphard Scales" ("Sensorimotor and Psycho-Social Developmental Grid"). The age span extends to 48 months. Altogether, the test instrument contains 10 different subtests with a total of 378 items. The test specifies whether the tasks concern both groups or partially sighted and blind children separately. The 10 subtests contain:

1. Gross motor: Mainly locomotion items for children aged from 11 to 48 months.

2. Hand motor — fine motor: Items for the manipulation of objects for children aged from 10 to 48 months.

3. Sensorimotor: Tasks for perceptive-motor coordination for children aged from 12 to 48 months.

4. Expressive Language: Items from birth to 48 months of age.
5. Speech Comprehension: Items from the 10th to the 48th month.
6. Social Behaviour: Items from birth to 48 months of age.

Finally, another 4 scales for daily living skills:

7. Eating: Items from the 1st to the 42nd month.
8. Putting on and taking off of clothes: Items from the 16th to the 48th month.
9. Washing: Items from the 20th to the 48th month.
10. Toilet: Items from the 15th to the 48th month.

The 90% standard from the Munich Functional Developmental Test was taken as a basis for a comparison score, that is, developmental retardations are assumed if the visually impaired children do not reach the 90% criterion of sighted children.

All three procedures are not strictly psychometric test procedures, that is, the authors deliberately avoid standardizing the test tasks and calculating normative data. The reason is understandable, as the variance in the developmental processes of visually impaired children would demand large sample surveys to obtain statistically sound normative data. Therefore, all the three procedures speak of comparative data, allowing only an estimate of the developmental stage of the individual child. In the Reynell–Zinkin Scales we obtain this estimate by comparing the individual child with a group of other visually impaired children – however, this group may be small. In the Oregon Project and the Würzburger Testinstrument, these estimates are obtained by reference to the age standards of sighted children. The comparison to age standards of sighted children is, however, a methodologically doubtful approach, as it assumes that the various aspects of development take a parallel course in blind and sighted children, that is, the developmental retardations of visually impaired children compared to sighted children are comparatively great in developmental areas like motor, cognition, language, social behaviour, orientation, and daily living skills. This assumption is neither in line with empirical results (e.g., Warren, 1984) nor with everyday experiences. The empirical examination of the Reynell–Zinkin Scales, for instance, shows that with 2- and 3–year–old visually impaired children developmental retardations are greater in areas with a stronger emphasis on perceptive–motor performances of coordination than in the language scales. This means that an exclusively intraindividual comparison as a starting point for early intervention like the one aimed at by the Oregon project and by the Würzburger Testinstrument leads to a misleading assessment of the actual developmental problems of visually impaired children. Let us assume, for instance, that a 4–year–old visually impaired child has a 2–year developmental retardation in the fine motor scale according to the skills inventory of the Oregon project, but only a 1 1/2–year retardation in the language scale. Then, according to the test authors, one would direct special attention to the intervention in the fine motor area, although when applied to the population of the visually impaired, the impairment in the language area must be considered as more serious than in the fine motor area. According to the empirical findings, a developmental retardation of 2 years in fine motor exercises must be considered relatively 'normal', whereas the apparently lesser developmental retardation of 1 1/2 years in the language area must be considered to give more cause for concern. With this way of ascertaining developmental retardations, the test authors indirectly reintroduce the comparison with the sighted population as a guide for assessment. Large developmental retardation means developmental retardation in comparison with the development of sighted children, and thus implies that the development of sighted children is taken as a standard for the necessity of early intervention.

With regard to the problem mentioned — adequate establishment of the developmental stage — the procedure used in the Reynell–Zinkin Scales has proved to be much better than the two other procedures. The developmental stage is assessed group–specifically and thereby allows a more valid statement about developmental problems that are specific to the blind and partially–sighted than is possible with the Oregon Test or the Würzburger Testinstrument.

The adequate choice of the comparative standard poses only one methodological problem when a developmental test is used with blind infants and preschoolers. However, two further methodological difficulties not sufficiently taken into account in previous constructions of developmental tests for blind children — the validity and instruction problems — appear to be even more serious and restricting.

3. Basic Methodological and Conceptual Difficulties in the Developmental Assessment of Blind Infants

3.1 Validity Problem

When constructing a special developmental test for blind and partially sighted children of preschool age, all test authors have up to now followed the same strategy, namely, choosing from current developmental tests for sighted children those test items which appeared to them to be the most useful for the assessment of the developmental stage of visually impaired children. To a minor extent, some tasks were modified or totally newly conceived. Such a transfer of tasks from general developmental tests is, however, only meaningful if the developmental aspect the task is to assess remains the same. Unfortunately this is frequently not the case, so that by using formally identical tasks, we assess something totally different in sighted compared to blind children, that is, the same task has a different validity for sighted and for blind children (Warren, 1984). In test–theoretical terms one speaks of "function fluctuation of an item", that is, the same task assesses a different developmental aspect in different groups or at different age levels.

The following two examples should make this point clear:

The subtest "Social Adaptation" in the "Reynell–Zinkin Scales for Blind and Sighted Children" mainly contains items from the "Maxfield–Buchholz Scale" (1957), which, again, is an adapted version for young blind children of the "Vineland Social Maturity Scale" (Doll, 1947), developed in the 1930s. The items in this subtest can be assigned to two classes: First, items which indicate early social–emotional bonds such as "Demands personal attention" or "Awareness of strangers", and secondly, items which indicate the independent accomplishment of daily routines such as "Holds cup when drinking" or "Eats with spoon." The question of validity — and thus the question of appropriateness of the items for visually impaired children — refers to the second class of items, that is, to those developmental tasks which assess the independent accomplishment of routines as an aspect of the social development of the child. In the original "Vineland Social Maturity Scale", this kind of task is used to determine to which degree children at a certain age are willing to execute socially desirable activities which are difficult for them because of their age.

Yet, when these items are used with blind children, we are, of course, testing something totally different; not the willingness to take on a routine, but their fine motor ability or, more precisely, their fine motor disability. Blind children in the second or third year of their life are mostly not capable of completing these fine motor tasks. Not being able to do so, does not mean, however, that they are retarded in their social development, but that they have difficulties in accomplishing fine motor activities of this kind, which is not astonishing when they are blind or when their vision is restricted.

The obvious simplest solution to this problem would be to change the age norms for blind children and to test this developmental aspect with blind children in their 4th or 5th year of life. This is not an adequate solution, however, because blind children in their 4th or 5th year of life are not comparable with 2- or 3-year-old sighted children because of their better cognitive, linguistic, and social performance. The only appropriate solution is to look for daily routines which are difficult but not impossible to accomplish for 2- or 3-year-old blind children and to use these to test their willingness to take on socially desirable activities. Then, and only then, do these tasks take into consideration the same underlying dimension of "Social Adaptation", and the tasks will have the same validity as those for sighted children.

Analagous examples of the inappropriateness of items can be drawn from the cognitive domain: Test authors use tasks with solutions that are highly dependent on sensorimotor ability. For instance, the Reynell–Zinkin Scale contains tasks like "Large and small boxes. Putting the correct lids on", or the Oregon–Test tasks like "Builds tower of 5–6 blocks", or the Würzburger Test-instrument tasks like "Unwraps objects." The test authors do not just want to assess motor skills with these tasks, but the cognitive ability to understand and solve the problem. It is evident that blind children are at a disadvantage on all three items, because the solution of the task is, to a great extent, visually influenced. Thus, these tasks say very little about the cognitive performance of blind children, but exclusively test their fine–motor ability — again, a totally different developmental aspect to that intended by the test authors.

It is extremely difficult to find an appropriate solution for this problem with tasks in the cognitive domain, because cognition in the first four years of life can almost exclusively only be tested by using tasks that require a manipulative–coordinative handling of objects. Cognitive performance can be tested at this age only in the form of a performance test and understandably not in the form of a verbal test.

Optimal tasks are those in which the loss of vision does not yield a disadvantage when solving the cognitive task. There are a few examples for such types of items. Hatwell (1966), for example, examined the ability of blind and sighted children to arrange several objects according to size, length, and weight. There were developmental lags in blind 5- to 10-year-old children ranging from one to three years in regard to the seriation of size and length. Yet, such a difference could not be found for the seriation of weights. The obvious reason is that vision is not a useful help for the arrangement of weights.

Warren (1984, p. 163), in reference to the study carried out by Tait and Ward (1982), mentions a further possible example of "blind-neutral items" for testing cognitive ability, namely, the recognition of jokes and riddles. Unfortunately, this type of task can only be used with older children. There are only a few tasks for young children up to the fourth year of life which do not show a visual-motor bias.

Up to now, no solution for this problem seems to be in sight. Optimal tasks would be those in which no group differences could be found between blind and sighted children, as, for instance, in the Hatwell comparison of weight. Yet, we usually find performance differences to the detriment of blind children, so that it is impossible to tell whether these differences indicate a retarded development of blind children or a handicap in dealing with the task.

It might be possible to rate empirically the proportion of the visual-motor component of the task by comparing the performance within the group of sighted children under two conditions − on one hand under a sighted condition, on the other hand under a blindfolded condition. If performance differences exist in such a comparison to the disadvantage of the blindfolded condition within the same children, then, such a result could be traced back to either these children's comparative lack of experience under this condition or to a high proportion of vision in respect to the solution of the task. However, if there are no performance differences, then such a result would indicate little visual influence on the solution of the task. Unfortunately, such a procedure is difficult to implement with younger children as the blindfolded condition cannot be realized practically. Therefore, it will be very difficult to obtain empirical proof in regard to "blind-neutral items" during the first years of life. Thus, we have to rely on a consideration of the content of items.

3.2   Problem of Instruction

If we analyze the type of tasks and the type of reactions which are expected from the children as "solution" in familiar developmental tests, we can see that the type of task as well as the expected solution changes drastically from the 1st to the 4th/5th year of life. This statement applies for general developmental tests for sighted children as well as for specific developmental tests for visually impaired children.

In the first year of life the spontaneous behavior of the children toward presented stimuli is observed; for instance:

1. their reflex activity (Munich Functional Developmental Test: "Walking automatism"),
2. their reactions to visually, auditorally, or tactually presented stimuli (Bayley Mental Scale: "Horizontal eye coordination: Red ring"; or Würzburger Testinstrument: "Follows sounds near the head"),
3. their fine– and gross motor performances that are largely considered to be determined by maturation (Reynell–Zinkin Scales: "Active grasp of object put into hand"; Griffiths: "Pulls himself up and stands afterwards, if he can cling to something.")

This kind of testing can be carried out relatively easily with blind children, too, and as Fraiberg's (1977) results show, there are only small differences between sighted and blind babies for most developmental aspects. Only at the end of the first year of life can differences be observed in self–initiated locomotion and hand coordination. These small developmental differences can be interpreted on the one hand as being due to the low influence of vision during the first months of life, and on the other hand due to methodological artefacts like the "bottom effect", that is, the developmental tests do not differentiate in this early span of life.

The assessment of the developmental stage becomes problematic within the second and third year of life, when we are no longer observing spontaneous behaviour, but when the children have to solve tasks according to instructions, for instance, Bayley Mental Scale: "Closes round box"; "Discriminates 3 objects: cup, plate, box"; or Oregon Test: "Moves self or object up or down on request ('Put your hand down' or 'Hold the spoon up high')"; "Puts together two parts of a shape to make a whole."

The verbal understanding of the instructions is so poor in this age range that the experimenter usually works a lot with demonstrations and gestures in front of sighted children in order to explain the task to them. The experimenter tries to stimulate the motivation of the infants with facial expression and gestures and clarifies the task to be accomplished by using demonstrations and gestural behaviour. This is either impossible or insufficiently possible with blind and partially sighted infants. The guidance of the hands is only a weak substitute for the lack of sight, and is often impeded by the infant's fear of being touched. The simplification or modification of the tasks for visually impaired children does not solve the problem properly, so that when interpreting the solution behaviour of visually impaired children at this age of life one is confronted with a decision that is difficult to solve. If failure of performance is the result, we do not know exactly whether there is a lack of ability or a lack of correct understanding of the instruction.

From the 4th and the following years of life onwards, this instructional problem diminishes, as the verbal understanding of the instructions increases and more and more verbal tasks can be used for an assessment of the developmental stage.

3.3   Conclusions from the Validity and Instruction Problems

The conclusion which one has to draw from these two conceptual difficulties is that it is difficult to make a valid statement about the development of visually impaired children, as the current developmental tests for blind infants and preschoolers have not paid enough attention to such principal problems. This statement should not create the false impression that the developmental retardations of visually impaired children, reported in the literature, are to be denied (Vander Kolk, 1981; Warren, 1984; Lewis, 1987). It would be unrealistic to assume that a developmental lag is not to be anticipated when one considers the sensory, physical, and social restrictions under which visually impaired children have to grow up. Yet, the question arises whether we judge the degree of the developmental retardation correctly. Maybe we overestimate the degree of developmental lag within the first years of life, above all in the second and third year of life, on account of insufficient tests.

The empirical findings in the literature can eventually be used to confirm this assumption. If we look at the findings on the developmental state of blind infants and preschoolers, we immediately notice the inconsistency of the results. This is not surprising when we consider the heterogeneity, the low sample sizes, and the differences between the procedures used. Nevertheless, cautious trends can be shown for the most frequently investigated field of development – cognitive development: Pronounced developmental retardations are found in the cognitive performance at preschool age and at the beginning of schooling (e.g., Reynell, 1978; Hatwell, 1966), and low or absolutely no differences can be shown in 11- to 12-year-old blind children (Gottesman, 1973; Smits and Mommers, 1976; Vander Kolk, 1977). Similar trends, that is, pronounced developmental differences at preschool age and low differences in adolescence and adulthood, are found for language development (Warren, 1984).

This finding is frequently interpreted as an indication that blind children catch up with sighted children in their cognitive development after the full acquisition of speech ability and through systematic schooling. An alternative explanation would be that test procedures are available for the older age groups that permit a fair comparison between sighted and blind children.

Only when we succeed in finding equivalent developmental tasks for blind infants and preschoolers that are not overloaded with visual–motor tasks, and when we succeed in designing the test situation in such a way that the demands of the tasks can be understood by the children, can we talk about a suitable developmental assessment for blind infants and preschoolers.

4. Description of the Bielefeld Developmental Test for Blind Infants and Preschoolers

4.1 Preliminary Analysis for the Construction of the Bielefeld Developmental Test

In a preliminary analysis, all the items from current developmental tests for sighted and visually impaired infants and preschoolers were classified according to two standpoints: First, we judged whether the particular item could be used for diagnosing the development of visually impaired children either: (1) without modification, (2) with modification, or (3) not at all. Second, we estimated which aspects of development each item assessed. Our goal was to find the largest possible pool of suitable tasks for assessing the development of blind infants and preschoolers. The following 14 developmental tests were subjected to this analysis:

- Bayley Mental and Motor Scale (Bayley, f1933, 1969)
- Bühler–Hetzer Test für das Vorschulalter (Bühler & Hetzer, 1932[1], 1977[4])
- Denver Entwicklungsskalen (Flehmig et al., 1973)
- Entwicklungskontrolle für Krippenkinder (Zwiener & Schmidt–Kolmer, 1982)
- Gesell & Amatruda Test (Knobloch et al., 1974)
- Griffiths Entwicklungsskalen (Griffiths, 1954; Brandt, 1983)
- Hawaii Early Learning Profile (Furuno et al., 1984)
- Kiphard sensomotorisches und psychosoziales Entwicklungsgitter (Kiphard, 1975)
- Münchener Funktionelle Entwicklungsdiagnostik für das 1. und 2./3. Lebensjahr (Hellbrügge et al., 1978; Coulin, et al., 1977)
- Oregon Test for Visually Impaired & Blind Children (Brown et al., 1978, 1979)
- Peabody Mobility Kit (Harley et al., 1981)
- Reynell–Zinkin Scales for Sighted and Blind Children (Reynell, 1979)
- Uzgiris & Hunt Developmental Scales (Uzgiris & Hunt, 1975)
- Würzburger Testinstrument für mehrfachbehinderte Blinde und sehbehinderte Kinder (Blindeninstitutsstiftung Würzburg, 1980)

When examining the more than 3,000 development items, we found that the current tasks in developmental tests could only be adopted without modification in a few areas of development, for example, the assessment of language development. In all other areas of development, such as sensorimotor, cognition, and social behavior, most of the tasks required sight or visually–guided fine motor skills. From the point of view of validity, such tasks assess different aspects of development in sighted and blind children. It was further noticeable that even in specific tests for visually impaired children (Oregon Test; Reynell–Zinkin Scales; and Würzburger Testinstrument) the instruction problem was not taken into account, that is, the form of test presentation selected was inadequate for blindness. Therefore, we constructed a new developmental test for blind infants and preschoolers in order to reduce the methodological problems mentioned.

4.2   Principles of Construction of the Bielefeld Developmental Test

The most important innovation in the construction of the Bielefeld Developmental Test compared to earlier developmental tests for blind infants and preschoolers is the subdivision of the developmental test into a general and a specific section. The general section should predominantly assess aspects of development that are "blind–neutral" and the specific section aspects that are "blind–specific." The contents of the general section deal with those aspects of development in which a primary relationship does not have to be assumed between blindness and developmental potential. To put this in other words: In these fields of development, a blind child who does not show any additional impairments and receives adequate education (including early intervention and schooling) should, in the long term, show comparable performances, abilities, and behaviors to a sighted child. These are the fields of cognition, language, social–emotional behavior, and neuromotor development.

In the specific section of the developmental test, in contrast, a differential assessment is made of those tasks in which sight is an essential precondition for the acquisition, execution, and refinement of the necessary skills. This primarily concerns visually–guided or –controlled skills such as spatial and geographical orientation, directed locomotion, and simple and complex fine motor actions. This specific developmental section should also reveal which alternative strategies the children apply in which way to overcome their perceptive–motor difficulties.

The division of the contents into a general and a specific section has consequences for the conception and selection of the items and the test material. In the general section the presentation of the items was designed so that sight would be of little importance for their solution. In the specific section, in contrast, the tasks were designed to reveal the problems that are specific to blindness.

The following measures were introduced in order to reduce the proportion of visual–motor skills in the general section:

1. Restriction of the test arrangement.
The majority of the standardized items in the general section are presented in a restrictive test arrangement that should facilitate the blind children's orientation through the spatial arrangement of the material. A test box was constructed for this purpose that serves as a "test space" in which the tasks can be performed. The goal of the test box and the additional aids to tactile and auditory orientation is to create a greater clarity for the blind child. The child should be informed where it has placed or should place objects in each situation.

2. Selection of suitable test material.
The most simple and clearly structured objects were chosen in the selection of the test material, for example, little boxes, cubes, and so forth; except, of course, in the tasks for testing exploratory behavior. Among everyday objects, things were chosen that would also be familiar to every blind child. In addition, many objects were chosen that make sounds when moved (sound producing objects). This not only will arouse the blind child's interest, but at the same time reveals to the child in which subdivision of the test box the object has been placed.

3. Blind–neutral test tasks.
In the selection of items for the general development section, value was placed on finding so–called "blind–neutral" developmental tasks, that is, tasks in which sight plays a lesser or nonexistent role. These are traditionally auditory tasks, such as recognition of the same human voices or bird calls or the recognition or continuation of series with acoustic signals. However, in the general section there are also verbal or tactile tasks which can be assumed to be blind–neutral, such as comparing the weights of objects or simple memory tasks using verbal material.

4.3   Brief Description of the Scales of the Bielefeld Developmental Test

The Bielefeld Developmental Test for Blind Infants and Preschoolers covers the age range from the middle of the first year of life to the end of the fourth year, but it also contains items for both younger and older children. The items in the single scales are ranked according to difficulty. The test comprises two sections containing a total of six scales:

I. General Section
Scale 1: Basic neuromotor skills
Scale 2: Cognitive development
Scale 3: Social–emotional development
Scale 4: Language development
II. Specific Section
Scale 5: Orientation and mobility
Scale 6: Daily living skills

The single scales assess the following developmental aspects in the different subscales:

Scale 1: Basic neuromotor skills
— Orienting reactions
— Postural motor system
— Hand coordination
This scale should assess basic developmental processes in the first year of life that depend on maturation. These include reflex activity (onset, disappearance, and persistence), orienting reactions, and locational and postural motor reactions. All these characteristics are only slightly affected by sight; neurological maturation processes are considered to be decisive for the behavior to be observed.

Scale 2: Cognitive development
— Object permanence and memory performance
— Classification and categorization performance
— Means and combination comprehension
This scale uses tasks in which the lack of sight is less of a handicap, for example, tasks with auditory stimuli, to assess the cognitive performance of blind children. The manipulative and coordination demands that are normally linked to such tasks are reduced through tactile and acoustic localization aids for the visually impaired child.

Scale 3: Social–emotional development
- Emotions
- Social interactions
- Control of impulsiveness

This scale emphasizes the assessment of emotional changes. The judgment of this aspect of development appears to be more important in handicapped children than nonhandicapped children. The scale additionally assesses interactive behavior and the learning of suitable social behavior.

Scale 4: Language development
- Language production
- Language comprehension

This scale primarily assesses expressive language development (language production) and is less comprehensive with regard to receptive language development (language comprehension). The subscale language production ranges from prelanguage phonation to the assessment of semantic structures. The subscale language comprehension only assesses more complex aspects of receptive language and, therefore, only covers older children.

Scale 5: Orientation and mobility
- Orientation
- Mobility

The problems specific to blind children in independent, goal–directed locomotion should be judged with this scale. The subscale orientation should firstly assess the infants' spatial perception of distance from and direction of objects and persons, and secondly, more complex orientation performances such as following a given route or going from one room in the family home to the next. The subscale mobility assesses the ambulatory performance of blind infants and preschoolers from the first independent movements to complex gross motor skills such as ascending a staircase, climbing, and so forth.

Scale 6: Daily living skills
- Basic manual skills
- Self–help

On the one hand, this scale assesses basic skills of hand coordination and the manual motor system, and on the other hand, complex everyday activities such as eating and drinking, washing, dressing, and undressing, The focus in all these tasks is to assess fine motor coordination performance.

Three different types of items are applied to assess the children's development: test, observation, and report items. Test items, in which the children are presented with a task in a standardized form, are used most frequently, for example, in all tasks assessing cognitive performance. Observation items relate to situations that occur frequently and are simple to assess, for example, whether a child already utters two–word sentences or moves independently through space. Finally, report items are used to assess tasks that cannot be performed or contents that are difficult to observe, for example, the investigation of a child's emotional utterances or the type of protective behavior in spatial locomotion.

The developmental test is performed in the parental home, as the familiarity of the environment can be considered an important requirement for suitable test behavior in visually impaired infants and preschoolers. The test will provisionally be administered to blind children aged between 9 and 48 months. We intend to test about 100 children who at the most can only perceive light but have no further serious disorders.

References

Bayley, N. (1933, 1969): Manual for the Bayley Scales of Infant Development. Berkeley: Institute of Human Development

Blindeninstitutsstiftung Würzburg (1980): Testinstrument zur Erfassung des Entwicklungsstandes mehrfachbehinderter sehgeschädigter Kinder. Würzburg: Blindeninstitutsstiftung

Brandt, I. (1983): Griffiths–Entwicklungsskalen (GES). Weinheim: Beltz (Original: Griffiths, B., 1954)

Brown, D., Simmons, V., and Methvin, J. (1979): The Oregon Project for Visually Impaired and Blind Preschool Children. Medford: Jackson Education Service District

Bühler, Ch., and H. Hetzer (1932, 1977): Kleinkindertests. Berlin: Springer

Coulin, S., Heiss–Begemann, E., Köhler, G., Lajosi, F., Schamberger, R. (1977): Münchener Funktionelle Entwicklungsdiagnostik 2./3. Lebensjahr. Experimentalfassung 1977. München: Institut für Soziale Pädiatrie und Jugendmedizin

Doll, E.A. (1947): The Vineland Social Maturity Scale: Manual of Directions. Minneapolis: Educational Test Bureau

Ferrell, K.A. (1986): Infancy and Early Childhood. In Scholl, G.T. (Ed.): Foundations of Education for Blind and Visually Handicapped Children and Youth. New York: American Foundation for the Blind, 119–135

Flehmig, I., Schloon, M., Uhde, J., and von Bernuth, H. (1973): Denver–Entwicklungsskalen; Testanweisung. Hamburg: Hamburger Spastikerverein

Fraiberg, S. (Ed.) (1977): Insights from the Blind. Comparative Studies of Blind and Sighted Infants. New York: Basic Books

Furuno, S., et al. (1984): HELP (Hawai Early Learning Profile) Palo Alto: VORT Corporation

Gottesman, M. (1973): Conservation Development in Blind Children. Child Development, 44, 824–827

Harley, R.K., Wood, Th., and Merbler, J. (1981): Peabody Mobility Kit for Blind Students. Chicago: Stoelting

Hatwell, Y. (1966): Privation Sensorielle et Intelligence. Paris: Presses Universitaires de France

Hellbrügge, Th., Lajosi, F., Menara, D., Schamberger, R., and Rautenstrauch, Th. (1978): Münchener Funktionelle Entwicklungsdiagnostik — 1. Lebensjahr. München: Urban & Schwarzenberg

Kiphard, E.J. (1975): Wie weit ist ein Kind entwickelt? Dortmund: Verlag modernes lernen

Knobloch, H., and Pasamanick, B. (1974): Gesell and Amatruda' Developmental Diagnosis (3rd edn.). New York: Harper & Row

Lewis, V. (1987): How Do Blind Children Develop? In V. Lewis: Development and Handicap. Oxford: Blackwell

Maxfield, K.E., and Buchholz, S. (1957): A Social Maturity Scale for Blind Preschool Children: A Guide to its Use. New York: American Foundation for the Blind

Norris, M., Spaulding, P.J., and Brodie, F.H. (1957): Blindness in Children. Chicago: University of Chicago Press

Reynell, J. (1978): Developmental Patterns of Visually Handicapped Children. Child Care, Health & Development, 4, 291–303

Reynell, J. (1979): Manual for the Reynell–Zinkin-Scales: Developmental Scales for Young Visually Handicapped Children. Part 1: Mental Development. Windsor: NFER–Publ.

Smits, B.W.G.M., and Mommers, M.J.C. (1976): Differences between Blind and Sighted Children on WISC Verbal Subtests. New Outlook for the Blind, 70, 240–246

Tait, P.E., and Ward, M. (1982): The Comprehension of Verbal Humor by Visually Impaired Children. Journal of Visual Impairment & Blindness, 76, 144–147

Uzgiris, I.C., and Hunt, J. McV. (1975): Assessment in Infancy. Ordinal Scales of Psychological Development. Chicago: University of Illinois Press

Vander Kolk, C.J. (1977): Intelligence Testing for Visually Impaired Persons. Journal of Visual Impairment & Blindness, 71, 158–163

Vander Kolk, C.J. (1981): Assessment and Planning with the Visually Impaired. Baltimore: University Park Press

Warren, D.H. (1984): Blindness and Early Childhood Development. New York: American Foundation for the Blind, 2nd Ed.

Zwiener, K., and Schmidt-Kolmer, E. (1982): Entwicklungskontrolle in der frühen Kindheit in ihrer Bedeutung für die gesundheitliche Betreuung und die Erziehung. Berlin: Volk und Gesundheit

Part Two

Risk Factors and Protective Factors in Childhood Development

Vulnerability and Resiliency: A Longitudinal Perspective

Emmy E. Werner

1. Introduction

As prospective studies of high–risk children are coming of age, we can begin to examine not only the differential course of youngsters exposed to a variety of risk factors and of low–risk comparison groups, but also the development of high–risk children who *did* and *did not* develop serious and lasting disabilities or disorders. The understanding of factors that pull children *toward* or *away from* increased risk at different stages of development can aid our efforts at primary prevention.

Beginning in the prenatal period, the Kauai Longitudinal Study has monitored the impact of a variety of biological and psychosocial risk factors, stressful life events, and protective factors on the development of a multiracial cohort of children who were born in 1955 and followed periodically until they reached adulthood (Werner, 1985; Werner and Smith, 1977, 1982).

We began by examining children's *vulnerability*, that is, their susceptibility to negative developmental outcomes after exposure to perinatal stress, poverty, parental psychopathology, and disruption of their family unit. As our study progressed, we also looked at the roots of *resiliency* in those children who successfully coped with such biological and psychosocial risk factors and maintained a sense of competence and control. It should be noted that *both* "vulnerability" and "resiliency" are probabilistic and relativistic concepts that do *not* preclude the likelihood of change in individuals over time.

2. The Setting of the Study

Kauai, "the Garden Island", lies at the northwest end of the Hawaiian chain, some 100 miles from Honolulu. It was settled in the 8th century by canoe voyagers from the Marquesas and the Society Islands and populated in the 12th and 13th century by migrations from Tahiti. The English seafarer, Captain Cook, "rediscovered" the island in 1778, and Christian missionaries established their first churches and schools there in 1820, at a time when Kauai was an independent kingdom. In 1835, the first sugar plantation was founded, creating an industry that has dominated the island's way of life ever since.

The 44,600 people who live on Kauai today are for the most part descendants of immigrants from Japan and the Philippines who came to work for the plantations. Many subsequently intermarried with the local Hawaiians. The Japanese, Filipinos, and Part–Hawaiians now account for three–fourths of the island's population. Portuguese from the Azores, Chinese, Koreans, and a few Caucasians make up the rest.

We chose Kauai as the site of our prospective study for a number of reasons: Here we found a population with low mobility, but with access to and coverage by medical, public health, educational, and social services that compared favorably with most communities of similar size on the U.S. mainland.

3. Methodology

From its conception, this has been an interdisciplinary study (Werner and Smith, 1977, 1982). Public health nurses recorded the reproductive histories of the women and interviewed them in each trimester of pregnancy, noting any exposure to physical or emotional trauma. Physicians monitored any complications that occurred during the prenatal, labor, delivery, and neonatal periods. Nurses and social workers interviewed the mothers in the postpartum period and when the children were 1 and 10 years old. They also observed the interaction of parents and offspring in the home. Pediatricians and psychologists independently examined the children at ages 2 and 10. They assessed their physical, intellectual, and social development, and noted any physical handicaps and learning or behavior problems.

From the beginning of the study we also recorded information on the material, intellectual, and emotional aspects of the family environment, including stressful life events that brought discord or disruption to the family unit.

When the children reached school age, their teachers evaluated their academic progress and classroom behavior. In addition, my colleagues and I administered a wide range of aptitude, achievement, and personality tests in the elementary grades and in high school. We also had, with permission of the parents, access to the records of the public health, educational, and social service agencies in the community, and to the files of the local police and family court. Last, but not least, we gained the perspectives of the individual members of the birth cohort when we interviewed them at ages 18 and at age 30.

While our focus in this study has been mainly on young people who appear *vulnerable* because of their exposure to biological and psychosocial risk factors, we could not help but be deeply impressed by the *resiliency* of most children. But our hopefulness was tempered by dismay when we noted the magnitude of the "casualties" which could have been prevented by early diagnosis and early intervention.

4. Results

4.1 The Reproductive and Caretaking Casualties

We noted that deleterious biological risk factors exerted their peak influence in the early weeks of pregnancy when 90% of the fetal losses in our study occurred. For 1,000 live births on Kauai, there were an estimated 1,311 pregnancies that had advanced to four weeks gestation.

These 1,000 live births yielded 865 surviving children at age 2 who were free of any observable physical defects and whose intellectual and social development had proceeded at a normal rate. By age 10, only 660 of these children were functioning adequately in school and had no recognizable physical handicaps or learning and/or behavior problems. By age 18, the number of survivors who had not developed any serious coping problems in the second decade of life (such as delinquencies and/or mental health problems) had shrunk to 615.

On Kauai, as on any battlefield, not all of the casualties died: Approximately *one out of every three* surviving children in this birth cohort developed learning and/or behavior problems during the *first decade of life* that interfered with their school achievement. By age 18, *one out of every five* youths had a delinquency record, and *one out of ten* had mental health problems that required in-or outpatient care.

The *majority* of the troubled children in this birth cohort had multiple problems and lived in conditions of chronic poverty and in a disorganized family environment. Among the *minority* who had been exposed to reproductive risk factors (such as anoxia, low birth weight, preterm birth), the quality of the caregiving environment markedly attenuated or exacerbated the effects of the biological insults.

At ages 2, 10, and 18, pre- and perinatal complications resulting in impairment of physical or psychological development were exacerbated when combined with unfavorable rearing conditions, that is, when children grew up in chronic poverty, and were brought up by parents with little education in a

family environment troubled by discord, divorce, or parental alcoholism or
mental illness. *Boys* who had been exposed to reproductive stress were more
vulnerable in such a disordered caregiving environment than *girls* who had
experienced pre/perinatal complications.

4.2   Vulnerable but Invincible Children

Two-third of the children who encountered *four or more* or such risk factors
before the age of 2 developed serious learning or behavior problems by age 10,
or had delinquency records or mental health problems by age 18. But unexpect-
edly *one out of every three* of the children who had experienced perinatal
stress, poverty, parental psychopathology, and disruptions of the family unit
developed, instead, into competent and caring young adults.

Looking back over the lives of these 72 resilient individuals, we contrasted
their behavior characteristics and caregiving environment with that of the high-
risk youths of the same age and sex who had developed serious coping problems at 10 or 18. We found a number of characteristics within the individuals,
within their families, and outside the family circle that contributed to their
resilience.

The 30 boys and 42 girls in this group had few serious illnesses in childhood
and adolescence and tended to recuperate quickly. Their temperamental characteristics elicited positive attention from family members as well as strangers. As
infants, *both* boys and girls were more frequently described by their caregivers
as "very active"; the girls as "affectionate" and "cuddly"; the boys as "good-
natured" and "easy to deal with". They had fewer eating and sleeping habits
that were distressing to their parents than did the high-risk infants who later
developed serious learning or behavior problems.

At 20 months, the resilient boys and girls tended to meet the world already on
their own terms. The pediatricians and psychologists who examined them noted
their alertness and autonomy, their tendency to seek out novel experiences, and
their positive social orientation, especially among the girls. They were also
more advanced in communication, locomotion, and self-help skills than the
children who later developed serious learning and behavior problems.

In elementary school, teachers noted that the resilient children got along well
with their classmates and were able to concentrate on their work. They had
better reasoning and reading skills than high-risk children who developed
problems, especially the girls. Though not especially gifted, the resilient chil-

dren used whatever skills they had effectively. Both parents and teachers noted that they had many interests and engaged in activities and hobbies that were not narrowly sex–typed. Such activities provided solace in adversity and a reason to feel proud.

In middle childhood and adolescence, many resilient youths took care of younger siblings. Some managed the household when a parent was hospitalized; others worked part–time to supplement the family income or to save for a college education. By the time they graduated from high school, the resilient youths had developed a positive self–concept and a strong faith in the control of their own fate. They displayed a more nurturant, responsible, and achievement–oriented attitude toward life than their high–risk peers who developed coping problems. The resilient girls were also more assertive, achievement-oriented, and independent.

The resilient boys and girls tended to grow up in families with four or fewer children, with a space of two years or more between themselves and their next sibling. Few had experienced prolonged separations from their primary care-taker during the first year of life. *All* had the opportunity to establish a close bond with at least one caregiver from whom they received plenty of positive attention when they were infants.

Some of this nurturing came from substitute parents, such as grandparents or older siblings, or from the ranks of neighbors and regular baby–sitters. Such substitute parents played an important role as positive models of identification, as did the example of a mother who was gainfully and steadily employed. Maternal employment and the need to take care of younger siblings contributed to the pronounced autonomy and sense of responsibility noted among the resilient girls, especially in households where the father was absent.

Resilient boys were often *firstborn* sons who did not have to share their parents' attention with many additional children. There were some males in the family who could serve as a role model (if not the father, then a grandfather, older cousin, or uncle). Structure and rules and assigned chores were part of their daily routine in adolescence.

The resilient boys and girls also found emotional support outside of their own family. They tended to have at least one, and usually several, close friends, especially the girls. They relied on an informal network of kin and neighbors, peers and elders, for counsel and support in times of crises. Many had a favorite teacher who had become a role model, friend, and confidant for them.

Participation in extracurricular activities played an important part in the lives of the resilient youth, especially activities that were cooperative enterprises. For still others, emotional support came from a youth leader, or from a minister or church group. With their help the resilient children acquired a faith that their lives had meaning and that they had control over their fate.

4.3   Ameliorative Factors versus Absence of Risk Factors

Among protective factors in the *first 2 years of life* that were important in counterbalancing stress, deprivation, or disadvantage, but *not* important among the children in this cohort in the absence of such circumstances were:
good health (for both sexes); autonomy and self-help skills (for males); a positive social orientation (for females) and emotional support provided by alternate caregivers in the family. For boys, being firstborn was an important protective factor; for girls, the model of a mother who was steadily and gain-fully employed.
These variables discriminated significantly between positive and negative devel-opmental outcomes in childhood and adolescence *only* when there was a series of stressful events in the children's lives or they grew up in chronic poverty. They *did not* discriminate between good and poor outcomes among middle-class children in our cohort, whose lives were relatively stress-free.
The number of ameliorative factors that discriminated between positive and negative developmental outcomes in this cohort increased with stress (in both middle- and lower-class children) and deprivation (among lower-class chil-dren). As disadvantage and the cumulative number of stressful life events in-creased, more protective factors in the children and their caregiving environ-ment were needed to counterbalance the negative aspects in their lives and to ensure a positive developmental outcome.

5. Objectives of the 30-Year Follow-Up

When we last interviewed the members of the 1955 birth cohort at age 18, we were aware that the maximum period for mental breakdown was still ahead of the high-risk youths (Werner and Smith, 1982). We did not yet know how well they would adapt to the demands of the adult world of work, marriage, and parenthood.
Since 1985, we have been involved in a follow-up of these resilient youth and of comparison groups of high-risk subjects from the 1955 birth cohort who had previously developed problems.

Our follow-up has two general objectives:

1. To trace the long-term effects of stressful life events in childhood and adolescence on the adult adaptation of men and women who were exposed to poverty, perinatal stress, and parental psychopathology, and
2. To examine the long-term effects of protective factors (personal competencies; sources of support) in childhood and adolescence on their adult coping.

We located some 80% (N: 545) of the survivors of the 1955 birth cohort. The majority of the men and women still live on Kauai. Among them are most of the former "problem children". Some 10% have moved to other Hawaiian islands. Another 10% live on the US mainland; some 2% live abroad, in Europe, Asia, Australia, and Oceania. Among those who moved away from Kauai are many of the resilient youths.

5.1   Instruments

The instruments administered in individual sessions at age 30 are: A checklist of stressful life events, Rotter's Locus of Control Scale, the EAS Adult Temperament Survey, and a structured interview.

The interview assesses the subject's perceptions of major stressors and sources of support in their adult lives, and their preferred coping strategies when confronted with adversity in school, at work, and in their relationships with their spouses or mates, their children, parents, in-laws, siblings, and friends. It concludes with a summary assessment of the person's state of health, satisfaction, and well-being at the present state of life.

In addition, we have access to the court records on Kauai and the other Hawaiian islands. These files not only contain major violations of the criminal law, but also information on domestic problems, such as desertion, divorce, delinquent child support payments, and spouse and child abuse. We also have access to the records of the Department of Health which registers marriage licenses, birth and death certificates, and maintains a statewide mental health registry.

We have follow-up data in adulthood on every member of the 1955 birth cohort with a criminal record or with a marriage that ended in divorce by age 30. We also have follow-up data on 86% of the resilient subjects and 90% of the teenage parents. We have follow-up data on 75% of the offspring of alcoholics, on 75% of the former delinquents, and on 80% of the individuals with mental health problems that required in- or outpatient care by age 18, or whose parents had received such care. We completed our data collection in the spring of 1988.

5.2 Long–term Consequences of Stressful Life Events in Child-hood and Adolescence

More than half of the stressful life events that significantly increased the like-lihood of having a criminal record or an "irrevocably broken marriage" by age 30 for members of this cohort took place in infancy and early childhood (see Tab. 1 and 2).

Tab. 1: Significant differences between M *with* and *without* a criminal record by age 30 (1955 birth cohort, Kauai)

Characteristics of home environment	M <u>with</u> criminal record (N: 25)	M <u>without</u> criminal record (N: 317)	p
<u>Birth to age 2</u>	%	%	
Chronic poverty	72.0	43.8	.01
Mother not married when M was born	24.0	10.4	.05
Prolonged disruptions in family during M's first year of life	12.0	3.6	.10
Prolonged separations from mother (year 1)	20.8	7.8	.10
Mother pregnant again or birth of younger sib before age 2	37.5	21.4	.10
Father absent permanently	20.8	4.5	.001
<u>Ages 2-5 yrs</u>			
Mother absent permanently	9.5	.7	.01
Conflict between parents	20.8	6.6	.01
Mother remarried; step-father moves in	16.7	1.4	.001
<u>Ages 6-10 yrs</u>			
Mother absent permanently	13.6	.3	.001
Father absent permanently	21.7	1.8	.001
Sister died	8.3	.3	.005
M changed schools	12.5	2.1	.02
<u>Ages 11-18 years</u>			
Father absent permanently	23.8	4.7	.001
Problems in relationship with father	23.8	10.1	.10

Tab. 2: Significant differences between Ss *with* and *without* a divorce record ("marriage irretrievably broken") by age 30 (1955 birth cohort, Kauai)

Characteristics of home environment	Females F with divorce (N: 32)	F without divorce (N: 323)	p
Birth to age 2	%	%	
Chronic poverty	51.6	30.3	.01
Mother not married when F was born	22.6	11.7	.10
Mother worked without adequate child-care	45.2	25.6	.05
Mother pregnant again or birth of younger sib before age 2	47.6	28.3	.10
Ages 2-5 years			
Mother permanently absent	10.0	1.7	.05
Father permanently absent	10.7	2.4	.10
Ages 10-18 years			
Father died	20.0	6.2	.10
Problem in relationship with father	35.0	13.0	.01
Teenage pregnancy	55.0	13.7	.001
Teenage marriage	25.0	5.0	.001
Teenage marital conflict	15.0	1.2	.005
Financial problems in teens	45.0	19.3	.01

Characteristics of home environment	Males M with divorce (N: 36)	M without divorce (N: 306)	p
Birth to age 2	%	%	
Mother not married when M was born	22.2	10.1	.05
Disruptions in family during M's first year	42.9	26.9	.10
Ages 2-5 years			
Father permanently absent	6.7	1.8	.10
Ages 6-10 years			
Mother died	3.3	.4	.10
Grandparent died	3.3	.4	.10
Close friend died	3.3	.4	.10

Among such stressful life events that had negative effects on the quality of adult coping for *both* men and women were:

1. the closely spaced birth of a younger sibling in infancy (less than 2 years after birth of the index child);

2. being raised by a mother who was not married at the time of the child's birth;
3. having a father who was permanently absent during infancy and/or early childhood;
4. experiencing prolonged disruptions of the family life and separations from the mother during the first year of life (that included unemployment of the major breadwinner, illness of the parent, major moves); and
5. having a mother who worked without adequate substitute child care during the first 12–20 months of the child's life.

A significantly higher proportion of males with a criminal record (that included promotion of harmful drugs, theft and burglary; assault and battery; rape and attempted murder) experienced such disruptions of their family unit in their early years, as did the men and women whose marriages had ended in divorce by age 30.

For the females, teenage pregnancies, teenage marriages, marital conflict, problems in their relationships with their fathers, and financial problems in their teens also significantly increased the likelihood of divorce by age 30; for the males, it was the absence of the natural father, as well as the death of the mother, or the departure of a close friend before age 10. Such events occurred in significantly greater frequency among children in this birth cohort who had been born and raised in chronic poverty.

Now let us turn to the other side of the vulnerability coin and examine some of the competencies and sources of support that characterized the resilient men and women in early adulthood.

5.3   Resilient Men and Women in their Early Thirties

We have follow-up data on 26 of the resilient men and 36 of the resilient women at age 30. All of these individuals had grown up in chronic poverty and had previously coped successfully with the effects of perinatal stress, parental psychopathology, and serious disruptions of their family unit (see Tab. 3 and 4).

Tab. 3:   Status and Goals of Resilient Ss (1955 birth cohort, Kauai) at age 30 (M: 26; F: 36)

*Marital Status	M%	F%
Married	50.0	86.2
Single	44.4	10.3
Divorced	5.6	3.4

**Children	M%	F%
None	55.6	20.7
One	16.7	20.7
Two	27.8	37.9
Three	----	13.8
Four or more	----	6.9

Complete Schooling beyond High School	M%	F%
Technical training	27.8	13.3
Jr. College	33.3	43.3
4 Yr College	38.9	40.0
Grad/Profess. School	11.1	3.3
No addtl. school	5.6	23.3

Current employment status	M%	F%
Professional	22.2	6.9
Semi-Profess./ Managerial	16.7	34.5
Skilled trade, Technical	38.9	31.0
Semi-skilled	16.7	13.8
Unemployed	5.6	13.8

Satisfaction with school performance	M%	F%
Did very well	37.5	58.3
Did adequately	56.3	41.7
Did not do well	6.3	----

Satisfaction with current work	M%	F%
Satisfied	76.5	72.4
Ambivalent	23.5	24.1
Dissatisfied	----	3.4

Goals for self	M%	F%
Career or job success	55.6	63.3
Self-fulfillment	33.3	20.0
Happy marriage	22.2	20.0
Close relations with friends, family	16.7	3.3
Social concerns	5.6	3.3

*Expectations from marriage	M%	F%
Permanency, security	61.5	72.0
*Intimacy, sharing	38.5	72.0
Children	38.5	16.0
Material comfort	15.4	4.0

----

* $p < .05$
**$p < .01$

Tab. 4:   Sources of stress and support of Resilient Ss (1955 birth cohort, Kauai) at age 30
          (M: 26; F: 36)

	M%	F%
Health Problems	M%	F%
(self-reported, stress-related)	58.8	36.7
Worries	M%	F%
Problems of family members	53.0	40.0
Finances, money	35.3	43.3
*Children	5.9	36.7
Spouse, mate	11.8	16.7
Work	23.5	6.7
Social issues	11.8	3.3
Problems of friends	5.9	----
*Sources of Support	M%	F%
Own determination, competence	66.7	60.0
Spouse, mate	33.3	46.7
Faith, prayer	22.2	40.0
Parents	27.8	16.7
Friends	16.7	30.0
Older relatives	5.6	16.7
Siblings	5.6	10.0
Co-workers	5.6	13.3
Teachers, mentors	5.6	3.3
Mental health professionals	----	6.7
Ministers	----	6.7
Can't thinks of any sources of support	5.6	----
Satisfaction with current status in life	M%	F%
Happy, delighted	29.4	50.0
Mostly satisfied	41.2	26.7
Mixed(somewhat satisfied,		
somewhat dissatisfied)	23.5	16.7
Mostly dissatisfied	----	3.3
Unhappy	5.9	3.3

----

* $p < .05$

It bears remembering that their fathers had worked as semi- or unskilled labor-
ers on the island's sugar plantations, and that they themselves joined the work
force during a serious economic recession in the USA. But, in spite of past and
present financial constraints, these young men and women, at ages 30–32, are
coping well with the demands of one of the most stressful periods in the adult
life cycle.

Both the men and women are highly achievement-oriented. With few exceptions, they have pursued additional education and they are currently in full-time employment, the women predominantly in semiprofessional and managerial positions, the men either in skilled trades and technical jobs or in professions. Three out of four among the resilient men and women are satisfied with their present employment status.

The majority of the men and women list "career or job success" as their primary goal for themselves at this stage of life, outdistancing other objectives, such as a happy marriage, children, or close relations with friends and family. A higher proportion of males than females consider "self-fulfillment" a primary objective in life.

The women in this group have made more transitions into multiple life trajectories than the men. Eighty-five percent of the women are married, have children, and work full time. In contrast, only half of the men are married and have children. The significant gender differences in life trajectories observed in this group may be in part a consequence of the spirit of Women's Liberation, but it may also represent realistic adaptations to economic stress (similar to those reported by Elder (1974) in *Children of the Great Depression* for an earlier generation.

There appears to be a greater reluctance among the resilient males in this cohort to make commitments to long-term relationships than among the females, perhaps a technique of distancing that had served them well in a troubled childhood (see Gruenebaum, 1982). Most of the resilient women (some three out of four) expect intimacy and sharing from such a relationship. Only a third of the men have similar expectations. A significantly higher proportion of the males than females reported that a breakup of a long-term relationship between 18 and 30 had been a source of great stress to them.

The greatest source of worry among the resilient men and women at this stage in their lives appears to be problems of family members, especially the health of parents or in-laws or divorces among parents or siblings. Work conditions are reported as major worries by a higher proportion of men; a significantly higher proportion of women tend to worry about their children.

The overwhelming majority of the resilient men and women at age 30 consider personal competencies and determination to be their most effective resources in coping with stressful life events. On Rotter's Locus of Control scale both sexes score more than two SD below the mean of the standardization group — in the *internal* direction.

But the resilient women draw on a significantly larger number of additional sources of support than the men that include faith and prayer, friends, siblings, parents-in-law, and co-workers. In contrast, the resilient men appear to rely almost exclusively on their own resources, with some additional support from spouses or parents. They less frequently derive emotional support from siblings and peer friends than women do. Co-workers are considered more often sources of stress for the men than the women, and less often sources of support.

The majority of the resilient men report health problems related to stress, whether ulcers, back problems, fainting spells, or problems with overweight. In contrast, only a third of the women report health problems — mostly related to pregnancy and childbirth (Emergency D and C; C-sections; toxemia of pregnancy; miscarriages; premenstrual syndromes).

But despite some continuing economic worries and the stress of multiple transitions into work, marriage, and parenthood, three out of four among the resilient men and women consider themselves happy or satisfied with their current status in life (only 6% rate themselves as unhappy or "mostly dissatisfied").

It appears from this preliminary analysis of our 30-year interview data that most of the individuals in this high-risk group that had coped successfully with adversity in childhood and adolescence are also competent in successfully dealing with transitions into adult responsibilities. But, as at age 18, the resilient women tend to weather stressful life events with less impairment to their health and fewer psychosomatic or "internalizing" symptoms than the men, and they also draw on more sources of social support. A high proportion of the men in this group appear to be reluctant to commit themselves to a sustained and intimate relationship with women at this stage of life.

6. Summary and Conclusions

Three relatively enduring constellations of protective factors emerge from our analyses of the developmental course of this cohort of multiracial children from infancy to young adulthood.

These factors are similar to those reported by Antonovsky (1987) and Rutter (1985) in Europe. They include: (1) Dispositional attributes of the individual that may have a strong genetic base, such as activity level, sociability, and intelligence; (2) affectional ties within the family that provide emotional support in times of stress either from a parent, grandparent, sibling, mate, or spouse; and (3) external support systems at school, work, or church that reward the individual's competencies and provide him with a sense of meaning and an internal locus of control.

The findings presented here suggest that such protective factors may have a more generalized effect on adaptation in childhood, adolescence, and young adulthood than specific risk factors or stressful life events. They may also have more cross-cultural universality than the risk factors that lead to pathology in a given culture (Werner, 1989).

The British child psychiatrist Rutter (1985), reminds us that many of the protective factors that enhance resilience in "high-risk" children operate through *both* direct *and* indirect effects, like chain reactions, over time. A major challenge for us is the examination of the individual links in such longitudinal chains.

In discriminant function analyses, in which we contrasted resilient and problem children and youths, we found that constitutional factors within the child (health, temperament) had their greatest impact in infancy and early childhood; problem-solving and communication skills, and alternative caretakers played a major role in middle childhood; and intrapersonal factors (internal locus of control; self-esteem) in adolescence (Werner and Smith, 1982).

What determined the range of developmental outcomes that we encountered in our study was *not* a single risk factor, but the *balance* between biological risk factors and stressful life events which heightened children's *vulnerability*, and the protective factors in their lives which enhanced their *resiliency*.

This balance changed not only with the stages of the life cycle, but also with the gender of the individual. Both our own and other American and European studies have shown that boys are more vulnerable than girls when exposed to biological insults and caregiving deficits in the first decade of life. This trend is reversed in the second decade, making females more vulnerable in late adolescence, especially with the onset of early childbearing. Judging from our follow-up data, in the early 30s the balance appears to shift back again in favor of the women.

As long as the balance between stressful life events and protective factors is manageable for an individual, she or he can cope. But when stressful life events outweigh the protective factors in his or her life, even the most resilient individual can develop problems; if not serious coping problems, then perhaps less visible "internalizing" symptoms, such as the health problems we have noted among the resilient males in their early 30s, and their reluctance to establish intimate committed relationships.

For clinicians, intervention in the lives of high–risk children and youth means an attempt to tilt the balance from vulnerability to resiliency, either by *decreasing* an individual's exposure to biological risk factors or stressful life events, or by *increasing* the number of protective factors (problem–solving skills, sources of support) that she or he can draw upon. For researchers, the challenge of the future is to discover *how* the chain of direct and indirect linkages is established over time that fosters escape from adversity for vulnerable individuals.

References

Antonovsky, A. (1987): Unraveling the mystery of health: How people manage stress and stay well. San Francisco: Jossey–Bass

Elder, G.H. (1974): Children of the Great Depression: Social change in life experience. Chicago: University of Chicago Press

Gruenebaum, H., et al. (1982): Mentally ill mothers and their children. Chicago: University of Chicago Press

Rutter, M. (1985): Resilience in the face of adversity: Protective factors and resistance to psychiatric disorder. British Journal of Psychiatry, 147, 598–611

Werner, E.E. (1985): Stress and protective factors in children's lives. In Nicol, A.R. (Ed.): Longitudinal studies in child psychology and psychiatry. Chichester, England: John Wiley and Sons

Werner, E.E. (1989): Protective factors and individual resilience. In Meisels, S.J., and Shonkoff, J.P. (Eds): Handbook of early intervention: Theory, practice and analysis. Cambridge, England: Cambridge University Press

Werner, E.E., and Smith, R.S. (1977): Kauai's children come of age. Honolulu: University of Hawaii Press

Werner, E.E., and Smith, R.S. (1982): Vulnerable but invincible: A longitudinal study of resilient children and youth. New York: McGraw–Hill

Mental and Physical Resiliency in Spite of a Stressful Childhood

Wolfgang Tress, Gerhard Reister, and Lutz Gegenheimer

1. Introduction

1.1 Long-Term Effects of Early Childhood Deprivation

A great number of findings from ethology, developmental physiology, deprivation research, and epidemiology basically agree that high psychosocial stress in early childhood has to be regarded as a predisposition to mental illness in adulthood.

1.2 Observations from Animal Research

The studies on apes by Harlow (1962, 1975) are well-known: New-born apes were raised without any maternal care and were later unable to nurse their own offspring. Other studies (Suomi, 1983) have shown how early social deprivation in young mice predisposes them to respond with physical illness to later experimental avoidance learning associated with small electric shocks. The morphological and biochemical effects of insufficient cognitive stimulation are known since the animal experiments by Krech, Rosenzweig, and Bennet (1966) and by Kandel (1983).

1.3 Observations in Children

The Mannheim Cohort Project (Schepank et al.,1987a, b), an epidemiological field study, found a highly significant correlation between high social and emotional stress in early childhood and later personality disorders. The shocking studies from R. Spitz (1945) on the effects of insufficient care and stimulation on the development of babies and infants in psychologically badly managed children's homes should also be mentioned. The children sustained irreversible damage if they were separated from their parents for more than 3 months. As a developmental psychologist, Spitz called the initial relationship a "bridge" that has to be built between the baby and its care person. This bridge permits initially nonverbal and later verbal interaction. Severe deprivation threatens the construction of this bridge. Attention should also be drawn to the lifework of John Bowlby (1969, 1973, 1980). His empirically founded "ethological attachment theory" underlines the primary relationship of the baby or infant to the mother. In their dependence on this primary relationship, children can be truly impaired by premature separations and intolerable grief.

Recent deprivation studies on children receiving good material care in children's homes (Meierhofer and Keller, 1974; Tizard and Hodges, 1978) leave no doubt about the far-reaching impairments of the child's personality that result from long stays in children's homes. Compensatory measures only have a good chance of success in the first year of life.

Of course, this highly significant correlation does not explain everything. Many aspects of further life decide whether dispositions formed in early childhood will become strengthened, lost, compensated, or manifest in later years.

Publications that aim to disprove this fundamental relation, such as the well-received monograph "Stellt die Frühkindheit die Weichen?" (Does early childhood set the course) by Ernst and von Luckner (1985), have to face the criticism (e.g., Fischer, 1986) that they interpret their research data in an extremely one-sided, even ideologically biased and methodologically unacceptable manner. Furthermore, the above-mentioned or comparable studies' use of the fact that a child has not displayed social or criminal disorders to confirm the assertion that this child has survived early trauma without disorder is not acceptable.

The deliberate one-sidedness neglects the possibility of psychosomatic illnesses or depressive developments. In fact, the children investigated by Ernst and von Luckner suffered remarkably frequently from depressions.

In addition, it is also not permissable to study only adolescents when trying to assess the guiding influence of early childhood; they are often still in early puberty when everything is in a state of change. Thus the above-mentioned and comparable studies fail in their efforts to disprove the hypothesis of a basic relationship between psychosocial impairment in childhood and psychogenic disorders in adulthood.

1.4   Psychological Resistance

Nevertheless, valid observations have been available for a long time that show that in individual cases an extremely detrimental childhood can be surmounted and overcome in a surprising manner. The concepts of psychological resistance ("psychological invulnerability" is only a rather imprecise description of this phenonomen) and protective factors are the two central terms used in this research.

Obviously, protective factors can only be effective when stressful life conditions are present. Then however, they largely protect the children concerned from developing the above–mentioned disposition toward psychological disorders in adulthood. Such protective factors should help to explain why the general relationship between a highly stressful early childhood and psychological disorders in adulthood does not manifest in a great number of individual cases.

The most outstanding study on the significance of protective factors during highly stressful childhood is the epochal, longitudinal study from Werner and Smith (1982) that has been running for 30 years on the Hawaiian island of Kauai. The authors followed the course of the lives of their children from birth. The majority of the former children who are now adults came from social classes with severe socioeconomic and educational deprivation.

As anticipated, social and personal development was a failure for those children who were exposed to severe biological, familial, and socioeconomic stress during the first two years of life (e.g., chronic poverty, poor upbringing and education of the parents, perinatal complications, psychopathological disorders in the parents, lengthy separations from the primary care person, short intervals to the birth of younger siblings, severe and repeated childhood illnesses, parental illnesses, developmental problems of siblings, chronic family quarrels, unemployment or absence of father, change of residence, divorce, separation from or death of parents or siblings).

1.5   Protective Factors

Nevertheless, a certain proportion of these highly impaired children attained an astonishing physical, mental, psychological, and social maturity. Their biographies contain the following protective factors that counteracted the high basic risk:

1. Enduring attention to the baby in the first months of life and a positive relationship of the physical parents to the child;
2. presence of additional care persons beside the mother;
3. the mother's involvement in activities outside the family home;
4. the availability of emotional support from peers and neighbors; and
5. clear structures and rules in the household and the family.

2. Epidemiological Field Study

In our own studies (Tress 1986a, b); we carried out further investigations into the question of protective factors in highly stressful early childhood in an epidemiological field study of a representative sample of adult citizens in the industrial and university town of Mannheim in West Germany.

The methodological and theoretical details of this research are given in Tress (1986b); the complete epidemiological material in Schepank et al. (1987a, b). This paper will only deal with the central aspects of the study.

The Mannheim Cohort Project (Schepank, 1987a, b) studied 600 representative adult citizens of Mannheim. For mostly descriptive purposes, the intention was to survey the distribution of psychogenic disorders (psychoneuroses, character pathologies, sexual deviations, psychovegative functional disorders) in a West German industrial and university town. The first interviews with these 600 persons (Study A) took place between 1979 and 1983. A follow–up study was carried out 3 years later (Study B). The evaluation of this study has just been completed.

In a psychoanalytical interview lasting between 2.5 and 3 hours, we used symptom checklists to document the relevant psychogenic symptoms. Then we asked about the history of illness and health behavior and gathered comprehensive information on the present living situation; this included behavior and experience in work, leisure time, and partnership, and sexual practices, dealing with possessions, and other items. Finally we encouraged the subjects to give an account of their early childhood, schooling, and adolescence containing all the elements that could be relevant for their psychogenesis. The subsequent analysis of the data took about 10 hours for each case.

2.1   The Case Definition Problem

The main problem in any epidemiological survey of clinical syndromes, which cannot be so definitively separated from the area of the healthy as, for example, a physical injury or a delirium tremens, is the question of case definition. In syndromes such as psychogenic disorders, in which severity follows a continuum that merges into the area of health, a clinically relevant cut–off point has to be made that is based on the level of severity of the syndrome.

This problem can be dealt with Schepank's Impairment Score (IS). The IS rates all psychogenic disorders (independent of their placement within the ICD categories 300 to 307) with respect to their impact on the person concerned revealed by the person's level of physical, psychological, and social impairment that can be identified on the following three dimensions:

1. The somatic dimension of subjective or objective physical impairment (0– 4 points),
2. the psychological (= experiential) dimension (0–4 points),
3. the dimension of interpersonal and communicational impairment (0–4 points).

The scores alloted to the subject on each of the three scales are added, giving a possible maximum of 12 points. This sum score is defined as the IS of the subject. One end of the scale, with a total score of 0 points, represents the ideal healthy person with no psychogenic impairment; the other end, patients with an extreme neurotic, psychosomatic, or characterological illness. Rating is carried out by experts on the basis of a detailed psychoanalytical examination.

The second classification that is important for our study refers to the stressful life events and circumstances during early childhood. In a global rating, the interviewer had to consider comprehensively all internal and external stressors during early childhood. Besides external factors such as absence of parents, psychopathology of parents, stress from siblings, illness, poverty, and so forth, the interviewer had to rate credibly reported experiences of disadvantage, humiliation, danger, not being wanted, and so forth, as internal stress.

This classification was also performed on a 5–point scale from 0 to 4, in which 0 represented no severe stressors; for instance, subject was child prodigy, both parents were present, father was employed with high earnings, mother was housewife, parents' relationship was clearly harmonious, no siblings.

A score of 4 in contrast stood for extreme stress; for instance, illegitimate, father unknown, mother seriously ill during subject's first year of life, care person was grandmother during this period, later residence in children's home for 4 years, hospital treatment for obscure stomach ache, subject returns to mother who has meanwhile remarried, alcoholic stepfather, child returned to children's home because of stepfather's cruelty.

For the purposes of this study, subjects were divided into two groups of either low or severe impairment on the basis of this rating. A test of reliability with seven interviewers produced a coefficient of kappa = 1.0.

2.2   Groups with Severe Stress during Early Childhood

The present study only concerns those subjects within the sample of 600 persons who had indicated severe stress in early childhood. This formed two extreme groups with definite, severe stress in early childhood: Group A containing persons who are now psychologically healthy; and Group B containing persons who now have severe psychogenic disorders.

Both groups belonged to the 11 to 12% of all subjects who were exposed to the worst developmental conditions at preschool age. Each group contained 20 subjects, equally distributed between the sexes. Their age range was between 25 and 45 years.

Tab. 1: Distribution of subjects according to average severity of impairment caused by psychogenetic disorders over the preceding 12 months and severity of psychosocial stress during the first 6 years of life

Score for early childhood stress	Average severity of impairment caused by psychogenic disorders (IS Scores for the last 12 months)			Totals
	0 - 3	4 - 5	6 - 12	
0 - 1	174 29.4 %	99 16,6 %	30 5.0 %	304 51.1 %
2	71 11.8 %	89 15.0 %	70 11.8 %	229 38.5 %
3 - 4	20 3.4 % Group A	22 3.7 %	20 3.4 % Group B	62 10.4 %
Totals	264 44,5 %	210 35.3 %	120 20.2 %	595 * 100 %

* Five of the 600 Subjects were not classified in relation to early childhood stress

2.3   Differences in Social Status and Morbidity

Only small differences were found in social class. Subjects who are now psychogenically healthy (Group A) tend to be members of the upper or middle social classes, while the subjects with present psychogenic disorders tend to be in the lower classes. This was not so at birth: The two groups did not differ regarding the social class into which they were born. The present differences in social status were completely due to the higher attractivity of psychologically healthy women in their search for a partner. Thus the class distinction was not the cause but the consequence of their better mental health.

Naturally, the two extreme groups clearly differed with regard to the types of

illness: The group with severe disorders mostly contained psychosomatic illnesses and character disorders.

2.4   Thirty Specific Aspects of Early Childhood

While we have previously only discussed high–level psychosocial stress in early
childhood, we will now compare 30 specific aspects of early childhood that
were included in the documentation of the interviews. These aspects were: sex,
age, illegitimacy, age difference between parents and between parents and
subject, completeness of parental couple, social class of family of origin,
presence of a substitute mother during early childhood before or after the
second year of life, absence of mother or father during the first year of life or
the following years, psychogenic illness of the mother or father, severe disorders in the parents' relationship, day nursery, residence in children's homes,
sibling–related aspects − particularly age gap to next sibling, neurotic symptoms during childhood, frequent changes of residence, high–stress single life
events during early childhood, and finally indications for the presence of a
stable, positive reference person during early childhood. This reference person
had to be constantly available as an emotionally concerned and loving adult
regardless of whether this was a parent figure, relative, or any other person in
the social environment.
Originally, it had not been intended to use such information in the computer
evaluation of the entire epidemiological research project.

2.5   Importance of Marked Age Gap to Father or Siblings and of
Stable Reference Person

Only 4 of the 30 aspects of psychosocial stress in early childhood showed
relevant and statistically significant differences between the extreme groups.
Marked differences that failed to reach statistical significance suggested that
subjects with present disorders were more frequently exposed to psychopatho-

logically suspect fathers, and additionally more frequently had to share bad living conditions in early childhood with a sibling with an age gap of less than 12 months.

However, two further aspects of early childhood discriminated decisively between the two extreme groups: The majority of the currently healthy subjects had been reared by their mothers alone (the classic broken–home situation!). However, above all aspects, a positive, stable reference person had been available to all the presently healthy subjects.

The central finding in our study was that 86% of all subjects could be assigned correctly to their extreme group purely on the basis of information on the completeness of the parental couple and the presence of a positive reference person.

Tab. 2:   Reduced model of conditions leading to psychogenic disorders in adulthood in regard to severe psycho–social impairment during childhood

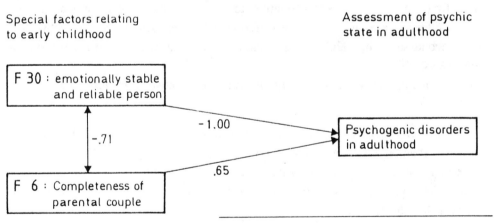

Special factors relating
to early childhood

Assessment of psychic
state in adulthood

F 30 : emotionally stable and reliable person

−.71

−1.00

Psychogenic disorders in adulthood

.65

F 6 : Completeness of parental couple

For the sample of the 22 probands with a stable reference person the correlation is : 66

Without the emotional support of a good reference person, not one of the children attained the present healthy group of subjects. However, when it was possible to identify such a helpful person, further development was dependent on the completeness of the parental couple: When the child lived alone with the mother, the expectancy of psychogenic health in adulthood was 90%. When the child grew up with both (not necessarily biological) parents, this expectancy was reduced to nearly 60%.

3. Second Study

Tress and Gegenheimer performed a replication of the results of our follow–up study (Study B, 1983–1986). Again we selected subjects from the random sample (Study B; $N = 528$) who had shown severe or extreme stress in early childhood in both studies *and* who belonged either to the group of severely ill or the group of mentally healthy persons. Additionally, persons belonging to the first group could be identified in one of the studies as risk subjects, that is, they had an IS of 4 or 5. Moreover, the dropouts in Study B were also taken into account. The sample classified according to these criteria contained 53 subjects: 18 healthy and 35 psychogenically ill persons.

In a first step, the 30 factors relating to early childhood were applied to test whether there were any significant differences between healthy and ill subjects.

In a second step, the validity of the ratings and diagnoses was examined for all interviews.

The following factors significantly discriminated between healthy and ill persons:

Factor 30 (emotionally stable and reliable reference person) $p = .001$
Factor 6 (completeness of parental couple) $p = .001$
These two factors also showed a negative intercorrelation.

Factor 23 (age gap of less than 1 year to next sibling) did not discriminate between healthy and ill persons.

Thus the replication study supported the reduced model of conditions leading to psychogenic disorders in adulthood.

Tab. 3: Reduced model: B–Study included

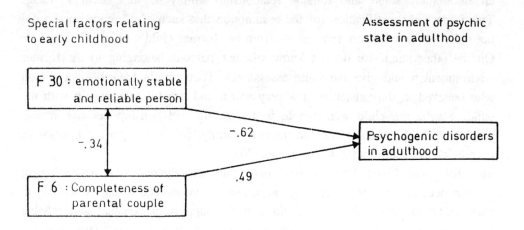

4. Discussion

Here we can only mention some aspects of the validity problems involved in retrospectively collected data. From a rather pragmatic point of view, it is only worth criticizing the retrospective collection of biographical data when statistically significant correlations emerge between certain biographical characteristics and the present psychosocial state of a person.

Although all the 30 factors of childhood impairment are certainly important, we shall confine our discussion to the central factor in our study: the stable reference person.

First of all, the interviewers had not been instructed to look particularly for such a person; they were told to gain a clear and comprehensive picture of the circumstances of early childhood in each case. These findings had to be recorded formally. The protocol of the biographical case history was used to seek definite indications for the existence of such a reference person. Our primary goal was to see whether or not a reference person was documented in the interview in which early childhood was discussed. If such a person could be identified, it seems to be legitimate to assume his or her real existence, even if the subject idealized this reference person.

But what about the subjects who did not report a stable reference person? Such an emotionally stable and reliable relationship simply did not occur to them. This is the only justification for the assumption that such a reference person did not exist — for whatever reasons — from the former child's point of view.

On the other hand, we do not know whether persons belonging to the former environment would give the same assessment. There might have been a person who believed in the existence of a very warm and trustful relationship with the child. Maybe the child was unable to realize this relationship because it was counteracted by a complete but chaotic family (cf. the significant negative correlation between Factor 6 and Factor 30).

Therefore we should like to emphasize that an advantageous psychological development in spite of completely detrimental psychosocial living conditions in early childhood can only succeed through the support of constant and reliable care from an available, stable, and beneficial reference person. This is not a surprising result; it is compatible with most previous studies.

From a psychoanalytical point of view and taking object–relation theories into account, the internalization of an early good object as the result of a sufficient self–object relationship can be regarded as the *basis* of later mental health.

The second result may confuse us at first sight. It is apparent that the absence of a father has a positive effect when psychosocial life conditions are detrimental during early childhood.

However, it should be considered that, as a rule, parents are unable to develop a constructive relationship under extremely stressful life conditions, but only a partnership fraught with battle and struggle. In such a tense and emotionally loaded family atmosphere full of disturbances and irritations, the child's chance of establishing a warm and safe relationship to one of the parents or to another person (often one of the grandparents) decreases drastically: The child would immediately enter into internal loyalty conflicts with one of the parents. Under these conditions, the offer of such a relationship would probably attract the child's open refusal. Therefore, in such a case, the absence of a father could be advantageous.

Thus epidemiology also confirms the concept of maternal care as a basis for the psychological development of every human being. Such a positive relationship is the basic requirement for a successful, healthy development even in a psychosocially deprived childhood. However, the basic family situation seems to play a decisive role, because the chances for affected children drastically decrease in emotionally loaded families. In this case, the internal and external loyalty conflicts are much lower for children who are reared by their mothers alone. Therefore, with psychosocially unfavorable living conditions, the absence of the father may well be a positive factor. We hope that investigations with comparable samples will provide comparable results.

References

Bowlby, J. (1969): Eine Analyse der Mutter–Kind–Beziehung (Attachment and loss. Vol I). Kindler, München 1975

Bowlby, J. (1973): Psychische Schäden als Folgen der Trennung von Mutter und Kind (Attachment and loss. Vol II). Kindler, München 1976

Bowlby, J. (1970): Verlust, Trauer und Depression (Attachment and loss. Vol III). Fischer, Frankfurt/M. 1983

Ernst, C., and v. Luckner, N. (1985): Stellt die Frühkindheit die Weichen? Enke, Stuttgart

Fischer, G. (1986): Empirische Forschung zur Wirkung von Taumata bei Kindern und Jugendlichen. Kritik und Information zu einem wieder aktuellen Thema. Psyche, 40, 145–161

Fischer, G., Ernst, C., and v. Luckner, N. (1986): Stellt die Frühkindheit die Weichen? Book review. Psyche, 40, 364–369

Harlow, H.F. (1975): Ethnology. In Freedman, A., Kaplan, H., Sadock, J. (Eds.): Comprehensive textbook of psychiatry, Vol. 1. William and Wilkins, Baltimore

Harlow, H.F., and Harlow, M. (1962): Social deprivation in monkeys. Science, Am., 207, 137–146

Kandel, E.R. (1983): From metapsychology to molecular biology. Explorations in the nature of anxiety. Am. J. Psychiatry, 140, 1277–1293

Krech, D., Rosenzweig, M.R., and Bennett, E.L. (1966): Environmental impoverishment, social isolation, and changes in brain chemistry and anatomy. Physical Behavior, 1, 99–104

Meierhofer, M., and Keller, W. (1974): Frustration im frühen Kindesalter. Huber, Bern–Stuttgart–Wien

Schepank, H. (1987a): Psychogene Erkrankungen der Stadtbevölkerung. Eine epidemiologisch–tiefenpsychologische Feldstudie in Mannheim. Springer, Berlin–Heidelberg–New York–London–Paris–Tokyo

Schepank, H. (1987b): Epidemiology of psychogenic disorders. The Mannheim Study. Results of a field survey in the Federal Republic of Germany. Springer, Berlin–Heidelberg–New York–Tokyo

Spitz, R. (1973/1945): Die Entstehung der ersten Objektbeziehungen. Klett, Stuttgart

Suomi, S. (1983): Models of depression in primates. Psychol. Med., 13, 465–468

Tizard, B., and Hodges, J. (1978): The effects of early institutional rearing on the behavior problems and affectional relationships of eight–year–old children. J. Child. Psychiat., 19, 99–118

Tress, W. (1986a): Die positive frühkindliche Bezugsperson. Psychother. Med. Psychol., 36, 51–57

Tress, W. (1986b): Das Rätsel der seelischen Gesundheit. Traumatische Kindheit und früher Schutz gegen psychogene Störungen. Vandenhoeck & Ruprecht, Göttingen

Werner, E., and Smith, R. (1982): Vulnerable but not invincible: A Study of resilient children. McGraw-Hill, New York

On the Concept of "Invulnerability": Evaluation and First Results of the Bielefeld Project

Friedrich Lösel, Thomas Bliesener, and Peter Köferl

1. Introduction

Prevention and intervention in childhood and adolescence require empirically well-founded knowledge about the etiology of the disorders under consideration. Without wishing to strain the fashionable concept of "paradigm change", in recent years we can see a new research. This can be illustrated by the following quotations:

> There is a regrettable tendency to focus gloomily on the ills of mankind and on all that can and does go wrong ... . The potential for prevention surely lies in increasing our knowledge and understanding of the reason why some children are *not* damaged by deprivation... . (Rutter, 1979, p. 49)
>
> Vulnerables have long been the province of our mental health disciplines but prolonged neglect of the "invulnerable child" — the healthy child in an unhealthy setting — has provided us with a false sense of security in creating prevention models that are founded more on values than on facts... . Were we to study the forces that move such children to survival and to adaptation, the long-range benefits to our society might be far more significant than are many efforts to construct models of primary prevention to curtail the incidence of vulnerability. (Garmezy, 1982, p. XIX)

The initial reports on invulnerable children were more programmatic conclusions from single-case observations (e.g., Garmezy and Nuechterlein, 1972; Anthony, 1974). Since then, a series of empirical studies have been published on factors that make it possible for children and adolescents to cope successfully with risk constellations and cumulative stressors (for an overview: Garmezy, 1985; Rutter, 1985; Werner, 1985; Cowen and Work, 1987). In the German-speaking world, however, up to now there has been little empirical research into the phenomenon of invulnerability (cf. Remschmidt, 1986; Ulich, 1988). There are recent retrospective studies on the differentiation between risk and protective factors (e.g., Dührssen, 1984; Tress, 1986), and some indications for differential vulnerabilities can be taken from longitudinal studies in developmental psychology (e.g., Meyer–Probst and Teichmann, 1984; Ehlers, Merz, and Remer, 1985). The focus of empirical research, however, is centered more on the field of the developmental psychology of "normal" coping with problems in adolescence (e.g., Fend, Schröer, and Richter, 1985; Olbrich and Todt, 1984; Seiffge–Krenke, 1986; Hurrelmann, 1987), although increased attention to the problems of developmental psychopathology can be detected (e.g., Silbereisen, Noack, and Reitzle, 1987; Fend and Prester, 1985).

A clear differentiation between the relevant fields of research is neither possible nor objectively appropriate. It is unmistakable that research on invulnerability has developed in close connection with the general upswing of transactional models or models of the individual as a productive processor of reality. As examples, we can mention here the models and findings from stress and coping research, socioepidemiology, and ecological psychology (e.g., Antonovsky, 1979, 1987; Dohrenwend, 1978; Dohrenwend and Dohrenwend, 1981; Lazarus and Folkman, 1984; Moos, 1984; Kobasa and Puccetti, 1983; for a summary Köferl, 1987). There is a multitude of constructs that are related to invulnerability, such as resilience, hardiness, adaptation, adjustment, mastery, plasticity, person–environment fit, or social buffering. However, as Prystav (1981) has shown for the concept of coping, the differentiation between processes, dispositions, patterns, resources, and outcomes is often insufficient. This leads to ambiguities in the meaning of specific terms and the representativity of concrete operationalizations.

The concept of invulnerability also contains the danger of other misunderstandings. It is used in a way that does not refer to the traditional medical understanding of vulnerability. From a medical perspective, vulnerability is understood as innate dispositions for specific illnesses or illness in general. Thus vulnerabilities are considered to be mostly independent of protective factors (Zubin and Spring, 1977). This is shown in the following simple model of the major factors influencing the development of psychiatric disorders.

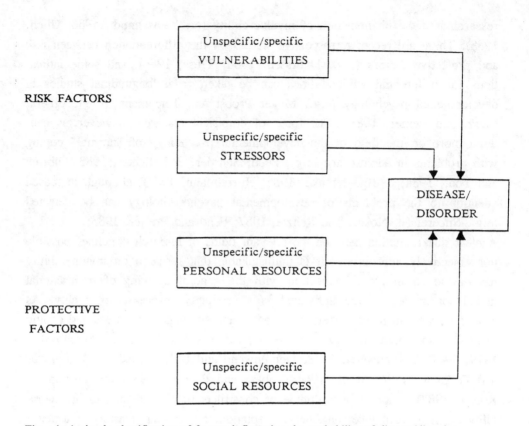

Fig. 1: A simple classification of factors influencing the probability of disease/disorder

However, in developmental psychopathology invulnerability is used in a way that includes protective factors (personal and social resources) that contribute to the *result* of mental health despite pronounced risk factors. What this means is that:

1. We are not dealing with some absolute or general "invulnerability", but only a relative immunity to stressful life events and circumstances.
2. It is not only genetic dispositions that are involved, but, in particular, protective factors from complex nature–nurture interactions.
3. The resistance to stress is not a fixed quality, but can vary across time and circumstances (cf. Rutter, 1985).

The concept is sometimes also misunderstood in the public health context. For example, in our own field contacts we have occasionally met defensive behavior that is based on the fear that a research concept of invulnerability would hinder efforts to change deprivating circumstances. Some popular idealizations ("super-kids", "vulnerable but invincible") may well have encouraged the perception that the relevant research could be used to oppose the development of health and social programs. But as, for example, Werner (1984), Garmezy (1987), or Cowen and Work (1987) have clearly indicated, invulnerability and similar concepts in no way suggest a lower social commitment to the psychological health of children and adolescents, but rather a stronger emphasis on primary prevention approaches within the natural context and also on the potentials of self-help (cf. also the concept of "empowerment": Albee, 1987; Cochran, 1987). For these and other reasons, we shall predominantly use the term "resiliency", meaning − in the sense of invulnerability − the effective coping with cumulative and severe stressful life events and circumstances.

1.1   Resiliency Research and "Traditional" Etiological Research

As, in recent years, some authors have noted a certain stagnation in the concepts of the individual as a productive processor of reality (Braukmann and Filipp, 1984), it seems necessary to consider the perspective of resiliency research in comparison to traditional deficit models. According to Rutter (1985) resiliency research is a *third phase* of research into child and adolescent disorders, which followed two deficit−oriented phases.

The *first phase* was essentially characterized by psychiatric and psychoanalytic approaches and can be traced back to the beginning of the 20th century. The dominant concepts were relatively nonspecific, but at the same time massive psychological effects evolving out of a spectrum of "negative" life experiences or events. The work of Bowlby (1951) on maternal deprivation and other fundamental concepts of the parent−child relationship can be considered as representative (cf. Toman, 1976). Though the borders with the first phase are rather blurred, the *second phase* is mostly concerned with research carried out during the 1960s and 1970s. It is characterized by the attempts to provide differentiated concepts on both − the not truly "causal" − "independent" and "dependent" variables and also the contexts of their relationships. For example, studies were done on the effects of different types of experiences of loss (Rutter, 1971), how variables differ in their risk potential for distinct kinds of developmental disturbances (Robins, 1966), or which differential constellations of parental education and family climate are particularly relevant for juvenile delinquency (Lösel, 1978).

Both phases of research have, methodologically speaking, explained a considerable proportion of the variance in the development of disorders (for summaries, see Garmezy and Rutter, 1983; Honig, 1986). In the field of juvenile delin-, quency as an example, numerous cross−sectional and longitudinal studies since Glueck and Glueck (1950) have repeatedly shown that the characteristics of a multiproblem milieu, such as parental criminality, poor parental supervision, cruel, passive, or neglectful attitudes, erratic or harsh discipline, mutual conflict, large family size, and socioeconomic disadvantages, correlate with the development of persistent delinquent careers (for summaries see Lösel, 1982; Rutter and Giller, 1983; Farrington, Ohlin, and Wilson, 1986; Loeber and Stouthamer−Loeber, 1986). Even long−term longitudinal studies report a substantial predictive power of risk variables (e.g., Farrington, Gallagher, Morley, Ledger, and West, 1986; Farrington, in press). At the same time, however a large part of the variance remains unexplained when base rates are taken into account. In many cases, delinquency is only a transitory phenomenon in the development of (male) adolescents, and the accuracy of predicting more persistent "criminal careers" on the basis of risk factors is rather limited (Petersilia, 1980; Gottfredson and Hirschi, 1986). Despite considerable problems in criminal career research (cf. Blumstein, Cohen, and Farrington, 1988) delinquency belongs, however, to those forms of deviance that can still be predicted *relatively* well (e.g., Robins, 1972; Gersten, Langner, and Simcha−Fagan, 1978; Rutter and Giller, 1983; Jesness, 1987).

In all, the empirical findings on risk or deficit variables are still not satisfactory with respect to the amount of explained variance. For example, in a meta−analysis, we have reappraised the German research on the relationship between various child and adolescent disorders and characteristics of family socialization. We assessed a total of 113 studies between the years 1971 and 1984. An effect size could be calculated as an indicator of the correlation between family characteristics and psychiatric disorders in 86 of the studies. The average effect size lay — depending on the analysis model used — between $r = .21$ and $r = .33$ (Binomial Effect Size Display from Rosenthal and Rubin, 1982). This shows that to turn our attention toward the "untypical cases" in traditional research (false negatives, false positives) is a necessary consequence if we want to explain more variance. Therefore studying the "false positive" group of resilient children is not so much an antipode to traditional deficit–orientated research but more its logical continuation.

1.2   On the State of Resiliency Research

In comparison with risk factors, systematic research into protective factors is rather underrepresented: However, well–known longitudinal studies, such as the studies on the Great Depression (Elder, 1974), the Menninger Coping Project (Murphy and Moriarty, 1976), the Berkeley Ego–Resilience Study (Block and Block, 1980; Gjerde, Block, and Block, 1986), the Harvard Preschool Project (White, Kaban, and Attanuci, 1979), the New York Longitudinal Study (Chess and Thomas, 1986) or the Study of Adult Development at Harvard Medical School (Felsman & Vaillant, 1987), have suggested significant factors. These are mainly: (1) *personal resources of the child* (such as autonomy, independence, empathy, task orientation, and diverse temperament factors), as well as (2) *social resources* (such as warmth, supportive mothers, open communication within the family, encouragement from the parents, agreement on moral values, and good peer–group relationships). However, some of the studies only deal with temporary stressors in intact, middle–class families. Two authors who have paid particular attention to such multiproblem milieus are Norman Garmezy (e.g., Garmezy, Masten, and Tellegen, 1984; Garmezy and Devine, 1985; Garmezy and Tellegen, 1984; Garmezy, 1987) and Emmy Werner (e.g., Werner and Smith, 1982; Werner, 1985, 1986).

> In two studies, Garmezy investigated about 600 students. He included four target groups and two control groups in his multiple group comparison design: (1) children of schizophrenic mothers, (2) children of depressed mothers, (3) children diagnosed with externalized disorders, and (4) children diagnosed with internalized disorders. The latter two groups

had been referred by school personnel to community child guidance clinics. One control group was matched for demographic variables and the other was randomly selected. Parent interviews, personality tests, and achievement tests were carried out alongside measurement of stress and competence and assessment of school data. The authors found two family-related mediators of competence and stress: family stability and organization, and family cohesion. Children with more advantageous family characteristics were more intelligent, more competent, and less likely to become disruptive under high levels of stress. Children with better assets (IQ, socioeconomic status, positive family attributes) appeared to be more socially competent and, under stress, more socially engaged with their peers.

Emmy Werner's most famous study was a highly detailed longitudinal investigation of 695 children from the 1955 birth cohort on the Hawaiian island of Kauai (Werner and Smith, 1982; cf. also Werner, in this volume). From the total sample, 72 children were selected who already indicated at least four serious risk factors during early childhood (e.g., poverty, psychotic parent member) but, nevertheless, had developed in a psychologically healthy way. They were perceived as "very active" and "socially responsive" infants, showed adequate problem-solving and communication skills as well as normal perceptual-motor development and displayed both "masculine" and "feminine" interests and skills. In late adolescence, they had higher scores on internal locus of control scales, a more positive self-concept, and a more nurturant, responsible, and achievement-oriented attitude toward life than the comparison group. At age 18, all were able to draw on a number of informal sources of support. Among the key factors on the part of environment were the age of opposite-sex parent, the number and age differences of children in the family, and the existence of alternate caregivers in the household such as grandparents (Werner, 1984).

In his comprehensive review, Rutter (1985) evaluates a series of characteristics and processes as being significant for resiliency, for example: the way in which children and adolescents deal with life stressors, and particularly the extent to which they act and do not just react; cognitions of self-efficacy and self-esteem as preconditions of a tendency to act; stable emotional relations to and positive experiences with others; temperamental characteristics that encourage successful coping and positive interactions with others; and a parental upbringing that encourages the child to cope with life events. Garmezy (1983), Remschmidt

(1986, 1988), or Felsman and Vaillant (1987), for example, have produced similar descriptions of personal factors (competences) and social factors (environmental conditions) that should be important for resiliency.

However, the previous assumptions and findings have raised theoretical, empirical, and methodological problems: The constructs used are derived from a wide range of theoretical contexts, so that their interconnection is based more on considerations of plausibility than on systematic deductions. This is nevertheless suitable for the state of research on resiliency, as it does — in the sense of problem–oriented research — not place too many preordained restrictions on the relevant phenomena (cf. Dörner, 1983). Furthermore, models of stress research that are relevant for resiliency phenomena still contain a lot of conceptual problems (cf. Garmezy, 1985). Even elaborated models such as the one from Pearlin (1987) contain ambiguous elements concerning the direction of effects; for example, whether personal mediators (coping, social support) should influence components of the self (and not vice versa as well). For practical purposes, more simple hypotheses seem to be adequate. According to these, the risks given at birth and the stressors accumulated later stand in a sort of balance that, depending on which way it is influenced, results in either psychological health or disorder (Werner, 1985; Remschmidt, 1986; cf. also the Diathesis–Stress–Model).

A further problem is that the risk and protective factors for the development of behavioral/emotional disorders cannot always be differentiated unequivocally. This problem is evident, for example, in the methodologically well–controlled study from Tress (1986; cf. also Tress et. al., in this volume):

> The data have been selected from the Mannheim Cohort Study dealing with diseases according to ICD–classifications 300–307. Based on a representative sample of the population of Mannheim, psychopathological developments within the 1935, 1945, and 1955 birth cohorts have been analyzed. Two extreme groups of 20 persons out of 600 persons have been specified. According to an objective index, both groups have been exposed to hard and stressful environments in childhood and infancy. One group, however, demonstrated no or very slight symptoms, the other group developed serious psychiatric disorders. The "strongest" protective factor has been the availability of a stable caregiver relation in early childhood.

However, the lack of a stable reference person simultaneously takes a significant role as a risk factor within the deficit models (see Bowlby, 1988). Very different findings can be anticipated depending on which side of the coin is regarded as a risk factor and which as a protective factor, and on how a "high risk" is defined. For this reason, Rutter (1985) argued in favor of a moderator concept, that is, factors should only be considered protective when they alone show an effect in the presence of stressors. In the empirical research on resiliency, it is accordingly also necessary to avoid an operational confounding of the risk factors with the protective factors.

A further problem of resiliency research is related to the range of validity or generalizability of existing results. A portion of the relevant studies are directed at coping with single critical life events in middle–class families in otherwise intact developmental contexts (cf. Cowen and Work, 1987; Ulich, 1988). However, several studies have shown that only a stronger accumulation of stressful circumstances or life events leads to a marked increase in the probability of behavioral/emotional disorders (e.g., Thomas and Chess, 1984). Some of the studies that have dealt with children and adolescents under cumulative risk loads in the sense of a particularly significant psychopathological multiproblem milieu have been carried out in rather specific cultural contexts (e.g., the Kauai study, Werner and Smith, 1982). Their generalizability to, for example, Western industrialized nations appears to be questionable. Other data of resiliency research are hard to compare with regard to the criteria of psychological disorder or health. To some extent, it cannot be excluded that although the resilient children have remained unrecorded in the externally more noticeable and easier to diagnose externalizing symptoms, they may well have developed disorders in the field of internalizing symptoms.

2. Concept for the Bielefeld Project

Our project was planned against the background of the research sketched above. Our main interest is in resilient adolescents who are (still) psychologically healthy despite high multiple exposure to stressful life events and circumstances as understood in the original concept of "invulnerability".

On the one hand, we are investigating how these adolescents differ from those who have developed disorders that reflect the typical risk constellations of "true positives". On the other hand, in the sense of the methodological problems reported, we want to test to what extent the findings on different criteria applied for risk factors and mental health/disorder remain stable. The risk factors were selected to be relatively accurate predictors of disorders in accordance with the present state of research. Thus we are trying to optimize the explanation of variance according to the traditional deficit model.

As we are interested in obtaining an approximation to the phenomenon of resiliency that is as naturalistic as possible and want to avoid research artefacts, the screening of subjects has been carried out with case–related interviews of educators, social workers, and teachers in social welfare institutions as well as schools. On the basis of this first recruitment, we undertake a validation through more objective measures of level of risk and health/disorder. The group of resilient adolescents determined in this manner are compared with an analogously recruited group who had developed disorders in line with the deficit model. The target population is the age group of 13 to 17 years. This age phase is particularly "sensitive" for developmental psychopathology. A longitudinal study with an onset in early childhood is not possible for economic reasons and is hardly acceptable for ethical reasons (nonintervention in the deviant group). The choice of this age group offers the possibility of follow–up studies with comparable instruments.

With respect to the resiliency construct, relevant personal and social resources were selected according to the state of research sketched above. Mischel's (1973) conception of a cognitive social learning theory of personality was chosen as a theoretical framework (cf. also Mischel, 1981). Accordingly, resiliency characteristics were expected in the following areas of *personal resources*: behavior construction competences (e.g., cognitive competences); coding strategies and personal constructs (e.g., constructs of social resources); behavior and outcome expectancies/evaluations (e.g., self–efficacy); self–regulating systems (e.g., self–esteem).

In addition, temperament characteristics were included. Recent findings have shown that factors of temperament appear to have a greater significance for

person-environment interactions than cognitive theories have at times presumed
(cf. Lerner, Palermo, Spiro, and Nesselroade, 1982; Strelau, 1984; Thomas
and Chess, 1984; Wolfson, Fields, and Rose, 1987). Although they are not
treated by Mischel, temperament factors, with their emphasis on the "how" of
behavior, can be subsumed under behavior-construction competences. To some
extent, this also applies for the *social resources*. Here we investigate characteristics of social support and social climate in the welfare institutions or families. As resiliency, in end effect, is always a result of the individual's differential processing of the environment, characteristics of the social environment can
be subsumed to Mischel's (1973) framework model as long as they involve the
coding and constructs of the respective person (and not judgments by others).
More details on the diagnoses of the groups, constructs, and methods will be
presented in the next sections. We will present two studies:

1. A *pilot study* in schools that was not only designed to develop and test the
   instruments for the diagnosis of risk factors and psychological health/disor-
   der, but also allowed us to make explorative evaluations on resiliency.
2. A first part of the current *main study*, in which resilient adolescents were
   investigated in social welfare and correctional institutions. As assessment is
   still continuing, the data which we will report on the main study should
   only be regarded as intermediate findings.

3. Pilot Studies

We carried out four studies in schools in North-Rhine Westphalia and in Lower
Saxony in order to develop and test our instruments. These were:

1. An assessment of 641 students aged between 12 and 16 years (6th- to
   8th-grade). We predominantly used instruments to assess stressful life
   events and circumstances and psychological health/disorder.
2. An investigation of 30 school teachers in which an instrument for teacher
   judgements on psychological health was tested on a subsample of the above
   sample of students.

3. An assessment of 115 students to test the reliability/stability of the statements on psychological health/disorder.
4. An assessment of 39 selected students to test the agreement between the teacher judgements and direct observation of behavior in the classroom.

In this paper, we will only report those results from the pilot studies which are relevant for a demonstration of the methods used in the main study (for further results, see, e.g., Lösel, Bliesener, Köferl, and Schmidtpeter, 1988).

3.1   Method

Instruments were applied to the following characteristics and constructs:

Stressful life events and circumstances. The 641 students completed a detailed questionnaire. Their answers were used to form a risk index which is intended to be suitable for standardizing and screening for the resilient and deviant groups in the main study. This instrument is divided into two sections: Part I refers to objective biographical events. Part II refers to more subjectively evaluated recent incidents and ongoing problem states in the family milieu. The selection of the single characteristics was oriented toward the risk factors pointed out in the literature (cf. Werner and Smith, 1982; Lösel, 1983; Rutter, 1983; Honig, 1986). The biographical part (47 items) contained questions on the occurence of events such as death of a parent, divorce/separation, hospitalizations, time spent in social welfare institutions, moving to another district, change in parental care person, socioeconomic deprivation, parental unemployment, and so forth. Questions were also included on the child's age at the time, the duration, and − when applicable − the frequency of the events. Part II of the instrument investigated characteristics such as extreme forms of punishment, subjective experiences of economic deprivation, tensions in the family, estimations of parental alcohol and drug consumption, and so forth (a total of 24 items). All of the items were selected from a larger pool using 3−point expert ratings (5 judges) on their empirically supported relevance as risk factors (the selection criterion was an agreement between at least four of the five raters). The single items in the two parts of the instrument were used to form risk indices (OBSTRESS, SUBSTRESS) that could then be summarized as a sum index (ALLSTRESS). The correlations between the subindices and the sum index were .59 for the former and .91 for the latter. While the distribution of OBSTRESS was slightly skewed to the right, SUBSTRESS showed a more marked skewness. The following distribution scores were found for the sum index: $M = 13.21$; $SD = 8.70$; $Mdn = 10$; and Range $= 0 - 52$.

Psychological health/disorder. In order to obtain a detailed assessment of the second classification criterion − psychological health or the lack of behav-ioral/emotional disorders − several versions of the well−established Achen-bach Child Behavior Checklist (CBCL) were adapted for German conditions (cf. Achenbach and Edelbrock, 1983, 1986; Achenbach, 1985; Achenbach, Ver-hulst, Baron, and Althaus, 1987; cf. also Achenbach, in this volume). The CBCL is designed for the assessment of child and adolescent disorders by one parent. Similar versions are available for information from teaching staff (Teacher's Report Form: TRF), from the adolescents themselves (Youth Self−Report: YSR), and for direct observation of behavior (Direct Observation Form: DOF). The various versions of the CBCL provide a profile of problem behavior differentiated according to age and sex. On the one hand, the scales capture empirically derived narrow−band syndromes (e.g., anxious, socially withdrawn, depressed, aggressive) that correspond to DSM−III criteria (cf. Achenbach, 1985; Remschmidt, 1983, 1985). On the other hand, they can be summarized for research purposes into rougher classifications of empirically derived broad−band syndromes (internalizing vs. externalizing syndrome). The TRF can be applied in the age range from 6 to 16, the CBCL from 2 to 16, the YSR from 11 to 18, and the DOF from about 6 years onward. In the pilot study reported here, we applied the YSR to our 641 students. In most of the scales it showed satisfactory reliabilities (see Tab. 1).

Tab. 1:   Consistencies and Intercorrelations of YSR—scales for boys and girls

	Internaliz. syndrome (I)					Externaliz. syndrome (E)		Boys N = 319
	Depressed	Unpopular	Somatic complaints	Self-destructive	Thought disorder	Delinquent	Aggressive	
	.82	.84	.70	.69	.72	.86	.84	Reliability
Somatic compl. (I)		.83	.65	.75	.68	.56	.57	Depressed (I)
Depressed	.71		.64	.80	.63	.60 / .65	.62	Unpopular
Unpopular	.51	.70		.54	.64	.53	.46	Somatic compl.
					.70	.56	.54	Self-destr.
Thought dis.	.62	.74	.53			.52	.48	Thought dis.
Aggressive (E)	.53	.71	.63		.69		.83	Delinquent (E)
Delinquent	.49 / .59	.61	.58		.66	.80		Aggressive
Reliability	.77	.90	.65		.74	.82	.82	

Girls N = 322	Somatic complaints	Depressed	Unpopular		Thought disorder	Aggressive	Delinquent	
	Internaliz. syndrome (I)					Externaliz. syndrome (E)		

Most scales correlated with each other. This shows that even broad–band and narrow–band syndromes do not represent distinctly separate classes. The inter-correlations of the scales within the broad–band syndromes, however, were higher than those between the syndromes. A further indication of validity was the correlation with the index of stressful life events and circumstances (accord-ing to sex and syndrome: .26 to .47). However, the correlations between YSR and TRF found in further pilot studies with smaller samples were low for both sexes (–.01 to .28 for the broad–band syndromes) and noticeably lower than the correlations between TRF and DOF (Lösel, Bliesener, Klünder, and Köferl, 1988). This indicates that not only the usual validity and reliability problems of the different data sources are involved, but also the highly different context to which the different informants refer. Insofar, our results are consonant with the meta–analysis of Achenbach, McConaughy, and Howell (1987) which proposes the perspective of the "multiple setting — multiple informant". For further findings on the YSR in our sample, see Lösel et al. (1987; Lösel, Bliesener, Klünder, and Köferl, 1988).

Social support. The concept of social support has received much attention in coping research, and is often considered to be an important protective factor (Barrera, 1986; Figley, 1986; Sarason, 1986). Nevertheless, there are a variety of definitions of the concept (e.g., Cobb, 1976; Kahn, 1979), different modal assumptions about its effects (Quast, 1985), and a great number of operationalizations (cf. Nestmann, 1988; Rock et al., 1984). However, it is possible to discriminate between two basic approaches: social support as actual, observable help from persons in the social environment, and social support as a subjective representation of received help (Baumann, 1987). These two approaches are not independent to the extent that in the latter sense, social support comprises episodic knowledge structures about actual helping performances (Morgan, 1986). Experiences with supporting persons in various problem situations are abstracted and cognitively represented as a personal construct in the sense of Kelly (1955).

To assess this subjective representation of social support, we developed a new procedure (FESU). Standardized problem situations were given according to different functions of support. These were: (1) emotional (i.e., the provision of love, trust, and empathy), (2) instrumental or material (i.e., loaning money or giving one's time or skills), (3) appraisal (i.e., giving evaluative feedback), and (4) informative support (i.e., giving advice or imparting knowledge).
For each situation, the adolescent had to report who they would ask for support in an unstructured response format. Further items related to the person- specific frequency and satisfaction with support. Various indices were developed from these answers. The indices for netsize, frequency, and satisfaction reached very good consistencies (.88–.90) and showed good stability over a retest interval of 2 weeks (.68–.76). In addition, we calculated a measure for the complexity of the representation of social support. This was done by weighting the frequency score for each person named with the situation–specific ranking of the naming. The variance of these weighted frequency scores was summed for all situations and for each person named. This index expressed whether the students differentiated between support persons and support situations, or whether their cognitive schema of helpers in their environment was more unstructured (cf. Kelly, 1955; Bieri, Atkins, Briar, Leaman, Miller, and Tripodi, 1966).

Social skills. In the pilot study, the Matson Evaluation of Social Skills with Youngsters (MESSY) was applied as a simple instrument for assessing personal resources (cf. Matson, 1986; Matson, Rotatori, and Helsel, 1983). The procedure is available in a self–report version for children and adolescents and a teacher–report version. The items in the self–report version are distributed across five factors (appropriate social skills, inappropriate assertiveness, impulsive/recalcitrant, overconfident, jealousy/withdrawal), and those in the teacher–report version into the two factors inappropriate assertiveness/impulsiveness and appropriate social skills. It was only possible to test the teacher– report version on a small sample of students, and the findings will not be further included here.

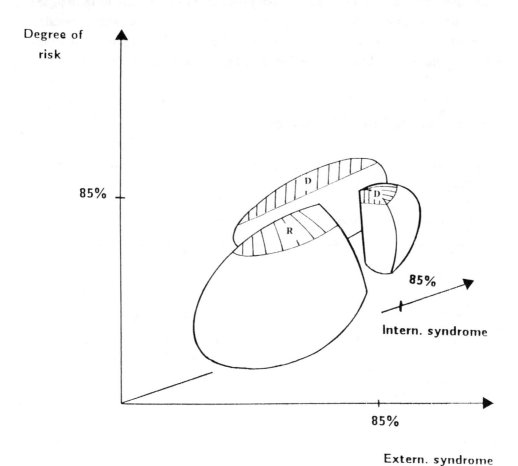

Fig. 2: Hypothetic distribution of resilients (R) and deviants (D) in normal population

Although the main purpose of the pilot study was to test the instruments for risk level and psychological health/disorder, the four areas of assessment also permitted explorative investigations into the resilience construct. For this purpose we created two subsamples (see Fig. 2).

A high risk index should be present in both groups: Therefore the top 15% who were most at risk were selected from the sample. The same procedure was used with respect to the behavior problems: Subjects with a symptom score above this cutpoint on either one or both broad-band dimensions were assigned to the deviant group ($N = 49$). All the remaining subjects who showed a symptom score below the 85th percentile on both the internalizing and externalizing scales of the YSR were assigned to the resilient group ($N = 48$).

3.2   Results and Brief Discussion

Tab. 2 contains mean comparisons for the *protective* factors assessed in the pilot study.

Tab. 2:   Comparison of resilients and deviants (pilot study)

	Expected direction R–D	Resilients (R) N = 48		Deviants (D) N = 49			
		M	sd	M	sd	t	p
Personal resources							
– Appropriate social skills	>	80.3	10.4	77.9	17.9	0.76	
– Inappropriate assertiveness	<	30.4	6.8	38.8	12.0	4.04	.000
– Impulsive/Recalicitrant	<	10.8	2.3	13.7	3.3	5.06	.000
– Overconfident	<	9.6	2.3	11.7	3.5	3.38	.000
– Jealousy/Withdrawal	<	8.4	1.9	11.8	3.2	6.28	.000
Social resources							
– Satisfaction with support	>	4.2	0.6	4.4	0.8	1.19	
– Frequency of support	>	3.6	0.6	3.8	0.6	1.09	
– Netsize	>	7.2	2.4	6.1	2.3	2.21	.015
– Complexity	>	9.5	4.4	7.9	4.5	1.79	.039

In the MESSY, the members of the "resilient group" appeared to be more appropriately assertive in social problems, less impulsive, less arrogant in their interaction with others, and less jealous and withdrawn. In contrast, no significant differences could be found on the dimension of appropriate social skills. There were also no differences found in the perceived frequency of social support or in the assessment of satisfaction. However, the resilients reported larger support networks (especially with respect to emotional, appraisal, and instrumental support situations). In addition, there was a contrast in the differentiation of cognitive structure: Resilients differentiated more strongly between persons and situations. Thus they reported the same persons in different support functions in a less uniform and a more situation–specific manner.

Overall, substantial relations are found with respect to both personal resources and social resources. The difference between the groups in the MESSY scales should, however, not be assigned too much weight. Similar to some other studies on resiliency, the indicators for the construct of social skills cannot be clearly separated from the characteristics that are relevant for the assignment to the groups of resilients or deviants. As there is a certain overlapping between the contents of the MESSY and the YSR, it is not surprising that its scales on skill deficits clearly differentiate between the two groups. In contrast, there is no significant t-value in the scale "appropriate social skills". Because of the problems with its discriminant construct validity, we dropped the MESSY from the main study.

With respect to social support, the findings differ for the single dimensions. The fact that the frequency and satisfaction scores do not differentiate between the two groups could be due, among others, to normative influences in the sense of social stereotyping or social desirability. This is supported by, for example, the generally high scores on satisfaction and the relatively low variances. In the size and differentiability of the social network there are, in contrast, the anticipated differences. The variances are also relatively larger here. In the group of resilients, a wider range of support persons across a wider range of situations is reported. This can be conceived as both specific support competences as well as a certain reciprocal substitution. Overall our results with a semistandardized, quantitatively assessable instrument are consistent with those findings from Emmy Werner that point to the importance of alternative caregivers.

4. The Main Study

As resiliency is not a mass phenomenon the search for resilients is very tedious. Therefore, in the first stage of our investigation, we approached social welfare institutions for children and adolescents, as an initial high level of risk can be assumed here. In a second stage, we are investigating schools where we cannot anticipate more than one resilient per class.

Up to now, we have approached 60 social welfare institutions. After a first contact through the post followed by an explanation of our purpose on the telephone and — whenever possible — a personal presentation of the project, we were able to study adolescents from 27 institutions. In 10 institutions we found no resilient subjects in our age group, in 14 we were unable to persuade the educators to participate, and in 9 cases there were structural problems (e.g., the institution had been closed down, large–scale staff changes) that prevented further investigation.

In every participating institution, we made an appointment with the staff of the institution. At this meeting, we presented the construct of resiliency in detail and discussed individual adolescents as in a case conference. The result of this case discussion was the naming of adolescents with a high–risk background who could be assigned to either the group of *resilients* or the group of *deviants* on the basis of the educators' naturalistic observations. After the adolescents and their educators had agreed to participate, we were able, up to now, to study 146 subjects in this way. From a total institution population of circa 1000, this involved 66 adolescents who were diagnosed as "resilient" and 80 who were diagnosed as being "deviant" (showing severe behavioral/emotional problems).

Both groups had a similar composition according to age and sex. The average age of the resilients was 15;5 years; that of the deviants 15;7 years (range in each case between 14 and 17 years). The sex distribution was roughly 3:2 (male:female).

The qualitative diagnosis from the case discussions with the educators proved to be valid according to the objective criteria of risk load. In our total index of stress characteristics, the resilients (R) had a mean of 29.09 ($SD = 14.94$) and the deviants (D) a mean of 27.40 ($SD = 14.32$). Thus both groups had a similar risk load, and the resilients' scores were even somewhat higher. In line with the requirements of the concept of resiliency, both groups had high loads compared to the general population. The mean of the ALLSTRESS index lay roughly on the 85th percentile of the unselected sample from the first pilot study ($N = 641$, see above). As for the second criterion of resiliency, the diagnosis of behavioral/emotional problems, the naturalistic group formation was also validated by quantitative data. In the TRF, which was later worked on by the educators, the deviants showed a mean of 42.71 in their externalizing score ($SD = 19.63$) and the resilients a mean of 26.02 ($SD = 15.06$). In contrast to this highly significant difference ($p < .001$), the scores for the internalizing syndrome were more similar with 15.80 (D; $SD = 7.91$) and 12.98 (R; $SD = 8.09$; $p < .05$). This confirmed the suspicion discussed above that the main feature of the perception of disorder was directed at antisocial symptoms, acting out, and so forth.

4.1   Assessment Instruments

The adolescents were given detailed interviews on their biography. They also carried out multidimensional tests and questionnaires on the following constructs: behavioral/emotional problems (YSR, see pilot study), life events and circumstances (risk questionnaire, see pilot study), intelligence, temperament, coping styles, self–oriented regulation, perceived social support, and educational climate. The data assessment was carried out in two sessions which each lasted between 90 and 120 minutes. In addition, we interviewed and gave questionnaires to the educators who were responsible for each adolescent (topics: the adolescent's biography, behavioral/emotional problems, coping behavior, and the educational climate in the institution).

A survey of all the methods used is given in Lösel, Bliesener, Köferl, and Schmidtpeter (1988). Up to now, we have mostly analyzed the instruments that permit a standardized evaluation. In the following, we shall limit ourselves to those features of personal and social resources that were reported by the adolescents. This presents the "hardest" test for the construct of resiliency, because the data were recorded in complete independence from the group assignments made by the educators. In contrast, for example, an educator's judgment of coping behavior (Stress–Response–Scale from Chandler, 1986) is to some degree confounded with his or her judgments of behavioral/emotional problems in the TRF.

Alongside the Achenbach Scales and the risk questionnaire, we used the following instruments to operationalize protective factors (personal and social resources):

Intelligence. We selected a short form of Horn's (1969) "Prüfsystem für Schul- und Bildungsberatung" (PSB). This test covers factors of verbal intelligence, reasoning, and technical ability following Thurstone's factorial model.

Temperament. The Dimensions of Temperament Survey (DOTS) from Lerner et al. (1982) includes dimensions on approach–avoidance tendencies in minor everyday stress situations, on rigidity (vs. flexibility) in expectancies regarding own and other behavior, on general mood, and on task orientation.

Coping styles. The adolescents' coping strategies were investigated with West-brook's (1979) Coping-Questionnaire in a modified German version from Seiff-ge-Krenke (1984). This contains items on various coping strategies, with particular emphasis on the factors: (1) active coping with problems using social resources, (2) economic handling of problems, and (3) problem–avoiding, fatal-istic behavior. As the resilience construct concerns relatively permanent strate-gies, we only used the version generalizing over situations.

Self-oriented cognitions. We constructed an instrument called the "Multidimen-sionales Selbstkonzept" on the basis of the Self–Description–Questionnaire (SDQ) from Marsh and O'Neill (1984; German translation from Hörmann, 1986), the hierarchic structure from Shavelson, Hubner, and Stanton (1976), and scales from Jerusalem and Schwarzer (1986). The instrument particularly contains the dimensions self–efficacy, helplessness, and general self–evaluation (= Selbstwertgefühl).

Specific personality characteristics. Further personality characteristics of self–regulation were assessed with the achievement motivation and ego strength scales from the "Mehrdimensionaler Persönlichkeitstest für Jugendliche" (MPT-J), a personality test for adolescents, from Schmidt (1983). We also incorporated the control scales on social desirability and correct test responses from this instrument.

Social support. We assessed the support from the social network with the same FESU used in the pilot study (see above).

Educational climate. We assessed the social and educational climate in the adolescents' direct environment with the "Familien–Klima–Skalen" (FKS) developed by Schneewind, Beckmann, and Hecht–Jackl (1985). We adapted these scales for conditions in social welfare institutions. The FKS is based on the Family Environment Scales from Moos (Moos, 1974; Moos and Moos, 1981).

4.2   Differentiation of Groups

As noted above, a major concern of our study was to test the consistency of findings in different operationalizations of resiliency. The naturalistic and qualitative diagnosis of the two groups thus only formed the starting point for a step–by–step specification of the groups in the sense of a multiple gating procedure (Loeber and Dishion, 1983). In the present paper, we compared groups of resilients and deviants in four steps defined according to different levels of strictness:

1. In the first step, the "naturally" diagnosed groups were compared (number of cases: resilients (R): $N = 66$; deviants (D): $N = 80$).
2. In a second step, the criteria of risk load were assessed more narrowly. In both groups, only those adolescents were retained who showed ALLSTRESS scores above the 90th percentile according to the norm data from the first pilot study (R: $N = 42$; D: $N = 50$).
3. In a third step, adolescents from the above groups were removed if, in the case of resilients, they were generally not below the 95th percentile in the narrow–band scales of the Child Behavior Checklist (TRF), or, in the case of deviants, if they were not at least once above the 95th percentile. This was performed regardless of whether these adolescents were either relatively free from behavioral/emotional disorders or clearly disturbed according to the qualitative judgments of the educators. Thus using this group definition, adolescents who, for example, were originally defined as resilient but had a

relatively high anxiety or withdrawal score were dropped (R: $N = 24$; D: $N = 26$).

4. In the fourth step, matched pairs of resilients and deviants were constructed from the above groups according to age, sex, and their quantitative levels on the risk indices (R: $N = 20$; D: $N = 20$).

4.3 Results and Brief Discussion

We compared the group means for the variables of personal and social resources at the four levels of differentiation. The results are presented in Tab. 3 and 4. As the number of cases in the four steps became increasingly small, we chose $p = .10$ as our level of significance. However, too much stress should not be placed on statistical significance, especially as this involves multiple testing of partially identical data sets. In our opinion, the consistency of the result patterns over the different definitions of resilient and deviant groups is of similar importance. For this reason, and also for reasons of clarity, we have not presented the single means and distributions in the tables, but emphasized the direction of the differences. In most of the variables, the expected direction of the differences is given; probable curvilinear correlations are not explicated.

An overview of the single findings shows the following: A series of variables that are assumed to be protective factors against stressors differentiate between the two groups. The extent of this differentiation cannot be explained just by "fishing for significance". All 74 significant differences show the expected direction. If nonparametric procedures (Mann-Whitney-U-test, Wilcoxon-test) are applied instead of the parametric t-tests this pattern of significance in general remains stable. Most of the nonsignificant differences also take the anticipated direction. In the personal resources, 53 of 56 comparisons take the expected direction; in the social resources, 80 from 84 (a total of 95%). However, only a portion of the findings prove to be also stable across the different types of group formation: A great number of differences between the analysis of the natural groups and the matched pairs are conspicuous here. Thus our multiple-gating approach to artefact testing shows that protective factors do not distinguish so clearly between the contrast groups as the sometimes quasi-typological use of the construct of invulnerability has suggested.

Tab 3 : Comparison of the personal resources in the various defined groups

	expected direction R D	"Naturalistic" group diagnosis 66/80 empirical direction R D	t	p	"Naturalistic" group at high risk 42/50 empirical direction R D	t	p	"Naturalistic" group at high risk, validated by TRF 24/26 empirical direction R D	t	p	Quantitatively matched pairs 20/20 empirical direction R D	t	p
Intelligence													
Verbal	>	>	1.57	*	>	1.44	*	>	1.39	*	>	1.21	
Reasoning	>	>	1.34	*	>	1.52	*	>	2.50	***	>	2.58	***
Technical	>	>	1.95	**	>	1.63	*	>	2.19	**	>	1.62	*
Temperament													
Approach/Withdrawal	>	>	0.78		>	1.19		>	1.96	**	>	0.74	
Flexibility	>	>	0.56		>	1.37	*	>	2.08	**	>	1.52	*
Quality of mood	>	>	0.01		>	0.12		<	1.21		>	0.73	
Task orientation	>	<	0.28		>	0.73		>	1.41		>	0.39	
Rhythmicity	>	<	0.84		<	1.25		<	1.43	*	<	1.64	
Coping behavior													
Active problemsolving	>	>	0.98		>	1.76	**	>	1.87	**	>	1.36	*
Economic handling	>	>	0.81		>	1.64	*	>	1.34	*	>	0.94	
Fatalism/Problem avoiding	<	<	1.04		<	1.70	**	<	2.23	**	<	2.20	**
Selfdirected regulations													
Self efficacy	>	>	1.13		>	2.18	**	>	1.87	**	>	2.37	**
Helplessness	<	<	1.03		<	0.98		<	2.61	***	<	2.45	**
Achievement motivation	>	>	1.53	*	>	1.49	*	>	1.43	*	>	0.73	
Self esteem	>	>	1.17		>	1.90	**	>	2.58	***	>	2.03	**
Method control scales													
Social desirability	=	<	1.18		<	0.18		>	0.15		>	0.53	
Correct performance	=	<	0.17		<	0.33		<	1.50		<	0.93	

* p < .10   ** p < .05   *** p < .01

Tab 4 : Comparison of the social resources in the various defined groups

	expected direction R D	"Naturalistic" group diagnosis 66/80			"Naturalistic" group at high risk 42/50			"Naturalistic" group at high risk, validated by TRF 24/26			Quantitatively matched pairs 20/20		
		empirical direction R D	t	p	empirical direction R D	t	p	empirical direction R D	t	p	empirical direction R D	t	p
Social support													
Frequency of													
emotional support	>	>	1.42	*	>	1.60	*	>	1.25		>	1.55	*
material support	>	>	0.67		>	0.20		>	0.39		>	0.06	
informative support	>	>	0.90		>	0.68		>	0.69		>	0.16	
appraisal support	>	>	1.28		>	0.78		>	0.41		>	0.01	
Netsize for													
emotional support	>	>	3.03	***	>	2.58	***	>	1.83	**	>	2.29	***
material support	>	>	3.39	***	>	3.01	***	>	2.12	**	>	2.69	***
informative support	>	>	2.27	**	>	2.06	***	>	1.22		>	1.53	**
appraisal support	>	>	3.06	***	>	3.15	***	>	2.08	**	>	1.85	**
Satisfaction with													
emotional support	>	>	1.99	**	>	1.22		>	1.12		>	0.59	
material support	>	>	1.67	*	>	1.92	**	>	1.73	**	>	1.08	
informative support	>	>	1.86	**	>	2.25	**	>	2.04	**	>	2.55	***
appraisal support	>	>	0.63		>	0.87		>	1.55	*	>	0.41	
Complexity	>	>	0.82		>	1.42	*	>	1.18		>	1.16	
Education climate													
Cohesion	>	>	1.19		>	0.63		>	0.46		>	0.33	
Openness/Frankness	>	>	2.68	***	>	1.88	**	>	1.37	*	>	1.86	**
Tendency for conflict	<	<	1.65	*	<	0.90		<	1.16		<	1.31	
Autonomy	>	>	1.99	**	>	1.95	**	>	2.69	***	>	2.90	***
Achievement orientation	>	>	0.46		<	0.28		<	0.40		<	1.10	
Planing of leisuretime	>	>	1.09		>	1.64	*	>	1.26		<	1.23	
Religious orientation	>	>	1.84	*	>	1.17		>	0.61		>	0.72	
Organisation		>	1.25		>	0.36		>	0.03		>	0.77	
Control	>	>	0.46		>	0.10		<	1.08		<	0.20	

* p < .10   ** p < .05   *** p < .01

As far as the contents of the results are concerned, there is a relatively large number of significant differences in the *personal* resources (35 from 56 mean comparisions). The methodologically more strict group definition thus led to more distinct differences than the natural group diagnosis. Resilient adolescents prove to be more intelligent than those who have become deviant. The more educationally dependent verbal intelligence plays a lesser role in this than the reasoning component. Resilients also report more active problem solving and less passive and fatalistic coping behavior. In their self–related cognitions, they experience themselves as being less helpless, more strongly self–effective, and have a generally more positive self–evaluation. The temperament factors prove to be less significant than expected, yet even here there are seemingly consistent indications for a more strongly approach–oriented and a more flexible behavior style. All these findings agree well with the assumptions reported in the literature on the construct of resilience. The findings in the methodological control scales do not suggest that the personality differences we observed are only due to questionnaire response styles and so forth.

In the instruments we used to assess *social* resources, there are in general somewhat fewer significant differences between the two groups than in the personal resources. Nevertheless, the findings here also support our assumptions on the construct of resiliency. The resilients consistently report a larger network of social support and a higher satisfaction with the support that they experience. This applies fairly uniformly for each of the four aspects of emotional, material, informational, and appraisal support that other empirical studies also mostly found to be not so clearly separated. In contrast, there are lower differences in the frequency of experienced social support and in its person– and situation–related cognitive discrimination (complexity). The differences are also less marked in the scales on perceived educational climate. Here, the resilients in particular report a more autonomy–oriented and more open climate in their institutional homes.

As far as the less distinct differences in the social resources are concerned, the following is one important consideration: In the operationalization of the risk or stress factors we included characteristics that could serve as protective factors in an inversed variable definition because of the above–mentioned artefact problem. The explanation of variance through social resources is thus on the one hand limited, on the other hand the group differences observed despite this indicate the relative validity of our procedure. A second important aspect concerns the institutional situation. We selected this setting in order to have a higher initial prevalence rate of stressors and thus of resilients and nonresilients. Characteristics that were related to the institutional situation could, however, provide a less powerful differentiation because the framing conditions are more homogeneous, and some constellations of social support and education climate equally confront resilients and deviants from one and the same institution. The significance of the size of the experienced network also has to be considered in the institutional situation, as alternative reference persons are probably more important here than in a stable family context.

As mentioned above, the analyses of standardized, quantitative variables reported in this paper only deal with a section of the total characteristics we assessed. Further educators' reports and interview data from the adolescents are not included. Nevertheless, we have attempted to estimate the efficiency of the separation between the two groups. We did this by calculating a hierarchical discrimination analysis. The efficiency of the separation was satisfactory: 83% of the cases were assigned correctly. This produces an increase in the efficiency of the separation compared to an assignment according to the a priori probability ($80/146 = 56\%$) of lambda$_b$ = .64 (Goodman & Kruskal, 1954). As expectable, the result is less favorable when − within methodological limits − a cross-validation is undertaken. We used a method similar to Tukey's Jackknife Method and estimated the error rate according to Lachenbruch and Mickey (1968). This produced an average of 76% correct assignments.

For the other steps of group formation, discriminant analyses are not meaningful as the sample size is too low. However, for purposes of comparison we performed a Manifest Dichotomy Analysis (Du Mas, 1968) for the matched pairs. In this the single variables are each assigned zero or one scores on the basis of median splits. An additive total index was formed from these scores. This index produced 80% of correctly assigned group members in the matched pairs. In judging such findings it should not be forgotten that the original group assignment and the protective variables are based on independent data sources. If, for example, we were to include the data on adolescents' coping styles reported by the educators that were not independent of the diagnosis of deviance, the efficiency of the separation would increase even more.

Even though they take the foreground in this first report of our findings, the mean comparisons in single variables and linear discriminant analyses in our project are only *one* among several methodological approaches. We consider that analyses of configurations or characteristic patterns are just as important (cf. Lösel, 1978). This is also underlined, for example, by the latest results from the Swedish research program Individual Development and Adjustment (Magnusson and Bergman, 1988). The expansion of the approach with variables as an analytical unit through an approach with persons as an analytical unit is particularly important for resiliency research because, to some extent, protective factors can only be expected in specific configurations of personal and social resources (cf. Rutter, 1985). Even if the study of "the person as a whole" (Magnusson and Bergman, 1988, p. 1) can indeed always only be meant in an ideal way, the first analyses of our data with HYPAG analyses (Wottowa, 1984) suggest the existence of differential patterns of selected protective variables. However, narrow limits are placed on analysis using HYPAG or configuration frequency analysis because of the mostly low sample sizes in resilients. This also applies for a further assessment of our groups, in which it is planned to study the stability of existing correlations over time.

References

Achenbach, T.M. (1985). Assessment and taxonomy of child and adolescent psychopathology. Beverly Hills: Sage.

Achenbach, T.M., and Edelbrock, C. (1983). Manual for the Child Behavior Checklist and Revised Child Behavior Profile. Burlington: University of Vermont, Department of Psychiatry.

Achenbach, T.M., and Edelbrock, C. (1986). Manual for the Teacher's Report Form and teacher version of the Child Behavior Profile. Burlington: University of Vermont, Department of Psychiatry.

Achenbach, T.M., McConaughy, S.H., and Howell, C.T. (1987). Child/adolescent behavioral and emotional problems: Implications of cross – informant correlations for situational specificity.Psychological Bulletin, 101, 213–232.

Achenbach, T.M., Verhulst, F.C., Baron, G.D., and Althaus, M. (1987). A comparison of syndromes derived from the Child Behavior Checklist for American and Dutch boys aged 6–11 and 12–16. Journal of Child Psychology and Psychiatry, 28, 427–453.

Albee, G.W. (1987). Powerlessness, politics, and prevention. The community mental health approach. In K. Hurrelmann, F.-X. Kaufmann, and F. Lösel (Eds.), Social intervention: Chances and constraints (pp. 37–52). Berlin/New York: De Gruyter/Aldine.

Anthony, E.J. (1974). The syndrome of the psychologically invulnerable child. In E.J. Anthony and C. Koupernik (Eds.), The child in his family: Children at psychiatric risk (pp. 529–544). New York: Wiley.

Antonovsky, A. (1979). Health, stress, and coping. San Francisco: Jossey–Bass.

Antonovsky, A. (1987). Unraveling the mystery of health: How people manage stress and stay well. San Francisco: Jossey-Bass.

Barrera, M. Jr. (1986). Distinctions between social support concepts, measures, and models. American Journal of Community Psychology, 14, 413–445.

Baumann, U. (1987). Zur Konstruktvalidität der Konstrukte soziales Netzwerk und soziale Unterstützung. Zeitschrift für klinische Psychologie, 16, 305–310.

Bieri, J., Atkins, A.L., Briar, S., Leaman, R.L., Miller, H., and Tripodi, T. (1966). Clinical and social judgement: The discrimination of behavioral information. New York: Wiley.

Block, J. H., and Block, J. (1980). The role of ego–control and ego–resiliency in the organization of behavior. In W.A. Collins (Ed.), The Minnesota Symposia on Child Psychology (Vol. 13) (pp. 39–101). Hillsdale, NJ.: Erlbaum.

Blumstein, A., Cohen, J., and Farrington, D.P. (1988). Criminal Career Research: It's Value for Criminology. Criminology, 26, 1–35.

Bowlby, J. (1951). Maternal care and mental health. Genf: WHO.

Braukmann, W., and Filipp, S.-H. (1984). Strategien und Techniken der Lebensbewältigung. In U. Baumann, H. Berbalk, and G. Seidenstücker (Eds.), Klinische Psychologie. Trends in Forschung und Praxis (Bd. 6) (pp. 52–87). Bern: Huber.

Chandler, L.A. (1986). The Stress Response Scale for Children. Revised Manual. Pittsburgh, PA: University of Pittsburgh.

Chess, S., and Thomas, A. (1986). Temperament in clinical practice. New York: The Guilford Press.

Cobb, S. (1976). Social support as a moderator of life stress. Psychosomatic Medicine, 38, 300–314.

Cochran, M. (1987). Empowering families: An alternative to the deficit model. In K. Hurrelmann, F.-X. Kaufmann, and F. Lösel (Eds.), Social intervention: Chances and constraints (pp. 105–120). Berlin/New York: De Gruyter/Aldine.

Cowen, E.L., and Work, W.C. (1987). Invulnerable children, psychological wellness and primary prevention. Manuscript submitted to publication.

Dörner, D. (1983). Empirische Psychologie und Alltagsrelevanz. In Jüttemann, G. (Ed.), Psychologie in der Veränderung. Weinheim: Beltz, 13–29.

Dohrenwend, B.S. (1978). Social stress and community psychology. American Journal of Community Psychology, 6, 1–14.

Dohrenwend, B.S., and Dohrenwend, B.P. (1981). Life stress and psychopathology. In D.A. Regier and G. Allen (Eds.), Risk factor research in the major mental disorders (DDHS Publication No. ADM 81-1086) (pp. 131–141). Washington, DC: US Government Printing Office.

Dührssen, A. (1984). Risikofaktoren für die neurotische Krankheitsentwicklung. Zeitschrift für psychosomatische Medizin, 30, 18–42.

DuMas, F.M. (1968). Manifest Dichotomy Analysis. Psychological Bulletin, 70, 221–230.

Ehlers, T., Merz, F., and Remer, H. (1985). Korrelate prä- und perinataler Risiken bei Sechs-bis Zehnjährigen. In L. Montada (Ed.), Bericht über die 7. Tagung Entwicklungspsychologie in Trier 1985. Trier: Universität Trier.

Elder, G.H. (1974). Children of the Great Depression: Social change in life experience. Chicago: University of Chicago Press.

Farrington, D.P., Gallagher, B., Morley, L., Ledger, R.J., and West, D.J. (1986). Cambridge study in delinquent development: Long-term follow-up. Second Annual Report to the Home Office. Cambridge: Institute of Criminology.

Farrington, D.P., Ohlin, L.E., and Wilson, J.Q. (1986). Understanding and controlling crime. New York: Springer.

Farrington, D.P. (in press). Later adult life outcomes of offenders and non–offenders. In M. Brambring, F. Lösel, and H. Skowronek (Eds.), Children at Risk: Assessment and longitudinal research. Berlin: de Gruyter.

Felsman, K.J., and Vaillant, G.E. (1987). Resilient children as adults: A 40–year study. In E.J. Anthony and B.J. Cohler (Eds.), The invulnerable child (pp. 289–314). London: Guilford Press.

Fend, H., and Prester, H.G. (1985). Jugend in den 70er und 80er Jahren: Wertwandel, Bewußtseinswandel und potentielle Arbeitslosigkeit. Zeitschrift für Sozialisationsforschung und Erziehungssoziologie, 5, 43–70.

Fend, H., Schröer, S., and Richter, P. (1985). Problemindikatoren und Entwicklungsbedingungen in der Adoleszenz. Familiäre Bedingungen depressiver Stimmungen und negativer Selbstkonzepte. In D. Albert (Ed.), Bericht über den 34. Kongreß der Deutschen Gesellschaft für Psychologie in Wien 1984 (Bd. 1) (419–422). Göttingen: Hogrefe.

Figley, C.R. (1986). Traumatic stress: The role of the family and social support system. In C.R. Figley (Ed.), Trauma and its wake: Vol. 2. Traumatic stress theory, research, and intervention (pp. 39–54). New York: Bruner/Mazel.

Garmezy, N. (1982). Foreword. In E.E. Werner, and R.S. Smith (Eds.), Vulnerable but invincible (pp. xiii–xix). New York: McGraw–Hill.

Garmezy, N. (1983). Stressors of childhood. In N. Garmezy, and M. Rutter (Eds.), Stress, Coping, and Development in Children, (pp. 43–84). New York: McGraw–Hill.

Garmezy, N. (1985). Stress–resistant children: The search for protective factors. In J.E. Stevenson (Ed.), Recent research in developmental psychopathology. Journal of Child Psychology and Psychiatry. Book Supplement No. 4 (pp.213–233). Oxford: Pergamon Press.

Garmezy, N. (1987). Stress, competence, and development: Continuities in the study of schizophrenic adults, children vulnerable to psychopathology, and the search for stress–resistant children. American Journal of Orthopsychiatry, 57, 159–174.

Garmezy, N., and Devine, V. (1985). Project Competence: The Minnesota studies of children vulnerable to psychopathology. In N. Watt, E.J. Anthony, L.C. Wynne, and J.E. Rolf (Eds.), Children at risk for schizophrenia (pp. 289–332). Cambridge: Cambridge University Press.

Garmezy, N., Masten, A.S., and Tellegen, A. (1984). Studies of stress–resistant children: A building block for developmental psychopathology. Child Development, 55, 97–111.

Garmezy, N., and Nuechterlein, K. (1972). Invulnerable children: The fact and fiction of competence and disadvantage. American Journal of Orthopsychiatry, 42, 328–329.

Garmezy, N., and Rutter, M. (1983) (Eds.) Stress, coping, and development. New York: McGraw–Hill.

Garmezy, N., and Tellegen, A. (1984). Studies of stress–resistant children: Methods, variables, and preliminary findings. In F. Morrison, C. Ford, and D. Keating (Eds.), Advances in applied developmental psychology (Vol. 1) (pp. 1–52). New York: Academic Press.

Gersten, J.C., Langner, T.S., and Simcha–Fagan, O. (1978). Developmental patterns of types of behavior disturbances and secondary prevention. International Journal of Mental Health, 7, 132–149.

Gjerde, P.F., Block, J., and Block, J.H. (1986). Ego centrism and ego resiliency: Personality characteristics associated with perspective–taking from early childhood to adolescence. Journal of Personality and Social Psychology, 51, 423–434.

Glueck, S., and Glueck, E. (1950). Unraveling juvenile delinquency. Cambridge: Harvard University Press.

Goodman, L.A., and Kruskal, W.H. (1954). Measures of association for cross classification. Journal of the American Statistical Association, 49, 732–764.

Gottfredson, M., and Hirschi, T. (1985). The true value of lambda would appear to be zero: An essay on career criminals, criminal careers, selective incapacitation, cohort studies and related topics. Criminology, 24, 213–234.

Hörmann, H.–J. (1986). Selbstbeschreibungsfragebogen SDQ–III–G. In R. Schwarzer (Ed.), Skalen zur Befindlichkeit und Persönlichkeit. Forschungsbericht 5 (S. 47–83). Berlin: Freie Universität Berlin, Institut für Psychologie.

Honig, A.S. (1986). Risk factors in infancy. In A.S. Honig (Ed.), Risk factors in infancy (pp. 1–8). New York: Gordon & Breach.

Horn, W. (1969). Prüfsystem für Schul- und Bildungsberatung P-S-B. Göttingen: Hogrefe.

Hurrelmann, K. (1987). The limits and potential of social intervention in adolescence: An exemplary analysis. In K. Hurrelmann, F.-X. Kaufmann, and F. Lösel (Eds.), Social intervention: Chances and constraints (pp.219–238). Berlin: de Guyter.

Jerusalem, M., and Schwarzer, R. (1986). "Selbstwirksamkeit" und "Hilflosigkeit" (Skalenbeschreibungen). In R. Schwarzer (Ed.), Skalen zur Befindlichkeit und Persönlichkeit. Forschungsbericht 5 (pp. 15–42). Berlin: Freie Universität Berlin, Institut für Psychologie.

Jesness, C.F. (1987). Early identification of delinquent-prone children: An overview. In J.D. Burchard, and S.N. Burchard (Eds.), Primary prevention of psychopathology: Vol.10. Prevention of delinquent behavior. (pp. 140–158). Newbury Park: Sage.

Kahn, R.L. (1979). Aging and Social Support. In M.W. Riley, Aging from Birth to Death. (pp. 77–91). Boulder Colo.: Westview Press, Inc.

Kelly, G.A. (1955). The psychology of personal constructs (Vol. 1). New York: Norton.

Kobasa, S.C., and Puccetti, M.C. (1983). Personality and social resources in stress-resistance. Journal of Personality and Social Psychology, 45, 839–850.

Köferl, P. (1987). Zur informations- und prozeßtheoretischen Integration von Streß–Modellen: Resistenz-, Plastizitäts- und Selbstregulationskonzepte. Forschungsbericht des Teilprojekts A2. Bielefeld: Universität Bielefeld, Sonderforschungsbereich 227.

Lachenbruch, P.A., and Mickey, M.R. (1968). Estimation of Error Rates in Discriminant Analysis. Technometrics, 10, 1–11.

Lazarus, R.S., and Folkman, S. (1984). Stress, appraisal, and coping. New York: Springer Publishing Company.

Lerner, R.M., Palermo, M., Spiro, A., and Nesselroade, J.R. (1982). Assessing the dimensions of temperamental individuality across the lifespan: The Dimensions of Temperament Survey (DOTS). Child Development, 53, 149–159.

Loeber, R., and Dishion, T.J. (1983). Early predictors of male delinquency: A review. Psychological Bulletin, 94, 68–99.

Loeber, R., and Stouthamer-Loeber, M. (1986). Family factors as correlates and predictors of juvenile conduct problems and delinquency. In M. Tonry, and N. Morris (Eds.), Crime and justice: Vol. 7. An annual review of research (pp. 29–150). Chicago: University of Chicago Press.

Lösel, F. (1978). Konfigurationen elterlicher Erziehung und Dissozialität. In K. Schneewind, and H. Lukesch (Eds.), Familiäre Sozialisation (pp. 233–245). Stuttgart: Klett-Cotta.

Lösel, F. (1982). Prognose und Prävention von Delinquenzproblemen. In J. Brandtstädter, and A. v. Eye (Eds.), Psychologische Prävention (pp. 197–239). Bern: Huber.

Lösel, F. (1983). Entwicklungsstörungen sozialen Verhaltens - Zusammenhänge zwischen Umweltmerkmalen, Erfahrungsdifferenzen, Persönlichkeitsdispositionen und Jugenddelinquenz. In H.–J. Kerner, H. Kury, and K. Sessar (Eds.), Deutsche Forschungen zur Kriminalitätsentstehung und Kriminalitätskontrolle (Bd. 6/1) (pp. 595–616). Köln: Heymanns.

Lösel, F., Bliesener, T., Köferl, P., Mittag, W., and Schmidtpeter, C. (1987) Familiale Belastung, Problemverhalten und soziale Unterstützung bei Kindern und Jugendlichen. Forschungsbericht des Teilprojekts A2. Bielefeld: Universität Bielefeld, Sonderforschungsbereich 227.

Lösel, F., Bliesener, T., Köferl, P., and Schmidtpeter, C. (1988). Invulnerabilität und Entwicklungsstörungen sozialen Verhaltens: Differentielle Bewältigung von Lebensbedingungen. (pp.38). Bericht an die Deutsche Forschungsgemeinschaft. Universität Bielefeld.

Lösel, F., Bliesener, T., Klünder, A., and Köferl, P. (1988). Behavior Disorders of German Adolescents: Applications of the Child Behavior Checklist and a Comparison with US – Self Report data. (pp.25). Research Report, University of Bielefeld, Special Research Unit 227.

Magnusson, D., and Bergman, L.R. (1988). Longitudinal studies: Individual and variable based approaches to research on early risk factors. Reports from the Department of Psychology, Nr. 674, University of Stockholm.

Marsh, H.W., and O'Neill, R. (1984). Self Description Questionnaire III: The construct validity of multidimensional self–concept ratings by late adolescents. Journal of Educational Measurement, 21, 153–174.

Matson, J.L. (1986). Matson Evaluation of Social Skills with Youngsters (Manuscript submitted for publication). Baton Rouge, LA: Louisiana State University, Department of Psychology.

Matson, J.L., Rotatori, A.F., and Helsel, W.J. (1983). Development of a rating scale to measure social skills in children: The Matson Evaluation of Social Skills with Youngsters (MESSY). Behaviour Research and Therapy, 21, 335–340.

Meyer–Probst, B., and Teichmann, H. (1984). Rostocker Längsschnittuntersuchung – Risiken für die Persönlichkeitsentwicklung im Kindesalter. Leipzig: Thieme.

Mischel, W. (1973). Towards a cognitive social learning reconceptualization of personality. Psychological Review, 80, 252–283.

Mischel, W. (1981). A cognitive social learning approach to assessment. In T. Merluzzi, C. Glass, and M. Genest (Eds.), Cognitive assessment (pp. 479–502). New York: The Guilford Press.

Moos, R.H. (1974). Family Environment Scale (FES). Palo Alto, CA: Stanford University, Social Ecology Laboratory.

Moos, R.H. (1984). Context and coping: Toward a unifying conceptual framework. American Journal of Community Psychology, 12, 5–36.

Moos, R.H., and Moos, B.S. (1981). Family Environment Scale (Manual). Palo Alto, CA: Consulting Psychologists Press.

Morgan, D.L. (1986). Personal relationships as an interface between social networks and social cognitions. Journal of Social and Personal Relationships, 3, 403–422.

Murphy, L.B., and Moriarty, A.E. (1976). Vulnerability, coping, and growth. New Haven: Yale University Press.

Nestmann, F. (1988). Die alltäglichen Helfer. Theorien sozialer Unterstützung und eine Untersuchung alltäglicher Helfer aus vier Dienstleistungsberufen. Berlin: de Gruyter.

Olbrich, E., and Todt, E. (1984) (Eds.). Probleme des Jugendalters. Berlin: Springer–Verlag.

Pearlin, L.I. (1987). The Stress and Strategies of Intervention. In K. Hurrelmann, F.–X. Kaufmann, and F. Lösel (Eds.). Social Interventions Potentials and Constraints. Berlin: de Gruyter, 53–72.

Petersilia, J. (1980). Criminal career research: A review of recent evidence. In N. Morris, and M. Tonry (Eds.), Crime and justice: Vol. 2. An annual review of research (pp. 321–379). Chicago: University Press of Chicago.

Prystav, G. (1981). Psychologische Coping-Forschung: Konzeptbildungen, Operationalisierungen und Meßinstrumente. Diagnostica, 27, 189–214.

Quast, H.H. (1985). Different perspectives in research on social support and stress. In R. Schwarzer (Ed.), Stress and Social Support, Research Report 4, Berlin: Department of Psychology – Educational Psychology – Freie Universität Berlin (pp. 45–82).

Remschmidt, H. (1983). Multiaxiale Klassifikation in der Kinder- und Jugendpsychiatrie. In H. Remscheidt, and M.H. Schmidt (Eds.), Multiaxiale Diagnostik in der Kinder- und Jugendpsychiatrie (pp. 11–42). Bern: Huber.

Remschmidt, H. (1985). Klassifikation kinder- und jugendpsychiatrischer Erkrankungen und Störungen. In H. Remschmidt, and M.H. Schmidt (Eds.), Kinder- und Jugendpsychiatrie in Klinik und Praxis: Bd. II. Entwicklungsstörungen, organisch bedingte Störungen, Psychosen, Begutachtung (pp. 21-27). Stuttgart: Thieme.

Remschmidt, H. (1986). Was wird aus kinderpsychiatrischen Patienten? Methodische Überlegungen und Ergebnisse. In M.H. Schmidt, and S. Drömann (Eds.), Langzeitverlauf kinder- und jugendpsychiatrischer Erkrankungen. Stuttgart: Enke, 1–14.

Remschmidt, H. (1988). Verlauf und Prognose kinder- und jugendpsychiatrischer Erkrankungen. In H. Remschmidt, and M.H. Schmidt (Eds.), Kinder- und Jugendpsychiatrie in Klinik und Praxis, Band 1, Grundprobleme, Pathogenese, Diagnostik, Therapie. Stuttgart: Thieme, 791–803.

Robins, L.N. (1966). Deviant children grown up. Baltimore: Williams and Wilkin.

Robins, L.N. (1972). Follow-up studies of behavior disorders in children. In H.C. Quay, and J.S. Werry (Eds.), Psychopathological disorders of childhood (pp. 414–450). New York: Wiley.

Rosenthal, R., and Rubin, D.B. (1982). A simple, general purpose display of magnitude of experimental effect. Journal of Educational Psychology, 74, 166–169.

Rock, D.L., Green, K.E., Wise, B., and Rock, R.K. (1984). Social support and social network scale: A psychometric review. Research in Nursing and Health, 7, 325–332.

Rutter, M. (1971). Parent–child separation: Psychological effects on the children. Journal of Child Psychology and Child Psychiatry, 12, 233–260.

Rutter, M. (1979). Protective factors in children's responses to stress and disadvantage. In M.W. Kent, and J.E. Rolf (Eds.), Primary prevention of psychopathology: Vol. 3. Social competence in children (pp. 49–74). Hanover, NH: University Press of New England.

Rutter, M. (1983). Stress, coping, and development: Some issues and some questions. In N. Garmezy, and M. Rutter (Eds.), Stress, coping, and development in children (pp. 1–41). New York: McGraw-Hill.

Rutter, M. (1985). Resilience in the face of adversity. Protective factors and resistance to psychiatric disorder. British Journal of Psychiatry, 147, 598–611.

Rutter, M., and Giller, H. (1983). Juvenile delinquency: Trends and perspectives. Harmondsworth: Penguin.

Sarason, B.R. (1986). Social support, social behavior, and cognitive processes. In R. Schwarzer (Ed.), Self-related cognitions in anxiety and motivation. Hillsdale, NJ: L. Erbaum, 77–85.

Schmidt, H. (1983). Mehrdimensionaler Persönlichkeitstest für Jugendliche (MPT-J). Braunschweig: Westermann.

Schneewind, K.A., Beckmann, M., and Hecht-Jackl, A. (1985). Das Familienklima-Testsystem (Forschungsbericht Nr. 8.1). München: Universität München, Institut für Psychologie.

Seiffge-Krenke, I. (1984). Problembewältigung im Jugendalter (Habilitationsschrift). Giessen: Justus Liebig-Universität, Fachbereich 06 Psychologie.

Seiffge-Krenke, I. (1986). Problembewältigung im Jugendalter. München: Urban & Schwarzenberg.

Shavelson, R.J., Hubner, J.J., and Stanton, G.C. (1976). Self-concept: Validation of a construct interpretation. Review of Educational Research, 46, 407–441.

Silbereisen, R.K., Noack, P., and Reitzle, M. (1987). Developmental perspectives on problem behavior and prevention in adolescence. In K. Hurrelmann, F.-X. Kaufmann, and F. Lösel (Eds.), Social intervention: Chances and constraints (pp. 205–218). Berlin: de Gruyter.

Strelau, J. (1984). Das Temperament in der psychischen Entwicklung. Berlin (Ost): Volk und Wissen.

Thomas, A., and Chess, S. (1984). Genesis and evolution of behavioral disorders: From infancy to early adult life. American Journal of Psychiatry, 141, 1–9.

Toman, W. (1976). Family constellation. New York: Springer, 1961 (3rd revised edition).

Tress, W. (1986). Die positive frühkindliche Bezugsperson — Der Schutz vor psychogenen Erkrankungen. Psychotherapie und medizinische Psychologie, 36, 51–57.

Ulich, M. (1988). Risiko- und Schutzfaktoren in der Entwicklung von Kindern und Jugendlichen. Zeitschrift für Entwicklungspsychologie und pädagogische Psychologie, 20, 146–166.

Werner, E.E. (1984). Resilient children. Young Children, 38, 68–72.

Werner, E.E. (1985). Stress and protective factors in children's lives. In A.R. Nicol (Ed.), Longitudinal studies in child psychology and psychiatry (pp. 335–355). Chichester: Wiley.

Werner, E.E. (1986). Resilient offspring of alcoholics. Journal of Studies on Alcohol, (submitted for publication).

Werner, E.E., and Smith, R.S. (1982). Vulnerable but invincible. New York: McGraw-Hill.

Westbrook, M.T. (1979). A classification of coping behavior based on multidimensional scaling of similarity ratings. Journal of Clinical Psychology, 35, 407–410.

White, B.L., Kaban, B.T., and Attanuci, J.S. (1979). The origins of human competence: Final report of the Harvard Preschool Project. Lexington, MA: D. C. Heath.

Wolfson, J., Fields, J.H., and Rose, S.A. (1987). Symptoms, temperament, resiliency, and control in anxiety-disordered preschool children. Journal of the American Academy of Child and Adolescent Psychiatry, 26, 16–22.

Wottawa, H. (1984). HYPAG : Ein neuer Ansatz zur Datenanalyse in der Marktforschung. Planung und Analyse, 11, 15–21.

Zubin, J., and Spring, B. (1977). Vulnerability — a new view of schizophrenia. Journal of Abnormal Psychology, 36, 103–126.

Later Adult Life Outcomes of Offenders and Nonoffenders

David P. Farrington

1. Introduction

In summarizing their study of the development of delinquency and crime in males, Farrington and West (1981) concluded that a constellation of adverse family background factors (including poverty, large families, marital disharmony, and ineffective child–rearing methods), among which parental criminality was often one element, tended to lead to a constellation of socially deviant features in the late adolescence and early adulthood (including drinking, drug use, reckless driving, sexual promiscuity, and aggression), among which criminality was again often one element.

West and Farrington (1973) found that juveniles who were later convicted differed significantly from their unconvicted peers in many factors measured at age 8-10. Official delinquents tended to come from low income families, and tended to have fathers with erratic job histories, including periods of unemployment. They tended to come from large–sized families, those in poor housing, and those with convicted parents. Delinquents tended to be suffering poor parental child–rearing behavior, including harsh or erratic discipline, and had parents who were in conflict with each other. They tended to have experienced broken homes or separations for reasons other than death or hospitalization. They also tended to have low intelligence and attainment, and to be troublesome and daring.

West and Farrington (1977) entitled their book "The Delinquent Way of Life" because they found that, at age 18, official delinquents were significantly different from the nondelinquents on almost every factor that they investigated. Delinquents drank more beer, they got drunk more often, they were more likely to say that drink made them violent, and they were more likely to get in trouble with the police after drinking. They smoked more cigarettes and had started smoking at an earlier age. They were more likely to be heavy gamblers. They were more likely to have been found guilty of minor motoring offenses, to have driven after drinking at least five pints of beer, and to have been injured in road accidents. They were more likely to have taken prohibited drugs such as marijuana or LSD, even though very few were convicted for drug offenses.

Official delinquents were more likely to have had sexual intercourse, especially with a variety of different girls, and especially beginning at an early age, but they were less likely to use contraceptives. They were more likely to be living away from home and did not get on well with their parents. They changed jobs more frequently and tended to hold relatively well paid but low status jobs. They were more likely to be tattooed. They were more likely to go out in the evenings and were especially likely to spend time hanging about on the street. They were more likely to go around in groups of four or more and were more likely to be involved in group violence and vandalism. They were much more likely to have been involved in fights, to have started fights, to have carried weapons, and to have used weapons in fights.

One aim of the present paper is to investigate how far convicted men still differ from unconvicted ones in later adulthood, at age 32. How far are the convicted men at age 32 recreating the same kinds of family environments for their children that they experienced at age 8? After reaching a peak in the teenage years, convictions decline markedly as men enter their 20s, suggesting that many men are reforming and becoming more conventional as they get older. Are the convicted men still significantly deviant in behavior and life style at age 32? Some convicted men desist from offending before age 21, while others persist into their 20s. Do the desisters become more conventional, like convicted men, by age 32, or are they still relatively deviant? How deviant are the persisters at age 32? A few men are latecomers to crime, in that they are not convicted until after reaching their 20s. Are the latecomers deviant like other convicted men, or are they more like the unconvicted men? These are the questions to be investigated in this paper.

2. The Cambridge Study in Delinquent Development

2.1 Description of the Study

This paper reports results obtained in the Cambridge Study in Delinquent Development, which is a prospective longitudinal survey of crime and delinquency in 411 males, mostly born in 1953. The study began in 1961–62, when most of the boys were aged 8–9. The major conclusions reached from data collected between ages 8 and 25 can be found in four books (West, 1969, 1982; West and Farrington, 1973, 1977 and over 50 published articles. The study was originally directed by Donald J. West, and it is now directed by David P. Farrington.

At the time they were first contacted, the boys were all living in a working-class area of London. The vast majority of the sample was chosen by taking *all* the boys who were aged 8–9 and on the registers of six state primary schools that were within a one-mile radius of a research office which had been established. In addition to 399 boys from these six schools, 12 boys from a local school for the educationally subnormal were included in the sample, in an attempt to make it more representative of the population of boys living in the area.

Most of the boys (357, or 86.9%) were white in racial appearance and of British origin, in the sense that they were being brought up by parents who had themselves been brought up in England, Scotland, or Wales. Of the remaining 54 boys, 12 were black, having at least one parent of West Indian (usually) or African origin. Twelve others were also rated at age 18 by our interviewers as having a nonwhite racial appearance, and these boys all had at least one parent from Cyprus (usually), Greece, or Turkey. Apart from these two groups, totalling 24 boys, all the other 387 boys in our sample were rated as white in racial appearance. Of the 30 white boys of non–British origin, 14 had at least one parent from the North or South of Ireland, and the remaining 16 boys had at least one parent from another country, such as Poland, Germany, or Australia.

On the basis of their father's occupations when they were aged eight, 93.7% of the boys could be described as working class (Categories III, IV or V on the Registrar General's scale), in comparison with the national figure of 78.3% at that time. This was, therefore, overwhelmingly a white, urban, working–class sample of British origin.

The boys were interviewed and tested in their schools when they were aged about 8, 10, and 14, by male or female psychologists. They were interviewed in the research office at about 16, 18, and 21, and in their homes at about 25 by young male social science graduates. The tests in schools measured intelligence, attainment, personality, and psychomotor coordination, while information was collected in the interviews about living circumstances, employment histories, relationships with females, leisure activities such as drinking and fighting, and offending behavior. The latest interview, in the men's homes at about age 32, is therefore the eighth personal face–to–face contact with this sample over a period of about 25 years.

In addition to interviews and tests with the boys, interviews with their parents were carried out by female social workers who visited their homes. These took place about once a year from when the boy was about 8 until when he was aged 14--15 and was in his last year of compulsory education. The primary informant was the mother, although many fathers were also seen. The parents provided details about such matters as family income, family size, their employment histories, their child–rearing practices (including attitudes, discipline, and parental agreement), their degree of supervision of the boy, and his temporary or permanent separations from them.

The boys' teachers also completed questionnaires when the boys were aged about 8, 10, 12, and 14. These provided information about the boys' troublesome and aggressive school behavior, their school attainments, and their truancy. Ratings were also obtained from the boys' peers when they were in their primary schools, about such topics as their daring, dishonesty, troublesomeness, and popularity.

2.2   The Men Interviewed at Age 32

Most efforts in the 2 years between December 1984 and November 1986 were directed toward locating and interviewing as many of the men in the sample as possible. Tremendous efforts were made to secure interviews, because (based in part on previous results obtained in this survey) it was believed that the most interesting subjects in any criminological project tended to be the hardest to locate and the most uncooperative. Surveys in which only about 75% of the target sample (or even less) are interviewed are likely to produce results which seriously underestimate the true level of criminal behavior. An increase in the percentage interviewed from 75% to 95% may lead to a disproportionate increase in the validity of the results. For example, in this survey at age 18, only 22.3% of the 318 who were easiest to interview were convicted men, in comparison with 35.9% of the 64 who were more difficult (excluding 7 men interviewed in penal institutions).

Eventually, after a great deal of detective work, every one of the men was located. Up to age 32, 8 of the men had died, and 20 had emigrated permanently. Of the remaining 383 who were alive and in the United Kingdom, 360 were interviewed personally (94.0%). Of the remaining 23, 19 refused (5.0%), and it was not possible to make personal contact with the remaining 4 (1.0%). Seven of the 20 emigrated men were also interviewed, either abroad or during a temporary return visit that they made to the United Kingdom, giving a total number interviewed of 367 of the 403 men still alive (91.0%). In addition, 9 emigrated men filled in self-completion questionnaires, and two cooperative wives of refusers filled in questionnaires on behalf of their husbands; in at least one case with the husband's collaboration and assistance. Therefore, interviews or questionnaires were obtained from 378 of the 403 men still alive (93.8%). For ease of exposition, this paper will refer to 378 men interviewed.

The median age at interview was 32 years 3 months. Seventy men were interviewed before age 32, 75 between 32 years 0 months and 32 years 2 months, 163 between 32 years 3 months and 32 years 5 months, 49 between 32 years 6 months and 32 years 11 months, and the remaining 21 after their 33rd birthday.

2.3   Categories of Offenders

Repeated searches were made in the central Criminal Record Office in London to try to locate convictions sustained by the men and by their relatives. The last search of the men was completed in June–July 1987 when the youngest men in the study (born in August 1954) were not quite 33. Hence, the conviction records of the men are reasonably complete up to the 32nd birthday, and probably also complete up to the date of the interview at age 32.

Over one third of the men (152, or 37.0%) were convicted for offenses committed up to age 32. In counting offenders, only crimes normally recorded in the Criminal Record Office were included. The most commonly included offenses were of burglary, theft, or taking vehicles, while the most common offenses that could not be included were motoring crimes such as speeding and drunken driving. The number of different offenders and the number of offenses committed peaked at age 17 (see Farrington, 1983).

Eighty-five men were first convicted as juveniles (age 10-16), 43 as young adults (age 17-20), and 24 as adults (age 21-32). Hence, of the 152 convicted men, 24 were termed latecomers to crime, since they were not convicted until after their 21st birthdays. Of the 128 men first convicted before age 21, 65 went on to be convicted again after age 21, and hence were termed persisters, in comparison with the remaining 63, who were termed desisters. In six of these 63 cases, death was a major cause of desistance.

In the remainder of this paper, the characteristics of different categories of offenders at age 32 are described. It was possible to interview 240 of the 257 unconvicted men still alive at age 32 (93.4%), 138 of the 146 convicted men still alive (94.5%), 22 of the 24 latecomers still alive (91.7%), 55 of the 57 desisters still alive (96.5%), and 61 of the 65 persisters still alive (93.8%). The major comparisons are as follows:

1. 138 convicted versus 240 unconvicted men.
2. 22 latecomers versus 240 unconvicted men.
3. 55 desisters versus 240 unconvicted men.
4. 61 persisters versus 240 unconvicted men.
5. 61 persisters versus 55 desisters.

Each feature measured at age 32 (such as home ownership) was compared with each measure of offending (such as convicted vs. unconvicted) in a 2 x 2 table. The significance of each relationship was investigated by calculating a value of chi-square (with Yates' correction for continuity) with one degree of freedom. The figures can be percentaged in two different directions; in the above example, the percentage of home owners who were convicted could be presented, or the percentage of convicted men who were home owners. For illustrative purposes, both methods will sometimes be used in the text, but the tables all show percentages in the second direction.

When many significance tests are carried out, 1 in 20 might be expected to be significant at the $p = .05$ level by chance alone. In comparing convicted and unconvicted men (Comparison 1 above), 23 out of 31 tests were in fact significant, far in excess of chance expectation. The corresponding figures for Comparisons 2, 3, 4, and 5 above were 2, 13, 23, and 10 significant (out of 31 tests in each case). Hence, the number of significant results was far greater than chance expectation in all comparisons except between latecomers and unconvicted men. The other possible comparisons involving latecomers also yielded few significant results (vs. desisters, 0 out of 31 tests significant; vs. persisters, 3 out of 31 tests significant). Hence, significant results involving latecomers may be due to chance. Also, some comparisons involving latecomers are invalid according to the rule-of-thumb criterion for chi-square that requires a minimum expected value of 5 in each cell of a 2 x 2 table.

The small number of significant results in comparisons involving latecomers is partly a consequence of the fact that the value of chi-square increases with the numbers being compared. Holding constant the strength of the relationship, comparisons between latecomers and unconvicted men are less likely to be statistically significant than comparisons between convicted and unconvicted men, and comparisons between latecomers and desisters are even less likely to be significant. Therefore, percentages should be inspected in the tables as well as levels of statistical significance.

3. Characteristics of Offenders at Age 32

3.1   Accommodation

Nearly half of the men interviewed (183, or 48.4%) were home owners, while 111 (29.4%) were renting from the local council, 25 (6.6%) were renting in the private sector, 16 (4.2%) were renting from a housing association, and 43 (11.4%) had some other arrangement. Those renting from the council (51.4%) and a housing association (56.3%) included the highest percentages who were convicted men, while only 26.2% of home owners and 28.0% of private renters were convicted.

Tab. 1 summarizes these results in more detail, and will act as a model for all subsequent tables. In the whole sample, 51.6% were not home owners and can be considered to be renting. However, this applied to 65.2% of convicted men and 43.8% of unconvicted men, a significant difference (chi-square = 15.32, 1 d.f., p<.001; all chi-square values quoted in this paper have 1 d.f.). The latecomers to crime — those first convicted after the 21st birthday — did not differ significantly from the unconvicted men in the percentage who were renting (54.5% versus 43.8%: chi-square = 0.56). The persisters — those who were convicted both before and after 21 — included 75.4% who were renting; significantly more than the unconvicted men (chi-square = 18.26, p<.001). However, the desisters — those convicted only before age 21 — included only 58.2% who were renting, and they were nearly significantly different from the unconvicted men (chi-square = 3.19, p<.10). The persisters, also, were nearly significantly less likely to be home owners than the desisters (chi-square = 3.15, p<.10).

Tab. 1: Offending Versus Accommodation

Percentage of:		Not home owner (51.6)	Poor home conditions (27.6)	Four or more addresses (13.3)	Unsat. accom. history (31.0)
(1) Unconvicted	(240)	43.8	23.9	10.5	25.8
(2) Convicted	(138)	65.2	34.2	18.1	39.9
(3) Latecomers	(22)	54.5	33.3	13.6	31.8
(4) Desisters	(55)	58.2	23.4	14.5	29.1
(5) Persisters	(61)	75.4	44.9	23.0	52.5
Comparisons:					
1 vs. 2		15.32***	3.38	3.82*	7.42**
1 vs. 3		0.56	0.37	0.01	0.13
1 vs. 4		3.19	0.00	0.39	0.11
1 vs. 5		18.26***	7.62**	5.64*	14.84***
4 vs. 5		3.15	4.01*	0.84	5.58*

All the comparisons by chi-square-tests; * p < .05   **p < .01   *** p < .001
Unsat. = Unsatisfactory; Accom. = Accomodation

The interviewers rated the home of each man according to whether it was considered to be dirty, smelly, damp, neglected, overcrowded, inadequately furnished, had vermin, or had structural problems. Tab. 1 shows that 27.6% of the men had poor home conditions according to at least one of these criteria. Persisters (44.9%) were the most likely to be living in poor home conditions — significantly more than the unconvicted men (chi–square = 7.62, p < .01), or than desisters (chi–square = 4.01, p < .05). Desisters (23.4%) were similar to unconvicted men (23.9%) in home conditions.

Most of the men (86.7%) had lived at between one and three addresses in the last five years, but 13.3% had been more mobile, living at four or more ad-dresses. Tab. 1 shows that 18.1% of the convicted men had four or more addresses, in comparison with 10.5% of those who were unconvicted, a result of borderline statistical significance (chi–square = 3.82, p = .05). Persisters (23.0%) were the most mobile, again significantly more than unconvicted men (chi–square = 5.64, p < .025).

In regard to accommodation, as with other aspects of life, a measure of success as opposed to failure was developed. The men considered successful were those with at least two of: home owner, no adverse ratings of home conditions, and not more than three addresses in the last five years. All these success criteria were developed *before* relationships with offending were known, so they were not designed to maximize any such relationships. Tab. 1 shows that 31.0% of men were considered unsuccessful, having an unsatisfactory accommodation history on this criterion. Convicted men were significantly more likely to have an unsatisfactory accommodation history than the remainder (chi–square = 7.42, p < .01). Persisters were the most extreme, since more than half of them (52.5%) had an unsatisfactory accommodation history. They were significantly different not only from unconvicted men (chi–square = 14.84, p < .001) but also from desisters (chi–square = 5.58, p < .025). Latecomers (31.8%) and desisters (29.1%) were not very different in accommodation from unconvicted men (25.8%).

3.2   Cohabitation

Over three–quarters of the men were living with either their wife (243, or 64.3%) or a female cohabitee (46, or 12.2%). There was a slight tendency for those living with a cohabitee to include more men who were convicted (43.5%) than those living with a wife (34.2%) or with neither (39.3%). Tab. 2 shows that there was no tendency for convicted and unconvicted men to differ in the proportion who were not living with a wife or cohabitee.

Tab. 2:   Offending Versus Cohabitation

Percentage of:		No wife or cohab. (23.5)	Divorced or sep. (19.6)	Doesn't get on with W/C (7.6)	Unsat. cohab. history (25.4)	Has struck W/C (14.5)
(1) Unconvicted	(240)	22.5	14.6	2.7	22.5	9.7
(2) Convicted	(138)	25.4	28.3	16.5	30.4	23.3
(3) Latecomers	(22)	27.3	27.3	6.3	27.3	12.5
(4) Desisters	(55)	21.8	27.3	7.0	23.6	14.0
(5) Persisters	(61)	27.9	29.5	29.5	37.7	36.4
Comparisons:						
1 vs. 2		0.26	9.56**	16.08***	2.51	8.84**
1 vs. 3		0.06	1.59	0.00	0.06	0.00
1 vs. 4		0.00	4.26*	0.84	0.00	0.30
1 vs. 5		0.51	6.47*	31.95***	5.13*	18.05***
4 vs. 5		0.29	0.00	5.95*	2.06	4.66*

All the comparisons by chi–square–tests; * p < .05   ** p < .01   *** p < .001
Cohab. = Cohabitee/Cohabitation;   Sep. = Separated
W/C = Wife or Cohabitee;   Unsat. = Unsatisfactory

About one fifth of the men (19.6%) had been divorced or separated from a wife by age 32. This applied to twice as many of the convicted men as of the unconvicted men (28.3% as opposed to 14.6%: chi–square = 9.56, p<.005). Latecomers (27.3%), desisters (27.3%), and persisters (29.5%) were equally likely to have been divorced or separated.

Most of the men who had a wife or cohabitee (92.4%) said that they got on well with her. However, convicted men were significantly more likely not to get on well with their wife or cohabitee (16.5% as opposed to 2.7%: chi–square = 16.08, p<.001). Persisters were the most extreme in this (29.5%).

They got on significantly badly with their wife or cohabitee, both in comparison with unconvicted men (chi-square = 31.95, p<.001) and in comparison with desisters (chi-square = 5.95, p<.025). Latecomers (6.3%) and desisters (7.0%) were not very different from unconvicted men (2.7%).

A combined measure of successful cohabitation history was also developed. The men considered successful had at least two of: living with a wife or cohabitee, never divorced or separated, and get on well with wife or cohabitee. Tab. 2 shows that persisters were the most likely to have an unsatisfactory cohabitation history (37.7%), and that they were significantly worse than unconvicted men (chi-square = 5.13, p<.025). Desisters (23.6%) were quite similar to unconvicted men (22.5%).

The men were also asked if they had hit their wife or cohabitee, and 42 of the 289 living with a woman said that they had (14.5%). Tab. 2 shows that convicted men were significantly more likely to have struck their wife or cohabitee than unconvicted men (23.3% as opposed to 9.7%: chi-square = 8.84, p<.005). Persisters, especially, included a high proportion (36.4%) who had used physical violence on their wives or cohabitees, and they were significantly worse than unconvicted men (chi-square = 18.05, p<.001) and than desisters (chi-square = 4.66, p<.05). Latecomers (12.5%) and desisters (14.0%) were not very different from unconvicted men (9.7%).

3.3   Difficulties with Children

Nearly one third of the men (119, or 31.6%) had no children, and these included a relatively low proportion who were convicted (21.8%). Of 259 men with children of their own, 58 (22.4%) had at least one child living elsewhere, and the remainder had all their children living with them. Twice as many of the men with children living elsewhere were convicted (69.0%) in comparison with those whose children were living with them (35.8%), a significant difference (chi-square = 18.82, p<.001). Tab. 3 shows that convicted men (35.7%) and especially persisters (46.3%) tended to be separated from their children. Even desisters were significantly more likely than unconvicted men to have children living elsewhere (27.9% as opposed to 12.2%: chi-square = 5.02, p<.025). This might have been a legacy from their criminal past.

Tab. 3:   Offending Versus Difficulties with Children

Percentage of:		Child living elsewhere (22.4)	Real problem with child (30.3)	Doesn't agree with W/C (18.1)	Difficulties with children (23.6)
(1) Unconvicted	(240)	12.2	32.7	14.5	16.3
(2) Convicted	(138)	35.7	26.8	23.8	33.0
(3) Latecomers	(22)	20.0	11.1	16.7	20.0
(4) Desisters	(55)	27.9	23.3	37.1	27.9
(5) Persisters	(61)	46.3	34.4	13.5	40.7
Comparisons:					
1 vs. 2		18.82***	0.46	2.39	8.95**
1 vs. 3		0.20	0.94	0.00	0.00
1 vs. 4		5.02*	0.58	7.70**	2.20
1 vs. 5		25.24***	0.00	0.00	11.99***
4 vs. 5		2.70	0.46	4.17*	1.21

All the comparisons by chi–square–tests; * p < .05   ** p < .01   *** p < .001
W/C = Wife or Cohabitee

Each man living with children aged 3–15 was asked about the following child problems: lying, stealing, running away, truancy, disobedience, fighting, temper tantrums, bullying, destructiveness, restlessness, bed–wetting, sleep disturbance, fears, and nervous habits. In practice, the wife or cohabitee (who was present in 137 cases) often helped in answering these questions. The men were asked to distinguish between problems and *real* problems. Nearly one third of the men with children (30.3%) said that their child had a real problem in one of the specified areas, but this was not significantly related to any category of offending. In fact, convicted men reported fewer real problems than unconvicted men. Unfortunately, this measure of child problems is unreliable, because it was the one factor on which the interviewers differed significantly.

The men were also asked about whether they usually agreed with their wife or cohabitee about how to control the children, and 81.9% said that they did. Tab. 3 shows that, rather surprisingly, desisters were the most likely not to agree (37.1%). They were significantly more in conflict with their wife or cohabitee than unconvicted men (chi–square = 7.70, p<.01) and than persisters (chi–square = 4.17, p<.05).

A combined measure of success with children was also developed. The men considered successful had at least two of: no children living elsewhere, no real problem with any child, and usually agree with the wife or cohabitee about how to control the children. (The men with no children, of course, were rated as "not applicable" on this measure.) Tab. 3 shows that significantly more of the convicted men had difficulties with their children (33.0% as opposed to 16.3% of unconvicted men: chi-square = 8.95, p < .005). Persisters (40.7%) were especially likely to have difficulties with children, while latecomers (20.0%) were similar to unconvicted men.

3.4   Employment

Two-thirds of the men (66.8%) were currently employed, and a further 16.2% were self-employed. Only 11.9% were unemployed or had casual work, and the remaining 5.0% were in other categories (e.g., working part-time). The unemployed men included 60.0% who were convicted, in comparison with 41.0% of the self-employed and 31.7% of the employed.

Tab. 4:   Offending Versus Employment

Percentage of:		Not now employed (11.9)	Social class IV or V (25.3)	Pay below £120 per week (25.8)	Unemployed 10 months or more (17.0)	Unsat. employment history (24.0)
(1) Unconvicted	(240)	7.5	25.0	22.1	10.0	18.3
(2) Convicted	(138)	19.7	25.7	33.0	29.4	34.1
(3) Latecomers	(22)	9.1	27.3	40.0	23.8	28.6
(4) Desisters	(55)	9.1	22.2	28.0	16.4	22.2
(5) Persisters	(61)	33.3	28.3	35.9	43.3	46.7
Comparisons:						
1 vs. 2		11.23***	0.00	3.96*	21.81***	10.89***
1 vs. 3		0.00	0.00	2.33	2.46	0.73
1 vs. 4		0.01	0.06	0.49	1.24	0.22
1 vs. 5		26.67***	0.13	2.71	36.04***	19.60***
4 vs. 5		8.54**	0.28	0.32	8.63**	6.42*

All the comparisons by chi-square-tests; * p < .05   ** p < .01   *** p < .001
Unsat. = Unsatisfactory

Tab. 4 shows that significantly more of the convicted men were unemployed than of the unconvicted men (19.7% as opposed to 7.5%: chi–square = 11.23, p<.001). The prevalence of unemployment was particularly high among persisters (33.3%), who were significantly worse than unconvicted men (chi–square = 26.67, p<.001) and than desisters (chi–square = 8.54, p<.005). Latecomers (9.1%) and desisters (9.1%) were similar to unconvicted men (7.5%).

The social class of the men's current or last job was classified on the Registrar-General's scale of occupational prestige. Only 16.5% of men were in Classes I or II (professional or managerial), 14.6% in Class III (skilled) non-manual, 43.6% in Class III manual, 18.1% in Class IV (semiskilled), and 7.2% in Class V (unskilled). Perhaps surprisingly, Class III manual contained the highest proportion who were convicted men (46.3%). Hence, low social class (IV or V) was not related to any category of offending (see Tab. 4).

About a quarter of the men (25.8%) who were being paid had a take–home pay below £120 per week; 31.9% received between £120 and £159, 27.6% received between £160 and £239, and 14.7% received £240 or more. Tab. 4 shows that convicted men were just significantly likely to have low take–home pay (33.0% as opposed to 22.1% of unconvicted men: chi–square = 3.96, p<.05). Late-comers (40.0%) were the most likely to have low take–home pay.

Two–thirds of the men (68.1%) had not been unemployed in the last 5 years, while 14.9% had been unemployed for 9 months or less and 17.0% for 10 months or more. The men who had been unemployed for 10 months or more included a particularly high proportion who were convicted (62.5%). Tab. 4 shows that nearly three times as many of the convicted men had been unemployed for a long period, in comparison with the unconvicted men (29.4% as opposed to 10.0%: chi–square = 21.81, p<.001). Persisters were particularly likely to have experienced long–term unemployment (43.3%) – significantly more than unconvicted men (chi–square = 36.04, p<.001) or desisters (chi–square = 8.63, p<.005).

A combined measure of success in employment was also developed. The men considered successful had at least three of: currently employed, social class I, II or III, take–home pay at least £120 per week, and unemployed less than 10 months in the previous 5 years. Tab. 4 shows that convicted men were significantly likely to have an unsatisfactory employment history on these criteria (34.1% of convicted men as opposed to 18.3% of unconvicted ones: chi–

square = 10.89, p<.001). Persisters were the most likely to have an unsatisfactory employment history (46.7%), and they were significantly worse than
unconvicted men (chi-square = 19.60, p<.001) and than desisters (chi- square
= 6.42, p<.025). Desisters (22.2%) were quite similar to unconvicted men
(18.3%).

3.5   Leisure Activities

Just over a quarter of the men (28.9%) went out less often than one evening
per week, while over half (54.0%) went out between one and three evenings
per week, and the remaining 17.2% went out four or more evenings per week.
The men who went out four or more evenings per week included the highest
percentage who were convicted (49.2%), in comparison with 32.3% of those
who went out between one and three evenings per week, and 37.7% of those
who went out less.

Tab. 5:   Offending Versus Leisure Activities

Percentage of:		4 or more evenings out per week (17.2)	Involved in fights (37.1)	Heavy smoker (27.2)	Drunk driver (52.6)
(1) Unconvicted	(240)	13.8	26.7	19.4	44.6
(2) Convicted	(138)	23.0	55.5	40.7	65.8
(3) Latecomers	(22)	28.6	45.5	38.1	41.2
(4) Desisters	(55)	20.4	49.1	51.9	70.8
(5) Persisters	(61)	23.3	65.0	31.7	69.2
Comparisons:					
1 vs. 2		4.42*	29.78***	18.55***	12.34***
1 vs. 3		2.24	2.64	3.02	0.00
1 vs. 4		1.01	9.52**	22.59***	9.57**
1 vs. 5		2.59	29.61***	3.51	8.99**
4 vs. 5		0.02	2.36	3.98*	0.00

All the comparisons by chi–square–tests; * p < .05   ** p < .01   *** p < .001

Tab. 5 shows that a significantly higher percentage of convicted men (23.0%) than of unconvicted ones (13.8%) went out four or more evenings per week (chi–square = 4.42, p<.05). Latecomers went out the most (28.6%).

Over half of the men (62.9%) had not been involved in physical fights — in which blows were struck — in the last 5 years. Fights in the course of work as a police officer, prison officer, or security guard, and men who were victims of mugging, were not counted. The percentage who were convicted increased with the number of fights in which a man had been involved: 25.7% of the 237 nonfighters were convicted, in comparison with 39.6% of 53 men involved in one fight, 59.5% of 42 men involved in two or three fights, and 66.7% of 45 men involved in four or more fights. Tab. 5 shows that a significantly higher percentage of convicted men (55.5%) than of unconvicted ones (26.7%) were involved in fights (chi–square = 29.78, p<.001). Even desisters (49.1%) were significantly more involved in fights than unconvicted men (chi–square = 9.52, p<.005). However, persisters (65.0%) were especially likely to have been involved in fights (chi–square = 29.61, p<.001).

Nearly half of the men (48.8%) spent nothing on smoking, while a quarter (24.0%) were moderate smokers — spending £1 per day or less, corresponding to a consumption of no more than 20 cigarettes per day — and the remaining quarter (27.2%) were relatively heavy smokers. The nonsmokers included 26.8% who were convicted, in comparison with 36.4% of the moderate smokers and 55.0% of the heavy smokers. Tab. 5 shows that convicted men were significantly more likely to be heavy smokers than unconvicted ones (40.7% as opposed to 19.4%: chi–square = 18.55, p<.001). Interestingly, desisters were the most likely to be heavy smokers (51.9%). They were significantly worse than unconvicted men (chi–square = 22.59, p<.001) and than persisters (chi–square = 3.98, p<.05).

About one sixth of the men (16.6%) were nondrivers. Just over half of the remainder (52.6%) had driven after drinking at least five pints of beer, or other equivalents of 10 units of alcohol, in the last 5 years. (One unit of alcohol corresponds to one half–pint of beer or cider, one single measure of spirits, or one glass of wine.) The consumption of 10 units of alcohol would almost certainly lead to a failure to pass the English breathalyser test, which sets a limit of 80 mg. of alcohol per 100 ml. of blood. The drunk drivers included a significantly higher percentage who were convicted than the remainder (47.0% as opposed to 27.0%: chi–square = 12.34, p<.001). Tab. 5 shows that a significant majority of convicted men (65.8%), desisters (70.8%), and persisters

(69.2%) were drunk drivers. However, latecomers (41.2%) were similar to unconvicted men (44.6%).

3.6 Substance Abuse

The men were asked what was the most they drank in any one evening (or daily drinking session), referring particularly to the last month. Nearly a quarter (22.7%) drank 5 units of alcohol or less or did not drink, while 32.5% drank between 6 and 10 units, 25.1% drank between 11 and 19 units, and 19.7% − the heavy drinkers − drank 20 units or more. The percentage who were convicted increased with the amount of alcohol consumed, from 21.2% of those who drank 5 units or less to 24.6% of those who drank between 6 and 10 units, 41.5% of those who drank between 11 and 19 units, and 67.6% of those who drank 20 units or more. Tab. 6 shows that convicted men, late-comers, desisters, and persisters were all significantly more likely than un-convicted men to be heavy drinkers. The persisters included the highest percentage who were heavy drinkers (45.0%).

Tab. 6:   Offending Versus Substance Abuse

Percentage of:		Heavy drinker (19.7)	Taken marijuana (18.4)	Taken other drug (9.5)	Substance abuser (11.7)
(1) Unconvicted	(240)	10.1	11.3	4.6	5.0
(2) Convicted	(138)	36.5	30.7	18.2	23.4
(3) Latecomers	(22)	36.4	9.1	4.5	9.1
(4) Desisters	(55)	27.3	25.5	12.7	18.2
(5) Persisters	(61)	45.0	43.3	28.3	33.3
Comparisons:					
1 vs. 2		36.65***	20.51***	17.31***	26.76***
1 vs. 3		10.57**	0.00	0.00	0.10
1 vs. 4		10.00**	6.33*	3.86*	9.44**
1 vs. 5		38.76***	31.59***	29.25***	37.52***
4 vs. 5		3.16	3.29	3.34	2.68

All the comparisons by chi-square–tests; * p < .05   ** p < .01   *** p < .001

Over one sixth of the men (18.6%) said that they had taken marijuana in the last 5 years, and 60.9% of these men were convicted, in comparison with 30.9% of the remainder; a significant difference (chi–square = 20.51, p<.001). Tab. 6 shows that even desisters were significantly more likely to have taken marijuana than unconvicted men (25.5% as opposed to 11.3%: chi–square = 6.33, p<.025). However, the highest percentage who had taken marijuana was among persisters (43.3%), who were significantly worse than unconvicted men (chi–square = 31.59, p<.001) and than latecomers (chi–square = 6.94, p<.01). Latecomers (9.1%) were similar to unconvicted men (11.3%).

Seven men said that they had taken heroin in the last 5 years, while 21 had taken cocaine, 22 had taken amphetamines, 13 had taken LSD, 10 had taken magic mushrooms, 5 had taken amyl nitrite, and 4 had taken barbiturates. All of these groups included high percentages who were convicted. Overall, 36 men (9.5%) had taken some drug other than marijuana, and most of these were multiple drug users. They included 69.4% who were convicted, in comparison with 32.8% of the remainder; a significant difference (chi–square = 17.31, p<.001). Tab. 6 shows that persisters were particularly likely to have taken other drugs (28.3% of persisters, in comparison with only 4.6% of unconvicted men: chi–square = 29.25, p<.001). Desisters were just significantly worse than unconvicted men (chi–square = 3.86, p<.05), while persisters were significantly worse than latecomers (chi–square = 4.02, p<.05). Latecomers (4.5%) were similar to unconvicted men (4.6%).

A combined measure of substance abuse was also developed. The men considered successful had at least two of: did not drink 20 or more units of alcohol in one session in the last month, no marijuana in the last 5 years, and no other drugs in the last 5 years. Tab. 6 shows that convicted men (23.4%), desisters (18.2%), and especially persisters (33.3%) included significantly higher percentages who were substance abusers than unconvicted men (5.0%). Latecomers (9.1%) were not very different from unconvicted men.

3.7   Self–Reported Offending

About a quarter of the men (24.1%) said that they had stolen something worth £5 or more from work in the last 5 years, and these men included a significantly high percentage who were convicted (52.7%, as opposed to 31.4% of the remainder: chi–square = 12.73, p<.001). Tab. 7 shows that desisters included the highest percentage who had stolen from work (41.8%, as opposed to 17.9% of unconvicted men: chi–square = 13.37, p<.001). Persisters were less extreme (31.1%), possibly because so many of them had long periods of unemployment in the last 5 years, but they were still significantly different from unconvicted men (chi–square = 4.43, p<.05).

Tab. 7:   Offending Versus Self-Reported Offending

Percentage of:		Theft from work	Tax evasion	Other self-report act
		(24.1)	(51.1)	(22.5)
(1) Unconvicted	(240)	17.9	47.1	14.2
(2) Convicted	(138)	34.8	58.0	37.0
(3) Latecomers	(22)	27.3	31.8	27.3
(4) Desisters	(55)	41.8	58.2	30.9
(5) Persisters	(61)	31.1	67.2	45.9
Comparisons:				
1 vs. 2		12.73***	3.73	24.82***
1 vs. 3		0.63	1.13	1.76
1 vs. 4		13.37***	1.78	7.64**
1 vs. 5		4.43*	7.10**	28.04***
4 vs. 5		1.00	0.66	2.14

All the comparisons by chi–square-tests; * p < .05   ** p < .01   *** p < .001

About half of the men (51.1%) had illegally evaded tax in the last 5 years by not admitting some earnings on which tax should have been paid, and these tax evaders included a near–significantly higher percentage who were convicted (41.5%, as opposed to 31.4%: chi–square = 3.73, p<.10). Persisters included the highest percentage who were tax evaders (67.2%, as opposed to 47.1% of unconvicted men: chi–square = 7.10, p<.01). Persisters were significantly more likely to be tax evaders than were latecomers (chi–square = 6.92, p<.01), who were rather unlikely to evade tax (31.8%).

The men were also asked about the commission of eight other specified offenses in the last 5 years. Nine (2.4%) admitted burglary, 11 (2.9%) admitted taking and driving away a vehicle, 8 (2.1%) admitted theft from a vehicle, 21 (5.6%) admitted shoplifting, 39 (10.3%) admitted obtaining government benefits by fraud, 4 (1.1%) admitted vandalism, 6 (1.6%) admitted theft from machines such as meters or telephone boxes, and 5 (1.3%) admitted stealing checks or credit cards and obtaining money with them. Overall, 85 men (22.5%) admitted at least one of these acts, and they included a significantly high percentage who were convicted (60.0%, as opposed to 29.6%: chi-square = 24.82, p<.001). Tab. 7 shows that even desisters included a significantly high percentage who were self-reported offenders on this criterion (30.9%, as opposed to 14.2% of the unconvicted men: chi-square = 7.64, p<.01). Latecomers were also high (27.3%), although not significantly so. However, persisters included the highest percentage who were self-reported offenders (45.9%).

3.8   Mental Health

The 30-item General Health Questionnaire was used to detect men with non-psychotic psychiatric disorder. According to Goldberg (1978), anyone scoring more than 4 on the GHQ could be identified as a probable psychiatric case. This was true of about a quarter (23.8%) of the men. The percentage who were convicted increased somewhat with the GHQ score, from 30.7% of 150 men scoring 0, to 33.7% of 95 men scoring 1–2, 44.2% of 43 men scoring 3–4, 44.2% of 43 men scoring 5–8, and 46.8% of 47 men scoring 9 or more. However, Tab. 8 shows that a GHQ score of 5 or more was not significantly related to any category of offending, although the percentage of convicted men with such a high score was almost significantly greater than the percentage of unconvicted men (29.7%, as opposed to 20.4%: chi-square = 3.68, p<.10). Latecomers were the most likely to have high GHQ scores (36.4%).

Tab. 8:   Offending Versus Mental Health and Social Failure

Percentage of:		GQH Score 5 or more or more (23.8)	Percentage fail- ure over 33 (24.6)
(1) Unconvicted	(240)	20.4	13.3
(2) Convicted	(138)	29.7	44.2
(3) Latecomers	(22)	36.4	40.9
(4) Desisters	(55)	25.5	32.7
(5) Persisters	(61)	31.1	55.7
Comparisons:			
1 vs. 2		3.68	43.36***
1 vs. 3		2.15	9.61**
1 vs. 4		0.41	10.62**
1 vs. 5		2.62	48.64***
4 vs. 5		0.22	5.30*

All the comparisons by chi–square–tests; * $p < .05$ ** $p < .01$ *** $p < .001$
GHQ = General Health Questionnaire

3.9   Social Failure

A measure of general social success or failure at age 32 was developed on the basis of nine criteria. The success criteria were as follows:

1. Satisfactory accommodation history.
2. Satisfactory cohabitation history.
3. Successful with children.
4. Satisfactory employment history.
5. Not involved in fights in the last 5 years.
6. Not substance abuser.
7. No self–reported offenses in the last 5 years (other than theft from work or tax evasion).
8. GHQ score 4 or less.
9. No convictions for offenses committed in the last 5 years.

Each man was scored according to the percentage of these nine criteria on which he was a failure. (Where a man was not known on one criterion, for example, if he had no children, the percentage score was based on eight criteria.) Previous work on this survey showed that men with a success score of 67% or greater (or a failure score of 33% or less) were also, independently, thought by the interviewers to be leading quite successful lives (Farrington, Gallagher, Morley, St Ledger, and West, 1987a, 1987b). Conversely, men with a failure score over 33% were considered by the interviewers to be relatively unsuccessful.

As might have been expected, the percentage of men who were convicted increased with the failure score. (To a small extent, this is artefactual, because conviction in the last 5 years was one of the nine criteria of failure. However, only 41 of the 138 convicted men were convicted in the last 5 years.) About a quarter of the men (90) had a failure score of 0, and these included 21.1% who were convicted, in comparison with 22.9% of 96 scoring 1-17, 36.4% of 99 scoring 18-33, and 65.6% of 93 scoring over 33. Tab. 8 shows that convicted men (44.2%), latecomers (40.9%), desisters (32.7%), and persisters (55.7%) were all significantly more likely to be classified as social failures than unconvicted men (13.3%). Persisters were the most likely to be general social failures, and they were significantly worse than desisters (chi-square = 5.30, p < .025).

4. Conclusions

Convicted men differed from unconvicted ones at age 32 in most aspects of life: in having more unsatisfactory accommodation, more divorce or separation from their wives, children separated from them, in conflict with their wife or cohabitee, more unemployment, lower take-home pay, more evenings out, more fights, more heavy smoking, more drunk driving, more heavy drinking, more drug-taking, more theft from work, more tax evasion, and more other types of offenses. Convicted men were nearly significantly different from unconvicted ones in the psychiatric disorder (GHQ) score.

Latecomers — those first convicted after the 21st birthday — did not differ so much from unconvicted men. They especially tended to be heavy drinkers, and they also tended to be divorced or separated, had the lowest take-home pay, went out most in the evening, were involved in fights, were heavy smokers, admitted many offenses (except tax evasion), and had the highest psychiatric disorder scores. However, they had satisfactory accommodation, got on quite well with their wife or cohabitee, were not currently unemployed, and were not drunk drivers or drug-takers.

Desisters — those last convicted before the 21st birthday — also did not differ so much from unconvicted men. They also tended to be heavy drinkers, as well as divorced or separated, with children living elsewhere, involved in fights, the heaviest smokers, the worst drunk drivers, drug-takers, and they admitted many offenses (especially theft from work). However, they had satisfactory accommodation and a satisfactory employment history.

In general, *persisters* — those who continued to commit offenses after the 21st birthday — were the most extreme. They were the worst in accommodation, divorce or separation, children living elsewhere, conflict with their wife or cohabitee, hitting their wife or cohabitee, unemployment, involvement in fights, heavy drinking, drug-taking, and self-reported offending (except theft from work). While latecomers and desisters were significantly high on general social failure, persisters were the worst.

In many ways, both offenders and nonoffenders became less deviant between 18 and 32, but the differences between offenders and nonoffenders were still apparent at age 32. However, they did not differ significantly in the probability of living with a wife or cohabitee, the social class of their jobs, child problems, or the psychiatric disorder (GHQ) score. As already indicated, the measure of real child problems may have been unsatisfactory, while convicted and unconvicted men were nearly significantly different on the GHQ. The lack of a relationship between adult offending and adult social class is interesting, because the social class of the fathers when the men were aged 8 was one of the few factors that did not significantly predict the men's juvenile offending. However, young adult offending at age 18 was significantly related to low social class of the man at age 18.

Differences between convicted and unconvicted men at age 32 in many respects replicated earlier differences between their parents. Just as low family income, poor housing, an erratic paternal job record, marital disharmony, and separation of a boy from his parents at age 8-10 predicted his later offending, so convicted and unconvicted men at age 32 differed in income, housing, employment history, the relationship with their wife or cohabitee, and having children living elsewhere. Farrington (1988) showed how far factors measured at age 8-10 predicted later life success at age 32.

Differences between convicted and unconvicted men at age 32 in many respects also replicated differences evident at age 18 — in having an unstable job record with periods of unemployment, heavy drinking, drunk driving, heavy smoking, fighting, drug-taking, spending evenings out, and committing a variety of offenses. Even divorce and separation might be considered to be related to sexual promiscuity evident at age 18.

The most interesting difference between relationships at 18 and 32 was in take-home pay. Whereas convicted men were significantly better paid than unconvicted ones at age 18, they were significantly worse paid at age 32. This probably reflects the fact that many convicted men took dead-end jobs with poor prospects (e.g., a laborer) after leaving school. These men were on the full adult wage at age 18, but this wage did not increase afterwards in relation to age. In contrast, unconvicted men at age 18 were more likely to continue studying or to take jobs with prospects of future advancement (e.g., a bank clerk) that were lowly paid initially but led to better pay in due course. By age 32, unconvicted men in jobs with prospects had overtaken convicted men in dead-end jobs. It is interesting that, in this survey, the peak age of offending coincided with the greatest relative amount of discretionary income for many men. The convicted men were relatively poor at age 8 and again by age 32, but they were relatively well-off at age 18 when they were committing the most offenses. This suggests that the link between poverty and crime is quite complex and possibly indirect.

As expected, the persisters were the most deviant at age 32. Latecomers and desisters were less deviant, but still significantly different from unconvicted men in behavior — especially in drinking and fighting. The most hopeful finding was that latecomers and desisters were not significantly different from unconvicted men in their accommodation and employment. Hence, offending that finishes early or starts late is not associated with social failure in all aspects of life. It is to be hoped that the satisfactory accommodation and employment of latecomers and persisters will eventually be followed by satisfactory social behavior.

References

Farrington, D.P. (1983): Offending from 10 to 25 years of age. In Van Dusen, K.T., and Mednick, S.A. (Eds.): Prospective studies of crime and delinquency. Boston: Kluwer-Nijhoff, 17–37

Farrington, D.P. (1988): Long-term prediction of offending and other life outcomes. In Wegener, H., Lösel, F., and Haisch, J. (Eds.): Criminal behavior and the justice system: Psychological perspectives. New York: Springer-Verlag, in press

Farrington, D.P., Gallagher, B., Morley, L., St Ledger, R.J., and West, D.J. (1988a): Are there any successful men from criminogenic backgrounds? Psychiatry, 51, 116–130

Farrington, D.P., Gallagher, B., Morley, L., St Ledger, R.J., and West, D.J. (1988b): A 24-year follow-up of men from vulnerable backgrounds. In Jenkins, R.L. (Ed.): The abandonment of delinquent behavior: The turnaround. New York: Praeger, in press

Farrington, D.P., and West, D.J. (1981): The Cambridge study in delinquent development. In Mednick, S.A., and Baert, A.E. (Eds.): Prospective longitudinal research: An empirical basis for the primary prevention of psychosocial disorders. Oxford: Oxford University Press, 137–145

Goldberg, D. (1978): Manual of the General Health Questionnaire. Windsor, Berks.: NFER-Nelson

West, D.J. (1969): Present conduct and future delinquency. London: Heinemann

West, D.J. (1982): Delinquency: Its roots, careers, and prospects. London: Heinemann

West, D.J., and Farrington, D.P. (1973): Who becomes delinquent? London: Heinemann

West, D.J., and Farrington, D.P. (1977): The delinquent way of life. London: Heinemann

Prediction of Writing and Reading Achievement — Some Findings From a Pilot Study

Renate Valtin

1. Introduction

In the theoretical and didactic discussion on the acquisition of written language, the learner's contribution to actively structuring and reconstructing the object of learning is currently being emphasized more strongly (Brügelmann, 1983). This paradigm has also led to a new approach to the analysis of reading, writing, and spelling difficulties. In the past, a functional deficit approach was mainly favored for the prediction of reading failure. The deficit approach (also sometimes known as the medical model) traced the causes of difficulty in acquiring writing skills to fundamental deficits in cognitive functions. This approach has since proven inadequate for a number of reasons (cf. Scheerer–Neumann, 1979, Valtin, 1978–1979, 1981).

In the present paper, I wish to introduce a *person–oriented approach* which views the acquisition of written language from the standpoint of cognitive developmental psychology. It takes account of the hypotheses formed by the learner during each subsequent acquisition phase, and of the cognitive models and private rules he or she sets up along the way. Too little attention has, so far, been paid to the circumstance that when children learn to read and write — in analogy to the way they learn to speak — they develop hypotheses and set up rules concerning written language, and actively structure the object of learning as they learn to master it. This process of structuring and construction is rendered especially difficult by the abstractness of written language, which abstracts both from the acoustic aspect of language and from the conversational partner. As the history of the development of written symbols shows, our alphabetic system is a relatively late human achievement based on advanced insights into the lexical, syntactic, and phonological structure of the alphabetic system. When children learn to write, they must reconstruct these linguistic insights possessed by the inventors of written language, and rediscover for themselves the rules by which it is coded (Downing, 1984). This process of reconstruction has two aspects:

1. A recognition of the communicative function of written language (which is a special form of language and not merely a set of symbols whose content is arbitrary); and
2. a recognition of certain linguistic units represented in our system of writing, such as sounds, words, and sentences.

Our alphabetic system requires a more highly developed ability to abstract than do the hieroglyphic and logographic systems.

My main thesis is that those who learn written language must acquire *cognitive clarity* with regard to its *function* (its particular symbolic form) and with regard to the *structural elements represented in alphabetic script* (cf. Downing, 1984). This cognitive clarity presupposes certain metalinguistic abilities which first graders cannot be expected to possess in any great degree: an ability to abstract from the context of action and meaning, to concentrate on the formal (phonetic) aspect of language, to divide semantic units into words, and to recognize certain segments of phonetic structure. Although first graders, being competent speakers and listeners, do know certain linguistic rules, these rules are *not consciously available to them*. Rather, they must gradually develop an awareness, in classroom instruction, of the structural elements represented in our form of language — sounds, words, and sentences. If the learner does not achieve cognitive clarity with respect to the function and structure of written language, or if instruction only produces cognitive confusion, difficulties in learning to read and write can result. Empirical findings from a pilot study are presented to support this view.

Some clarifications regarding the terms language awareness and phonemic awareness seem necessary. Valtin (1984a, b) has analyzed these rather vague concepts into their conceptual components. Based on newer German research (especially Andresen, 1985) she presented Leontev's model of speech as a theoretical framework. This model allows a differentiation between various forms of awareness as well as a suggestion as to their developmental order and their relation to the learning of written language. It claims that the child acquires the linguistic notions of word and phonemic mainly through instruction in reading and writing (spelling) in school. Anglo–American studies on phonemic segmentation as well as some newer European studies provide evidence that phonemic synthesis and analysis develop as a function of various factors: general cognitive level, preschool reading ability, performance level at the beginning of school, and length of reading instruction. Although no direct experimental evidence is available, the results are consistent with the view that phonemic segmentation develops largely as a consequence of learning to read, and that the two interact with each other. If some children already possess phonemic segmentation abilities (mainly because of some preschool reading ability), this may facilitate the first stages of learning to decode words. Children with no or low phonemic segmentation abilities when entering school may generally acquire these by learning during the first months of school. Although it is possible to train segmentation abilities prior to reading instruction, as Russian studies and the project by Lundberg presented in this book show, there seem to be some arguments against this procedure. First, phonemes may not be identified simply through auditory perception or articulation. Second, by means of acoustic and articulatory analysis of speech sounds, the child will not become aware of the relevant speech units which are represented by graphemes. At best, the child will arrive at allophones. According to German linguists (Eichler and Bünting, 1976), a German adult speaker produces about 120 to 150 perceptually discriminable speech sounds in his speech, whereas only 38 to 40 phonemes have the function of indicating a difference in meaning. The child must learn what class of speech sound corresponds to a specific phoneme. Third, the child may learn a wrong spelling strategy while relying too much on phonetic cues. In Germany, the spelling teaching method "spell as you speak" is still widely in use, and is undoubtedly responsible for many spelling errors. The children must shift from phonetic transcriptions to a transcription of deeper structures of language. Fourth, this technique seems to be uneconomic because segmentation training with visual markers, especially letters, is more effective. Ehri (1984) has provided evidence that letters were helpful in enabling learners to distinguish the correct size and identity of the sound units.

2. The Study

2.1   The Sample

Two school classes, one of 5-year-old preschoolers and one of first graders, were observed, interviewed, and tested over the period of a year by education students (one for each class). The preschoolers, at their own request, learned to write letters and single words as if playing a game, without systematic, formal instruction. In the 1st-grade class, instruction followed the reading and writing course of the *Bunte Fibel*, a book based on an analytic and synthetic procedure. Both classes originated from urban areas of Berlin in which almost every social stratum is represented. Complete data were gathered for 25 children in the 1st-grade class, and for 15 of the total of 22 children in the preschool class, whose attendance fluctuated considerably. The overall results of the investigation have been described elsewhere (Valtin et al., 1986).

2.2   Instruments

In the investigation, the following instruments were used in the course of the school year:

When starting school:
LARR (Linguistic Awareness in Reading Readiness, Downing et al., 1984)
Segmentation test: What is written in a written sentence? (Ferreiro, 1979)
Interview about the concept of reading, writing, and words.

After 3 months:
Identification of writing strategy (dictation of three sentences):
1. Ich bin ein Junge/Mädchen   (I am a boy/girl)
2. Ich heiße ...   (My name is ...)
3. Oma und Opa lesen   (Grandma and grandpa are reading)

After 6 months:
Segmentation test (Ferreiro, 1979)
Interview about the concept of a word ("Can you give an example of a word?
Which word is longer *Kuh* or *Piepvögelchen*? Is *in* a word? Can you give an
example of a letter, a word, or a sentence?)

After 8 months:
Interview about the concept of reading and writing

After 10 months:
Identification of writing strategy (see above)

After 11 months:
Oral reading of a text.

In the present paper, I shall concentrate on the data for those pupils who were
the most backward of their groups at the end of the school year.

2.3   Characterization of the Backward Pupils

Backward pupils were defined as those who were weakest in their class at the
end of the school year in terms of *strategies to convert spoken into written
language*. In order to determine these strategies, we dictated the following three
sentences to the first graders after 3 and 10 months of instruction:

1. "Ich bin ein Mädchen/ein Junge"   (I am a girl/a boy);
2. "Ich heiße ...."   (My name is ...); and
3. "Oma und Opa lesen"   (Grandma and Grandpa are reading).

The preschoolers had to write these sentences after 8 months of school.
The backward 1st-grade pupils were characterized by their having reached, at
best, a semiphonetic stage by the end of the first school year. In other words,
these children showed first signs of having grasped that our written language is
sound-oriented. They reproduced the most important sounds, and frequently

represented at least every syllable with a letter. Almost all the dictated words
were reproduced, although many of the children left the word *und* out of the
sentence *Oma und Opa lesen*. In the first dictation, most of the children used
uppercase letters and ran words together in disregard of their boundaries.

Daniel, for example, wrote the three sentences as follows after 10 months of
instruction:

Daniel L.   26. 6. 85

isch   E BBi Aelok
         HoH Daniel
isk

Oraa OBa lesen

After 3 months of instruction, Daniel had converted the three spoken sentences
into sequences of letters without any recognizable phonetic connection, although
he did place his name in the correct place in the sentence.

10.12.84
OANiEL·L

1. MR()ZL

2. R/ZOANiEL·L

3. Z()7NUl

Carsten's first attempt to convert the three sentences likewise resulted in sequences of letters, although he did succeed in writing his own name and the word *Oma*. However, his sentences remained incomplete.

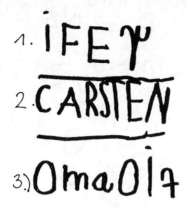

1. IFEᵞ

2. CARSTEN

3.) OmaOI٦

The second time, Carsten managed to write words, or rather word–like configurations, but these stood in no phonetic relation to the dictated sentences.

Carsten, June 1, 1985:

eif daf ein bein   Ich bin ein Junge

eif daf ine   Ich bin ein Carsten

CARSTEN.

ein Auto Cin CARSTEN.   Ich heiße Carsten

Oma lesr Omf.

Oma und Opa lesen

In the preschool class, our backward pupils had, at best, reached the stage of prephonetic writing by the end of the school year, that is, they produced lines of capital letters which evinced only rudimentary connections with word sounds.

Example: *Wolfgang*

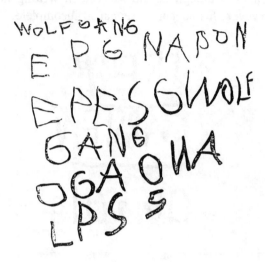

The backward writers in the 1st–grade class were also invariably backward readers, as a reading test at the end of the school year indicated. In this test, the children were asked to read aloud a short story with which they were unfamiliar.

Significant Spearman rank–order correlations were found between reading and writing. In the 1st–grade class ($n=25$) the level of spelling after 10 months correlated with the reading speed of an unfamiliar story at the end of the school year (–.60) and with reading errors (–.73).

2.4   Functions of Written Language

To ascertain how much knowledge of reading and writing the children had before starting school, we employed the Linguistic Awareness in Reading Readiness test by Downing et al. (1983). This paper–and–pencil test was administered to small groups during the first week of school. In the subtest, "Recognizing Literacy Behavior," the weaker pupils had difficulty in distinguishing between the activities of reading, writing, and painting, and were unable to identify numbers as symbols that can be read.

The LARR test results for the first school year showed a significant correlation with spelling level at 10 months (.50), with speed in reading an unfamiliar story (-.34), and with reading errors (-.43).

2.5   Metalinguistic Abilities

Segmenting Test (based on Ferreiro, 1979)

At the start of the school year, a procedure developed by Ferreiro was used to test whether our pupils were capable of associating the elements of a given written sentence with the elements of oral speech. This procedure enabled us to draw conclusions regarding the ideas children form about the relationship bet-ween written and spoken language. Each child was individually interviewed. The investigator began by writing the following sentence for the child in large capitals:

VATER SIEHT DIE KATZE
(Father sees the cat)

The investigator then read the sentence aloud, pronouncing it in a normal manner without emphasizing the individual words, and then asked the pupil to repeat it. When he or she had done so, the interviewer asked, "Did I write father (*cat, sees, the*) somewhere?" If the child was unable to associate the word with components of the text, the interviewer pointed them out and asked, "And what is this?" Finally, the child was requested to repeat the sentence again. An analogous procedure was followed with the (handwritten) sentence

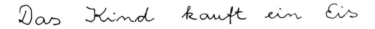

(The child buys an icecream)

In this case, the interviewer inquired about the words in this sequence: *Ice-cream, child, buys, an, the.*
Ferreiro (1979) observed certain levels in the reply patterns of the Mexican preschool children she investigated, and we found these levels in our sample as

well. They ranged from Level 1, a complete inability to segment a spoken sentence; Level 2, an inability to correctly identify text segments; Levels 3 and 4, an ability to identify certain segments (first nouns, then noun–verb combinations); to Level 5, in which the child was able to correctly identify all elements including articles. This reply pattern results from the fact that children initially tend to believe that only certain words, such as nouns, are visually represented in written language. The average preschooler thinks that articles are not represented.

The backward pupils in our sample were all characterized by being on Level 2 at the start of the school year and showing no particular progress when the test was repeated after 6 months of instruction. To cite a few examples: Carsten, age 5, thought that *father* and *cat* did not occur in the sentence *Father sees the cat*, but that *father sees* did. Six months later his skill had scarely improved. Carsten now associated the spoken word *father* with "father sees the cat" and the remainder of the sentence with "The child buys an icecream". When shown the second sentence, he began to segment it, although he interpreted the article and the noun as a single word and associated the remainder of the sentence as follows:

"Show me where the words are"

```
  THE      CHILD    BUYS     AN     ICE
 ╱ │         │        │      ╲       │
The child   buys   himself    icecream
```

When asked what the final, unidentified component meant, Carsten replied, "The one with the bear", referring to another sentence employed in the investigation.

Five–year–old Manuel thought that the written sentence "Father sees the cat" contained only *father* and *cat*, but not *sees* and *the*. Asked what the final, unidentified word meant, he said, "a mouse". However, it was not only the slow pupils in our sample who associated unidentified elements with additional units of meaning (one child associated the first, unidentified word in the sentence "The child buys an icecream" with the text "The child goes into the shop" and its last word with "The child, it liked the icecream").

Daniel, a 6–year–old in the 1st–grade class, solved this task at the beginning of term by employing a right-to-left strategy, that is, by pointing at each question from right to left to the written words. Apparently he could not conceive that the sequence of written words conformed to that of the spoken words. Six months later he associated the following words and word sounds with the sentence:

```
       Vater    sieht    die    Katze
         |        |               \
         |        |                \
       Vater    sieht   'ne Kat-   -ze
```

Although he had now apparently realized that a correspondence existed between spoken and written sequence, he still had trouble segmenting the sentence correctly. In the second sentence he was unable to identify any of the segments in the sentence.

Of all the procedures used in our investigation, this resulted in the most significant findings. All of the first graders, who after 6 months of schooling were unable to make correct associations between the oral and written words, belonged to the group of poor writers (and poor readers) in our sample. They evidently had not yet understood that the sequences of spoken and written words correspond; moreover, as a further investigation revealed, they were unable to divide a sentence into words. After 6 months of instruction the children were asked how many words the sentences "Vater sieht die Katze" and "Das Kind kauft ein Eis" contained. None of the preschoolers and only two first graders were able to answer this question correctly. Our backward 1st-grade writers all belonged to the group of children who completely failed in this part of the investigation. Their difficulty in counting the words in a sentence arose, on the one hand, from an inability to segment it according to linguistic units. An example was Carsten, age 6. He thought the sentences contained only two words each, Sentence 1 *Vater* and *sieht die Katze*; and Sentence 2, *Das Kind* and *das Eis*. Nadine counted *sieht die* and *kauft ein* as one word each.

On the other hand, the children's wrong answers may be explained by the fact that rather than counting words, they replied by giving separate sounds, although these sounds seldom agreed with the first letters of the words. Six-year–old Oliver, for instance, thought the first sentence contained five words, which he called *V, A, T, S, K*. Daniel believed it contained seven words, but gave only five units, *V, T, S, T* and *Z*.

This conceptual confusion between sounds and words brings us to the next section of our investigation. But before moving on to it, a few correlations should be given.

The segmentation test administered at the start of term correlated significantly, in the case of the first graders, with the following variables: LARR test (.78), spelling level after 10 months (.59), segmentation test after 6 months (.47), reading speed at the end of the school year (–.57), and reading errors (–.66). The segmentation test given after 6 months correlated with the LARR test (.46), with spelling level after 3 months (.41) and after 10 months (.65), with reading speed (–.60), and with reading errors (–.61).

2.6   Awareness of Such Linguistic Units as Letters, Words, and Sentences

When the school year began, none of the backward writers in our sample were able to give an example of a word or explain what a word is. After 6 months in class, all of them still belonged to that group of children who had trouble with our questions relating to the concept "word", particularly with the questions, "Can you give an example of a word? Which word is longer, *Kuh* or *Piepvögelchen*? Is *in* a word? Can you give an example of a letter, a word, or a sentence?" (This last question was asked a week later). The backward writers could either give no examples or confused the terms. Oliver, age 6, for example, replied to the question "Do you know what a word is?" by saying "no", but justified his reply that *Piepvögelchen* was longer than *Kuh* by saying that *Piepvögelchen* had two words in it. Oliver belonged to the group of children who had no consistent conception of words but who attributed varying dimensions of significance to them depending on the context. Carsten, age 5, explained that "A word is when someone says something to you", and gave the logical example, *Guten Tag*. A week later, he gave *A* as an example of a letter and *Katze* as an example of a sentence, but was unable to give an example of a word.

Carsten, age 6, when the sentences "Vater sieht die Katze" and "Das Kind kauft ein Eis" were read aloud to him, decided that each had two words. When the same two sentences were presented to him in writing a few minutes later and he was asked about the number of words they contained, he gave the correct number, adding spontaneously that he could see it by the spaces.

Wolfgang, age 5, replied to the question, "Do you know the difference between a letter, a sentence, and a word?" by saying "A sentence is something completely different from a word. A word is a lot of letters together, a sentence is also a lot of letters together." As an example of a letter, he gave *A*, of a sentence *Mai*, and of a word *Mai* again. Like various other children in our sample, Wolfgang had difficulty in strictly applying his own criteria, giving *Mai* as an example for both a word and a sentence. But he did not think the word *in*, which like *Mai* comprises two sounds, was a word at all, saying *In* is not a word, because it's so short. A word is much longer."

In sum, we were able to conclude that the backward writers in our sample had no secure conception of the terms word and sentence, either systematically confusing them or giving them different meanings depending on the context in which they were mentioned.

That school beginners do not yet have a mature conception of the word as a linguistic unit, was also observed by Januschek, Paprotté, and Rohde (1979). They too found that children attribute varying meanings to the word *word*. From the data given here, it would appear meaningful to distinguish at least two variant meanings of the concept "word": a *figurative* meaning, oriented to external, visual characteristics; and an *operative* meaning, which presumes conceptual knowledge. Thus a few of the school beginners in our sample were quite capable of identifying words in the sequences of graphic signs of the LARR test (which included letters and numbers), apparently judging them by the length of the symbol. For instance, they correctly identified *Elefant* as a word, but not *zu*, which has only two letters. However, these children were not identical with those who were able to give an example of a word. That figurative and operative conceptions of the word should be distinguished from one another can also be seen from the fact that no significant statistical correlation was found between an ability to identify words visually (figuratively) and achievements in our oral survey on the word concept (e.g., giving examples of words, comparing the length of words, etc.).

To cite some of the correlations we found: During the first school year the figurative conception of words (seven items from the LARR test related to the identification of a written word) correlated with the results of segmentation tests after 3 months (.59), and after 6 months (.63), with level of spelling after 3 months (n.s.), and 10 months (.66), with reading speed (−.37), reading errors (−.52), and with operative conception of words, that is, items of the oral survey (.26 n.s.).

The operative conception of words showed significant correlations with the following variables: segmentation tests after 3 months (.34) and after 6 months (.55), spelling level after 3 months (.47) and 10 months (.70), with reading speed (−.53) and reading errors (−.54).

2.7   Strategies of Writing on the Text Level

Up to now, we have discussed only conversion of spoken to written language on the sentence level, concluding that our backward writers first developed only a rudimentary awareness of the phonetic nature of writing and its representation of all essential speech sounds; and second, that they had difficulty in segmenting sentences into words. Some of them left out words; particularly functional words.

Let us now turn to strategies of writing on the text level. The preschoolers were asked after 3, and again after 10 months in class, to write a letter. On the first occasion, they were to tell Martin, a pupil who was ill at home, that some of the fish in the classroom aquarium had died. In their second letter, the children were to tell a friend about the mice they kept in the classroom. In terms of form, the children's letters all showed certain similarities. They all contained three elements: the child's own name, drawings, and scribbles or sequences of letters. When they read their letters aloud, however, it became evident that the symbolic content differed from the message it was intended to convey. Three basic categories of letter could be distinguished; those of the backward pupils generally fell into the first two categories.

*1. Letters whose content consisted of a commentary on the drawings, which
   represented the recipient or activities associated with him.*

Example: Charly

(Q: What did you write in your letter, Charly?)
"Charly."
(Q: And why did you write it backwards?)
"Because it was in the corner."
(Q: And what did you draw here — a little blue man?)
"Martin is big."
(Q: Why did you draw him so big?)
"So I could color him better."
(Q: And this here — the green drawing?)
"Martin is just getting into the bathtub."
(Q: And here?)
"Martin's a snowman."
"And the sun's not shining any more (it's down in the corner because it's just
going down)."

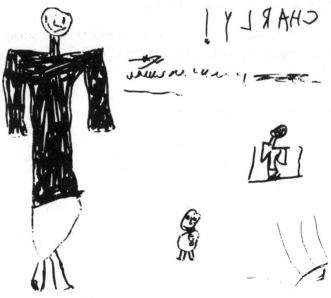

2. *Letters whose content was formulated in indirect speech. The four children who employed this linguistic mode were all among the slower pupils in the class.*

Example: Carsten

Carsten drew a large church and made scribbles and wrote sequences of letters along the upper and lower edges of the sheet. When asked what he had written, he replied:

"Carsten, that Martin should get well soon and that he should come back to preschool soon − and that he should come to the football club soon, and that we won 10:0."

(Q: And what did you write here, near the 5?)

"That he should come to see me soon, 5 Elisenstraße."

(Q: What did you draw here?)

"A church."

(Q: Why?)

"So he could be glad I drew him a picture."

Like Carsten, four other children wrote numbers that stood for a unit of communicative meaning. Meike, for example, wrote a 7, "so you can tell that Martin is 7."

Another example is from Tanja

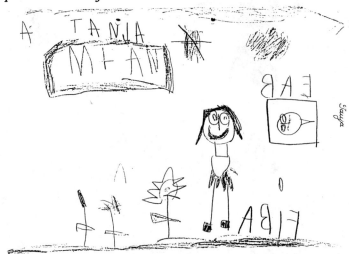

(Q: Tanja, what did you write?)
"Oh, what is this! I don't know any more ....That the fish is dead (drawing of a dead fish in a box) ... that the flowers — I don't know any more; that this is Tanja."

3. *Letters that were read aloud in direct speech and which, in most cases, contained such formal elements of a letter as introduction, salutation, and return address. This type of letter was written primarily by the better pupils.*

Example: Niklas

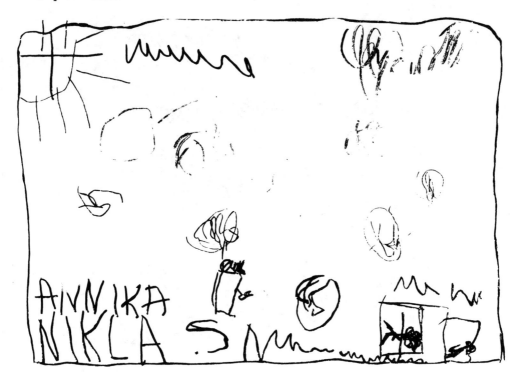

Dear Martin,
The sun is not shining, it is raining instead.
(Q: Is that why you crossed out the sun?)
"Yeah, sure."

(Q: And what else did you write?)
"Don't get a shock, because the fish are dead. Here are the dead fish, and here are only a few left over." (i.e., live fish)
(Q: And what is this here?)
"Dear Martin, kind regards from Annika (Niklas' sister) and Niklas."

The good writers in our sample already possessed considerable awareness of the mode of speech used in letters — direct speech in complete sentences. The backward writers, by contrast, apparently had not yet achieved this insight. In the second letter, written 10 months later (about the mice in the classroom), the backward writers typically continued to employ indirect speech and/or incomplete sentences.

Tanja read this letter of hers aloud as follows: "All the different things the mice eat; that the baby mice have arrived; that some of 'em died."
The texts of the other backward pupils comprised a mixture of complete sentences and sequences of nouns, and sometimes only of the latter.

Example: Carsten

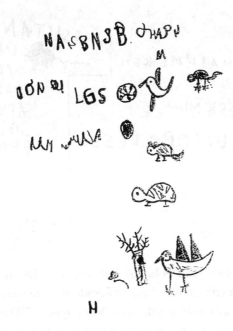

His letter reads: "A mouse, sunflower seeds. A mouse asleep, a cucumber (drawing), a little apple, a bird (drawing), mouse (drawing), a mouse feeding."

Manuel wrote two lines in capital letters (or letter–like shapes) and read his letter aloud as follows: "A mouse, father mouse, straw, nut."

Here is a final example, written by a good pupil. This, like most of the competent writers' letters, employs complete sentences.

Example: Mila

MILA

ISHCB(NAINMEHCEN

I HCHASE MILA

OMAUNOPALESEN

DSISTANEMAU
UNDMAU s
VRIST
KAROT
APVEL
SALAT
PROT

SONE
NRUN
ENEU
RNER

DASINDM
SEBEBE

Mila's spelling strategies (left column) indicate that she managed to achieve an almost complete phonetic conversion, although she showed very little tendency to segment her sentences into words. Her letter reads: "This is a mouse and the mouse is eating carrots, apples, lettuce, bread, sunflower seeds. These are baby mice."

Mila was the only pupil in the preschool class to reveal an incipient awareness that sentences can be segmented, though she actually made word divisions only rarely. Only one of our preschoolers remarked, when writing her letter, "There should be spaces between the words somewhere; you're not supposed to run it all together." Nevertheless, in her letter she ran articles and nouns together, omitted the words *in the* from the phrase *in the houses,* and left gaps within words.

Example: Oda

DIMSE HM AINAFL
HOIT HDI MOI SF
OT ABK
DIM OIS SAFE

HOS AN

Oda's text reads: "The mice have an apple. Today the mice got their food. The mice sleep in the houses."

We also had access to letters written by the first graders in our sample after they had started second grade. Those by the backward writers were characterized by two traits — the use of incomplete sentences and/or sentence units not segmented into words.

Example: Carsten

Like many preschoolers in their scribble letters, Carsten began his letter with his own name which he put before the introduction "Dear Grandma and Grandpa." Although the following sentence, "Grandma and Grandpa in their garden", is related in meaning to the recipients, it is not formulated in a personal manner and is, moreover, incomplete.
Some of the other pupils' letters also revealed that they were still having considerable difficulty in properly segmenting sentences.

Example: Oliver

Oliver was not able to divide the sentences "Wie geht es dir?" (How are you?)
and "Geht es dir gut?" (Are you well?) adequately into words. However, he
did choose a highly original form for his message, providing boxes with *yes*
and *no* for the recipient to check, questionnaire style.

In conclusion, the scribble letters and the first true letters by the backward
writers in our sample were characterized by two principal features: (1) The
mode of speech employed: either incomplete statements, some of which comprised sequences of nouns only, or indirect speech; and (2) an erroneous
segmentation of sentences in which functional words were often omitted, the
sentences were not divided into words, or the division was incomplete.

3. Summary

In this investigation it was observed that many children when they began
school, and some after several months of instruction, did not yet possess cognitive clarity with regard to the function and features of written language. They
did not yet have, for example:

1. an awareness of the social function of written language;
2. the knowledge that all parts of speech, not only nouns and verbs, are represented in a sentence, and that the sequence of written words matches that
   of spoken words;
3. an ability to divide into words a sentence read aloud to them;
4. the insight that letters are written in direct, coherent speech (and not in
   indirect speech or lists of nouns);
5. an awareness of the fact that the words of a text are separated by spaces or
   gaps; and
6. a knowledge that words and sentences represent linguistic units.

Some of the instruments used in this investigation — especially the segmentation test by Ferreiro but also the dictation used for the identification of the
writing strategies of the child — seem to yield valuable information for teachers
as regards the pupil's insight into function and features of written language.

References

Andresen, H. (1985): Schriftspracherwerb und die Entstehung von Sprachbewußtheit. Opladen: Westdeutscher Verlag.

Brügelmann, H. (1983): Kinder auf dem Wege zur Schrift. Konstanz: Vaude.

Downing, J. (1984): Task awareness in the development of reading skill. In J. Downing, and R. Valtin (Eds.): Language awareness and learning to read. New York: Springer, pp. 27–55.

Downing, J., Ayers, D., and Schaefer, B. (1983): Linguistic Awareness in Reading Readiness (LARR) test. Windsor, England: NFER–Nelson.

Eichler, W., and Bünting, K.-D. (1976): Deutsche Grammatik. Kronberg, Germany: Scriptor.

Ehri, L.C. (1984): How orthography alters spoken language competencies in children learning to read and spell. In J. Downing, and R. Valtin (Eds.): Language awareness and learning to read. New York, Berlin: Springer.

Ferreiro, E. (1979): Qu'est-ce qui est écrit dans une phrase écrite? Une réponse psychogénétique. Institut Romand de Documentation Pédagogique, Recherche 1979 (Nr. 5).

Januschek, F., Paprotté, W., and Rohde, W. (1979): Zur Ontogenese sprachlicher Handlungen. Osnabrücker Beiträge zur Sprachtheorie, 10, pp. 37–69.

Scheerer–Neumann, G. (1979): Intervention bei Lese–Rechtschreibschwäche, Bochum: Kamp

Valtin, R. (1978–79): Deficit in reading or deficit in research. In Reading Research Quarterly, Vol. XIV, No. 2, pp. 201–221.

Valtin, R. (1981): Zur Machbarkeit der Ergebnisse der Legasthenieforschung. In R. Valtin, U. Jung, and G. Scheerer-Neumann: Legasthenie in Wissenschaft und Unterricht. Darmstadt: Wissenschaftliche Buchgesellschaft.

Valtin, R. et al. (1986): Kinder lernen schreiben und über Sprache nachzudenken: Eine empirische Untersuchung zur Entwicklung schriftsprachlicher Fähigkeiten. In R. Valtin, and I. Naegele (Eds.): "Schreiben ist wichtig": Grundlagen und Beispiele für kommunikatives Schreiben(lernen). Frankfurt, Arbeitskreis Grundschule.

Valtin, R. (1984): The development of metalinguistic abilities in children learning to read and write. In J. Downing, and R. Valtin (Eds.): Language awareness and learning to read. New York, Berlin: Springer.

Valtin, R. (1984b): Awareness of features and functions of language. In J. Downing, and R. Valtin (Eds.): Language awareness and learning to read. New York, Berlin: Springer.

The Bielefeld Longitudinal Study on Early Identification of Risks in Learning Read and Write: Theoretical Background and First Results.

Helmut Skowronek and Harald Marx

1. Introduction

When we started to plan the present project, in 1984, the discussion about dyslexia or (in German) "Legasthenie" had arrived at a state that for German speaking countries was aptly reflected in a report by the Deutsche Forschungs-gemeinschaft (DFG) "Zur Lage der Legasthenieforschung" (1978). The critical discussion of the concept of 'Legasthenie' and the underlying theoretical models had uncovered various substantial and methodological weaknesses. On the other hand, around 1965 and particularly in the USA, research on the normal processes of learning read and write was increasing. It was based on comparable criticisms of traditional research on dyslexia and was stimulated by then recent developments in psycholinguistics, developmental psychology and human information processing (Kavanagh and Mattingly, 1972).

1.1 Phonological Processing — Prerequisite of Learning to Read?

In traditional research on backwardness in learning to read, which aimed at discovering basic perceptual or cognitive deficiencies, the idea prevailed that impairment in the visual perception of forms in general and of letters specifically are causally related to these difficulties. Errors in spatial orientation (e.g., confusing b with d) typically made by poor readers were long seen to support this suggestion. It has since become clear, however, that the percentage of these errors in good and poor readers is practically the same, and that they may be classified as naming inaccuracies (Angermaier, 1977). Many studies that were thought to demonstrate visual deficiencies in poor readers are not free from confounding effects that may be caused by group differences in comprehending instructions, in verbal encoding ability, in attentional and memory processes, and/or in previous experience with written language. The more the experimental tasks succeed in isolating visual processing, the more the differences between good and poor readers decrease (Vellutino, 1979). One of the first signs of the new orientation was to be found in the now classic book by Vernon (1957) on "Backwardness in Reading" in which she pointed out the significance of both visual and auditory skills in learning to read. Interestingly, the German author Bosch claimed as early as 1937 that skills in processing oral speech are of utmost significance: "... the most general precondition for learning to read is a certain distancing from speech..., which enables the learner to see through the language analytically, to the degree required by the structure of the letter script, thus first understanding the composition from parts of speech, then recognizing how it is determined by certain articulatory aspects ..." (Bosch, 1937, p. 93, our translation). Obviously what is meant by "distancing" or "objectivation" of speech is closely related to what has become known since about 1970 as "linguistic awareness" or "phonological awareness" (Mattingly, 1972).

According to this view that phonological awareness plays a vital role in learning to read, the learner has to direct his attention to the (formal) phone aspect of language and to discriminate suitable elements to successfully acquire the sound letter correspondences constitutive of the alphabetic script. Otherwise these correspondences would appear arbitrary to the learner. If he cannot use phonological awareness to a sufficient degree to analyze the stream of speech sounds he eventually will run into troubles with reading, sooner or later. The volume "Toward a Psychology of Reading", edited some years after the general hypothesis about the relation of phonological awareness and learning to read had been levelled (Reber and Scarborough, 1977), summarized the relevant theoretical considerations and empirical results up to that time. Although the correlative nature of early findings about relations of phoneme segmentation or rhyme production to reading achievement precluded any inference on causal direction, the idea that phonological awareness causally precedes learning to read became prevalent. Serious doubts concerning this view were first raised by Morais,

Carey, Alegria and Bertelson (1979) who on the basis of findings from adult illiterates claimed, to the contrary, that the ability to segment the stream of speech is not the prerequisite but the result of learning to read.

The debate since then has led to important qualifications. It became clear that individual longitudinal correlational studies which were thought to demonstrate the causal role of phonological awareness fail to control for preexisting reading skill — acquired spontaneously or by stimulation in kindergarten. When, for instance, the study done by Lundberg, Olofsson and Wall (1980) was re-analyzed by controlling for initial reading level (Wagner and Torgesen, 1987) the correlations of measures of phonological awareness and reading achievement became insignificant. To avoid tautological inference — reading is predicted by reading — deliberate controls are necessary. Most of the relevant studies fail to consider the alternative causal direction — from reading to phonological aware-ness. Yet, the question of learning to read and write seems to be too complex as to be answered adequately by finally deciding on one of the two directions. Processes in learning to read are so extended in time until adequate comprehen-sion of text is achieved that many intermediary stages of interweaving of phonological awareness and reading skill have to be conceived of. "The question we must now ask is both more complex and more to the point: which aspects of phonological processing ... are causally related to which aspects of reading ... at which point in their codevelopment, and what are the directions of these causal relations?" (Wagner and Torgesen, 1987, p. 209).

1.2   Different Forms of Phonological Processing

On average, 19% of the adult illiterates studied by Morais et al. (1979) re-sponded correctly to phonological awareness tasks. Obviously, some amount of phonological processing is acquired independent of formal learning processes. On the other hand, one can think of higher degrees of difficulty; for example, replacing phonemes within words that will not be mastered before exact alpha-betic strategies have been acquired as a consequence of advanced teaching.

Morais, Alegria and Content (1987) themselves offer suitable differentiations for

unpacking the global concept of phonological awareness: awareness of phonological strings, phonetic awareness, and awareness of phonemes. (Below, in
classifying our own screening tasks we will distinguish between phonological
awareness in a narrow vs. a broad sense.) The fully developed ability to segment phonemes "requires awareness that utterances are phonological strings.
This implies that one is able to disregard meaning for a while" (Morais et al.,
1987, p. 425). This initial sensitivity for and focusing on the phonological form
of oral language is certainly manifest in 4– to 5–year olds.

On the other hand, segmenting the stream of speech sound, which may be
observed in playing with language, for example, separating syllables and
rhyming, during the final preschool year, is phonetic in nature. This phonetic
type of segmentation probably occurs at the surface level and is controlled by
articulatory properties of speech; thus phonemes as abstract linguistic elements
are not yet implied. Evidence from linguistic and psychological sources supports
the idea of an intermediate level between the syllable and the phoneme (Treiman 1987): Experimental findings in recall of nonsense syllables suggest that
they are separated in short–term memory into units of onset and rhyme. According to Bradley and Bryant (1983) comprehending and producing rhymes by
5–year olds presupposes awareness on an intermediate level of analysis of
speech between syllable and phoneme. Obviously phonological processing of
this type is normally achieved before children enter formal reading instruction.
Finally, to be able to segment speech into the abstract linguistic units of
phonemes seems to presuppose, as a rule, the progressive mastery of the alphabetic system and orthography. That children, even after major advances in first
reading and writing, have difficulties in correctly analyzing consonant clusters
at the beginning of words, e.g. /bl/, demonstrates that this advanced stage of
phonological processing is also reached gradually, by way of many intermediary
and content–specific steps.

Besides phonological awareness and its unpacking into developmental stages we
have to distinguish further component processes of phonological processing that
are significant for learning to read (Wagner and Torgesen, 1987). First, there is
phonological recoding in lexical access, that is, representing the written symbols
in a sound–based, or 'phonological' code, to get at the meaning of words
decoded. A common task to assess this process is rapid naming of colors,

objects, and other stimuli (Denckla and Rudel, 1976). To be sure, the skilled reader will pass from the graphic pattern of written words to their lexical meaning by direct matching, but in the early stages of learning to read, or in the case of highly unfamiliar words, phonological recoding seems to be an important path to the lexicon. Second, there is phonetic recoding to retain information in working memory. This process, too, pertains to representing the written symbols in a sound–based form that is close to speech. For the beginning reader, effective storing of sounds corresponding to the letters has to be maintained until the sounds have been blended into a word. Therefore, phonetic recoding seems to be vital in the early stages of reading (Baddeley, 1982). Furthermore, recoding phonetically might be important in comprehending sentences (Perfetti and McCutchen, 1982).

1.3   Processes of Visual Attention in Learning to Read

In learning to read, apart from phonological processing of speech visual informations also have to be encoded and integrated, for example, letters as visual units and the left–to–right sequence of writing. Early approaches, which emphasized general visual processing in the acquisition of literacy, viewed, as mentioned above, learning disabilities in reading and writing as a consequence of deficits in visual processing.

According to this view Frostig (1972) constructed training units for dyslexic children that included materials on form perception and field dependency. The training improved visual performance in general, but did not produce the expected specific effects on reading and writing (Elkind, Larson and Doorninck, 1965).

In a similar vein, Kagan (1965) and Wagner (1976) looked at impulsivity as a general style of information processing that contributes to difficulties in learning to read. Training impulsive children to act in more reflective ways and so to improve their reading and writing performance also had no specific effects (Edler, Ostrau, and Schulze, 1977). Consequently, visual skills have to be examined as subject–specific skills, that is specific to learning processes in reading and writing (Kohlers 1970). Marx (1985) has demonstrated that reading development is influenced by the way in which the visual information of graphic symbols is processed and in which specific processes of visual attention are applied.

2. The Bielefeld Longitudinal Study

2.1   Characterizing the Bielefeld Longitudinal Study

The Bielefeld study differs in some ways from earlier longitudinal studies, particularly in the selection and assessment of predictors. Research by Butler (1979), Butler, Marsh, Sheppard, and Sheppard (1985), Badian (1982, 1986), and Bradley and Bryant (1983) — to mention but a few — is restricted regularly to one initial assessment and one or several criterion measurements in a sample that is not differentiated into subgroups. The selection of predictors was, in most cases, carried out in an empiristic way, on the basis of correlational results reported in relevant research. Either skills from different sensory modalities (e.g. Badian, 1982; Butler, 1979; Wendeler, 1986; Satz and Friel, 1978; Satz, Friel, and Goebel 1975; White, Batini, Satz, and Friel 1979), very specific aspects of one modality or dimension (e.g., Lindgren, 1978; Rourke and Orr, 1977; Wolf, 1984, 1986), or even a single variable from a relevant dimension (e.g., sound categorization from phonological awareness; Bradley and Bryant, 1983) were chosen. As a rule, the second measurement occured at the end of first grade or, at least, after instruction in basic skills of reading and writing had taken place. In many cases assessment of predictor variables was not replicated in a second measurement; only general criterion performance (by reading and spelling tests, teacher ratings, marks) was assessed. Variables that correlated significantly with at least one of the criterion measures were interpreted as valid predictors of reading and orthographic writing.

To infer in this general way is doubtful for several reasons. As for the predictors, the single measurement before school entrance precludes assessments of stability or reliability of predictors. Whether allocation of children to risk and nonrisk groups, according to first screening, was valid — if it was done at all in advance rather than a posteriori — cannot be ascertained. Consequently, the contribution of development or instruction to change in the predictors remains undiscovered.

In contrast to these approaches, the present longitudinal study selects the predictors according to a theoretical rationale. Essentially, prediction is based on two domains of performance, operationalized by various types of tasks. All predictor variables and some supplementary variables are repeated before school entrance, after a 6-month interval, with two subgroups. Children are allocated to the risk group by explicit classification on the basis of screening data, not on the basis of correlational evidence. Repeated measurement of the predictors enables us to infer ex post, whether the prediction of reading difficulties is dependent on the time of measurement, and whether the different predictors bear different weights at different times.

To assess the impact of formal instruction, all further measurements, planned in 6-month intervals up to fourth grade, include several predictor variables as well as various criterion variables.

2.2 Principles in Constructing the Bielefeld Screening Battery

We shall not present a detailed report on the many pilot studies and revisions we made (cf. Mannhaupt and Jansen, in press), but simply point out the major principles in selecting and constructing the screening procedure with various types of tasks:

1. For practicability and economy, the administration of the screening should take about 30 to 35 minutes.
2. The different tasks in one subtest should be completed before the child becomes bored.
3. The individual subtests should each contain roughly the same number of items and take about the same time.
4. Subtests should only be included that discriminate well in the lower third of the distribution.
5. Tasks should be constructed in a way that allows for administration in an enlarged or modified form in subsequent measurements.

6. Besides adding up to a sum score the individual subtests should allow some inspection of the strategies and ways of processing information in the individual child.
7. Repeated measurements and the changing number and quality of correct answers should reveal developmental changes.
8. The various subtests should contain demands on the child which are probably related to different stages in the processes of learning to read or that influence the development of component skills — without being criterion performances in themselves.

Up to number 4 the principles match the criteria which have been formulated for screenings as global selective procedures (Lichtenstein and Ireton, 1984). Principles 5 and 7 derive from the claim of the present study to tap general developmental changes and specific individual differences by specific types of tasks and by overlapping of different subtests. Principle 6 reflects the intent to allow for multiple interpretation of the numerous data from the screening.
Finally, Principle 8 underlines that the predictors are based on a theoretical rationale and turns against the practice — to be observed in some most recent longitudinal studies (Mann et al., 1987, Experiment 1; Vellutino and Scanlon, Experiment 1) — of including variables as predictors which can be scarcely distinguished from variables to measure reading skills.

2.3 Characterization of the Screening Tasks

The predictor variables in the Bielefeld Screening Battery contain four grades of tasks with mostly phonological components (cf. Wagner and Torgesen, 1987). In addition, it uses visually presented material to include tasks that test different aspects of attention. The level of knowledge for written symbols is recorded as a control variable (cf. Tab. 1). In the following, the construction principle of each task is explained along with its theoretical background, and different ways of analyzing the data are demonstrated.

Tab. 1: Domain classification and indices of the Bielefeld Screening Test including the variables used for determining risk and their risk point limits taking into account either the probabilities of random assignments (R) for answers rated as correct or the empirical distribution (D)

Domain	Screening task	Number of items	Variable rated	Number (N), mean (M), and standard deviation (s) for the total sample			Risk point limit and method of determination
				N	M	s	
Phonological awareness in a broad sense	Recognition of rhyming word pairs	10	Correct decision	1120	8.32	1.85	< 7 (R)
	Syllable segmentation	10	Correct pronunciation	1116	7.79	2.37	< 7 (R)
Phonological awareness in a narrow sense	Phoneme-word matching (initial phoneme)	10	Correct decision	1114	7.86	2.05	< 7 (R)
	Phoneme blending (with picture)	10	Correct decision	1120	4.68	1.96	< 7 (R)
			Decision with same vowel	1120	8.88	1.32	
Phonetic recoding	Repeating pseudowords	10	Correct repetition	1115	6.12	2.11	< 4 (D)
Attention to visual sequences of symbols	Word matching	12	Identical alternative 75-100%	1120	8.53	2.86	< 8 (R)
			identical alternative Median processing time (averaged)	1120	10.13	2.06	< 3.76 (D)
				1118	7.41	3.88	

Tab. 1/Continued

Domain	Screening task	Number of items	Variable rated	Number (N), mean (M), and standard deviation (s) for the total sample			Risk point limit and method of determination
				N	M	s	
Lexical recoding speed	Rapid naming of the colors of objects	24	Uncorrected error	1104	0.47	1.59	
			Naming time 1	1102	50.59	19.58	> 63 (D)
Distraction or interference	Rapid naming of the colors of color-incongruent objects	24	Uncorrected error	1092	1.08	2.99	
			Naming time 2	1085	78.68	29.44	
			Naming time difference 2-1	1084	28.68	19.68	> 40 (D)
Memory for object attributes	Knowledge of object colors	8	Correct naming	1104	7.88	0.57	< 7 (D)
Knowledge of written symbols	Naming letters/ numbers	25	Correct naming of letters/ phones (without "o")	1118	4.19	6.06	
		9	Correct naming of numbers (1-9)	1118	6.32	3.07	

2.3.1   Assessment of Different Aspects of Phonological Processing

Alongside the acquisition of grapheme–phoneme pairs, the phonological segmentation, combination, and short–term retention of acoustically received or
self–produced sound elements or units belong to the skills that are constantly
required in both reading and writing after the pseudoadaptive (cf. Marx, 1985)
or logographic (cf. Frith, 1985) phase of reading. Each of the tasks described
below tests single aspects of these skills in the auditory domain.

Phonological awareness in a broad sense

Tasks that require the ability to cope with the phonetic aspects of spoken language (e.g., recognizing rhyming word pairs) are labeled phonological awareness tasks in a broad sense in the following. As a rule, the demands of these
tasks relate to language performances that are contained in concrete game
sequences with which the child is familiar.

The recognition of rhyming word pairs
This task stresses the aspect of reception and in contrast to Bradley and
Bryant's (1983, 1985) "sound categorization" only requires one form of categorization, thus greatly reducing memory load. Pairs of words are spoken out
loud to the child (e.g., *boat − coat* or *boat − chair*), and the child has to
decide whether the endings of the two words in a pair rhyme. The number of
correct solutions is recorded. In addition, guessing strategies can be analyzed
from the response tendencies.

Syllable segmentation
This task requires a production performance. A series of nouns is spoken out
loud to the child (e.g., *basket* or *shuttlecock*). The child has to break these
words down into syllables with the help of hand clapping. Only the child's oral
pronounciation is evaluated. In addition to the correct/incorrect rating in
completely correct segmentations, it can be seen whether the child knows how
to separate speech rhythm from meaning - particularly in critical, three − syllable nouns that are made up of two semantic units.

Phonological awareness in a narrow sense

Speech performance in which it is necessary to operate explicitly with phonological structures that show neither semantic nor speech–rhythmic references, are labeled phonological awareness tasks in a narrow sense.

Phoneme–word matching

As in the recognition of rhyming word pairs, this task stresses speech reception. The child has to decide whether an isolated vowel that is spoken out loud sounds the same as a vowel that is placed at the beginning of a semantically meaningful word (e.g., "Can you hear an /i/ in *Igel* ?" or "Can you hear an /i/ in *Auto* ?"). As in the categorization of alliteration in Bradley and Bryant (1983, 1985), the beginning of the word becomes the critical decision area in phoneme–word matching. However, in our case, the comparison is more simple in that a single vowel phoneme has to be related to a syllabic vowel of a word. The number of correct decisions is recorded.

Phoneme blending

This requires a production performance. In contrast to syllable segmentation, in which the child has to break up words into speech units, this task demands an abstract blending of artificially separated auditorily presented words (e.g., *Zange* as /ts/ − /ange/) into meaningful complete words. In order to facilitate this abstract performance, or even to render it first possible, four picture alternatives are presented for each item (e.g., *Zange, Pinsel, Zebra, Schlange*). These show two possible alternatives to the correct answer in which either the first (*Z–ebra*) or second (*Schl–ange*) element agrees with the test item. The third, incorrect alternative if correctly named (*Pinsel*) possesses no phonetic similarity to the auditorily presented sequence of phonemes. The child's task is to assemble the phonetic units to form a word and point out the correct picture alternative. Only the spoken series of phonemes is rated. In addition to a correct/incorrect evaluation, it is also possible to make a graded evaluation according to the phonetic similarity.

Phonetic recoding in short–term memory

To assess phonetic recoding for the retention of information in short–term or working memory, most research uses the memory span for lists of words,

numbers, or letters (cf. Baddeley, 1986; Wagner and Torgesen, 1987) or articulation speed in repeated utterances or loud reading of words (cf. Vallar and
Baddeley, 1982; Wagner, Balthazor, Hurley, Morgan, Rashotte, Shaner, Simmons, and Stage, 1987). A further possibility of measuring phonological
processing within this field is introduced with the task used here: repeating
pseudowords. This task is related to studies on the effect of word length (e.g.,
Baddeley, Thomson, and Buchanan, 1975; Baddeley, Lewis, and Vallar, 1984).

Repeating pseudowords
This task requires the short–term retention and recall of series of syllables of
varying length that are joined together to form a pseudoword (e.g., *zippelzak* or
bunitkonos). First of all, it tests memory span, but second, the precision in
articulating unknown terms. The ten items were selected from Predictor Probe
2 (a group of items for testing auditive differentiation performance and motoric
speech coordination taken from Tiedemann, Faber, and Kahra, 1985). A criticism of this task is that acoustic misunderstandings can occur as early as stimulus encoding, and these can be taken over in the articulatory loop in the phonological coding. Although, according to Baddeley (1986), it is the articulatory
coding and not the phonetic similarity that is responsible for the phonological
misinterpretation, because of the unfamiliarity of the pseudowords it cannot be
ruled out that incorrect performances are due to both difficulties in stimulus
encoding and/or are due to the repetition. The assessment is limited to counting
the completely correct repetitions.

2.3.2   Determining Different Aspects of Attention and Access to Memory

Particularly in the initial phase of learning to read, it is important for the child
to learn to discriminate between relevant and irrelevant information in the
written material (Marx, 1985) and apply its resources with controlled attention.
The child must internalize the spatio–temporal structure of written language by
painstakingly checking the position and number of letters as well as whether
they are written in upper or lower case. Single grapheme–phoneme combinations and possibly also written form–word combinations must additionally be
automatized and rapidly recalled during a corresponding stimulus presentation,
and interfering information should have as little influence as possible.

Attention to visual sequences of symbols

A first clue as to how preschool children use their resources is provided by assessing the precision with which the children attend and process unfamiliar sequences of symbols that vary in their ease of discrimination. In this task, which is performed without time restrictions, the quality of the solutions is essentially decided by the application of resources. More difficult tasks can be solved just as well as easier ones through a correspondingly higher application. If, in contrast, the test phase is held constant independent of the difficulty of the task, or only a limited amount of information is attended to, then incorrect decisions are made (cf. Norman and Bobrow, 1975).

Word matching task
In this task, the child is presented with a series of small cards one at a time. A four-letter, meaningful word (standard) is printed in the middle of the upper half of each card, and four meaningful words (alternatives) are presented, clearly separated, in a row in the middle of the lower half. The alternatives have either 100, 75, 50, or 25% agreement with the standard with regard to the letters and their position (e.g., *Bein — Bein/ Wein/ Garn/ Ruin*). Each standard is presented four times with the same alternatives placed in a different one of the four possible positions. The child's task is to look for the alternative that is identical to the standard and point to it. The child can perform the task at the speed of its choice. A recording is made first of the number of correct choices and second of the reaction time to the first answer (using a stopwatch rounded off to the nearest one-tenth of a second). When an alternative is chosen, it can be seen whether attention has been paid to the internal structure of the sequences of symbols, and whether the position was significant for the correct solution from the row of alternatives. Taking the quality of performance into account, the reaction time informs whether and for how long a child is prepared to pay attention to written symbols. To some extent, it is also possible to deduce test strategies.

Memory for attributes

According to the phonological coding hypothesis (Vellutino and Scanlon, 1987, Experiment 2), problems in naming can be traced back to weak representations of phoneme attributes of a name that is associated with the visual stimulus. The testing of typical colors of objects from memory offers a good way of determining how well and precisely children have stored specific attributes of well-known objects as belonging to the object, and whether — in a mostly automatic form — these are available to them.

Knowledge of object colors
First, a pretest is given to see whether the child can at least repeat without mistakes the names of objects (lettuce, plum, lemon, tomato), which are spoken out loud once and presented as colored drawings in their typical colors, and whether the child can afterwards name the color of the objects unaided. Then the colored drawings are covered up, and the children are twice (before and after the presentation of the rapid naming of the colors of objects) asked to name the colors of the four objects ("What is the color of a ... lettuce/plum/lemon/tomato?"). The number of correct namings of colors in both memory tests is recorded. With children who have initial problems with the classification of colors, it can be assumed that they are at least able to use their short–term store adequately if the memory recall is correct.

Lexical recoding speed

Poor readers cannot recall the names of objects or colors as quickly as good readers (Denckla and Rudel, 1976; Wolf, 1984, 1986; Blachman, 1984). However, this in no way applies generally (Perfetti, Finger, and Hogaboam, 1978; Stanovich, 1981; Stanovich, Feeman, and Cunningham, 1983).

Rapid naming of the colors of objects from uncolored line drawings.
This task, in contrast to studies that test the recoding from and to lexical memory, does not test the name of a directly present object or feature, but tests a feature that can only be recalled through the correct recognition of the form of the object. The child's task is to report as quickly as possible the correct colors of objects on a DIN–A4 answer sheet with seven lines for each of four objects. A stopwatch (rounded off to the nearest second) is used to measure the time after the first line, which is withheld from analysis as a practice trial, and ends with the child's last naming of a color. In addition, all uncorrected false namings of colors and the number of colors named by the experimenter, which are always given if the color response is withheld for more than 5 seconds, are recorded. The rapid naming of colors of objects presented as black and white

line drawings provides information on the speed of access to lexical memory as long as the color classifications have not already been learnt during the practice trials. At the same time, this task serves as a control test for the next task.

Distraction of attention or interference

For the rapid recall of information from memory it is also decisive whether and how the child deals in a given situation with the irrelevant stimulus information in which the relevant information to be processed is embedded (cf. Ackermann, 1986). More or less marked distraction effects occur when the processing of interfering stimuli cannot be avoided because of their spatial arrangement or semantic closeness (Stroop, 1935; Neumann, 1980), or are not avoided because of their subjective importance (Odom, Cunningham, and Astor-Stetson, 1977; Rosenthal and Allen, 1980).

Rapid naming of the correct colors of objects with incongruent colors.
In this table, the child also has to recall the correct color of the object from memory, and additionally ignore the presented color that does not belong to the object. Therefore the child has to dismiss a stimulus that is directly available, belongs to the response category, and is relevant to the task, and attend to the color that corresponds to the presented form. The procedure and evaluation of this task is the same as in the rapid naming of the colors of objects. The differences in the number of mistakes and processing time between the inter-ference condition and the control condition without color distraction particularly provide information on the type and extent of distraction of attention.

Knowledge of Written Symbols as a Control Variable

Although many authors include the knowledge of letters as one of the best predictors of reading and writing achievement, we use it as only a single and additionally very weak indicator for the knowledge of written language.

Naming of letters/numbers

The children are presented with a table on which all the letters of the alphabet and the numbers 1 to 9 are presented in a random sequence. They have to name all the symbols that they know. The number of correct namings of letters or phones and numbers is recorded. Further analysis could consider the mistakes on a vowel versus consonant basis.

2.4   Screening Procedure

The Bielefeld Screening Battery was performed twice with an interval of almost 6 months. The assessments at Timepoint 1 were carried out in 84 of the 107 kindergartens in Bielefeld by 20 trained experimenters between October and December 1986. The assessments at Timepoint 2 took place between March and May 1987 in the same institutions, but each experimenter was sent to a different institution in order to avoid experimenter effects. Two subsamples from the original sample participated in the second assessment. The tests consisted of four sessions per child in which the first session was a repetition of the Bielefeld Screening Battery.

The sequence of the single tasks was arranged so that all the acoustically presented tasks using a cassette recorder were interspersed with visual tasks whenever possible. The experimenter used practice items to explain each task to the child. (If the items were presented with a cassette recorder, then at least the last practice item was played through the cassette recorder). Positive feedback and repetitions of the instructions and/or single items were restricted to the practice phases. The first answer to the test items was noted in each task, and no feedback was given. Only in syllable segmentation did the children have to repeat their responses if there was an incongruence between hand–clapping and voicing syllables. In such cases, the experimenter should only pay attention to oral pronounciation.

3.   First Findings and Discussion

3.1   The Original Sample

Description. After sending requests to over 1,800 guardians, we obtained permission for 1,214 children to participate in our study. From 1,168 children who were accessible during the period of the study, 48 had to be excluded from the analysis for various reasons (e.g., passing the age limit, speech and testing problems). The average age of the 1,120 children subjected to analysis was 70.06 months ($s = 3.69$); 558 were boys and 562 were girls. German was not the mother tongue in 86 children (7.7%) (particulary Turkish children and children of emigrants from Eastern Europe).

Representativity. One goal of the first assessment was to obtain the largest possible and, at the same time, a representative original sample. The high participation of kindergartens (78.5%) and their fairly even distribution across the sponsors of the institutions and the social geography of Bielefeld permit an initial positive conclusion on the representativity of the original sample. To test the hypothesis of a positive or negative selection, especially in the kindergartens with a participation rate of less than 50%, we formed four groups of different participation rates (up to 50%, from 51 to 67%, from 68 to 84%, and above 84%) and compared their performance on the dependent variables in the screening. The totally nonsignificant differences between the groups exclude systematic selection effects and can be assessed as an empirical support for the representativity of the original sample.

Performance. Tab. 1 presents the original sample's scores on the dependent variables in the screening battery. It is noticeable that the distributions in the measures of phonological awareness in a broad sense are skewed to the right and indicate ceiling effects that can also be seen in the scores in phoneme–word matching (cf. also the maximum frequencies in Tab. 3). Marked shifts in the means to the upper third of performance can also be seen in the task repeating pseudowords, the word matching task (identical decision), and in the knowledge of object colors. In the latter, however, 16 children were not taken into account because they had such enormous difficulties in naming colors that the task was broken off. Whereas phoneme blending was clearly the hardest task among the phonological tasks despite the assistance of pictures, the low number of uncorrected namings of false colors in both presentations and the high number of correct solutions in the word matching show that children in this age group were able to direct their attention adequately when the presentation of the tasks gave them unlimited processing time and material. However, they could not cope if — as in the case of phoneme blending – they had to make a forced choice because of either the subjective importance of the pictorial distractor (cf. Odom et al., 1977), the restricted time available in a tape–recorded presentation, and/or simply because of a restriction of resources (a lack of the preconditions for solution).

The children's poor performance in color recognition, the increases in mistakes in processing the incongruent object table, and the marked fluctuations in processing times or the above–mentioned skewed distributions of phonological measurements can be conceived as a confirmation of Construction Principle 4 (Creation of differentiation possibilities in the lower third of the sample). In each screening task, a number of children could not cope with the demands placed on them and/or the highly structured test situation (e.g., dissenters). (It should be noted that the reasons for the discrepancies in the number of subjects in the precision and speed parameters in the word matching task were technical (the stopwatch was broken), while the discrepancies in rapid naming were due to the content. When a child named all objects with, for example, only one or with random color names, the time taken was regarded as an inadequate attempt to solve the task and was subsequently dropped from analysis.)

The, on average, very slight knowledge of anything more than four letters — for example, naming letters in an upper case alphabet (median = 2.0!) — is in marked contrast to the findings in Anglo–American literature (cf. Share et al., 1984; Ehri and Wilce, 1987; Vellutino and Scanlon, 1987). This low level of knowledge can be evaluated as an indication that the performances in the phonological awareness tasks were not confounded with preschool reading experience (cf. Wagner and Torgesen, 1987) in the majority of the children.

3.2   Selecting the Subsamples

Our goal was to select a subsample from the original sample that was of man-ageable size for the longitudinal study but remained representative. The size of the original sample and the apparent lack of selection effects permitted the selection of a representative subsample from our original sample. Because of limited resources, we restricted ourselves to a selection rate of about 15%. Taking into account the age and sex distribution, 171 preschool children were randomly placed in the representative subsample.

A further subsample was assembled from the remainder of the total sample by using an initially purely statistical cut–off to select subjects with scores in the lower 15% range. Tab. 1 presents the means and standard deviations of all the variables used to determine risk as well as the cut–off scores for setting the risk point limits; these were either based on probability theory or empirically calculated. The performance of the children shows that the construction princi-ples of the screening battery could not be realized on the task level in all the tests. It was necessary to make changes in the analysis so that we could use all the phonological awareness tasks in a narrow sense in addition to the phonological awareness tasks in a broad sense that appeared to permit a differentiation in the lower area. Construction Principle 6 was used in the case of phoneme blending. A differentiation could be achieved here by lowering the requirements for a correct solution (the naming of an alternative containing the same auditorily presented vowel was rated as a correct response).

Every uncompleted or inadequately completed task was also rated with a risk point. Through the type of task situation or the lowering in the demands, all the phonological awareness tasks as well as the number of solutions accepted as correct in the word matching task were restricted to the narrow area between the random probability of success and the ceiling effect. In the timed measurements and the phonetic recoding, the cut–off was set according to the empirically found distributions.

All preschool children who were beyond the risk point cut–off in four or more dependent variables in different fields –taking into account the 15% border of problem cases that can be anticipated — were labeled as children at risk. In addition, through calculating discriminant analyses with the empirically anticipated basis rate of 15:85, all the children who belonged to the bottom 15% of the sample according to the discriminant function but were not labeled risk children were placed in the risk sample as borderline cases. In this way, 169 children from the remainder of the total sample were labeled either risk cases or borderline risk cases.

3.3   Starting Point for the Prediction and Changes in Performance that are not Due to the Effects of Schooling

These 169 subjects combined with the 35 risk or borderline risk cases in the representative subsample formed the starting point for the prediction. Under the admittedly criterion–dependent assumption of a roughly 15% incidence of reading and writing difficulties, problems should occur in 15% of our representative sample and in all the children in our risk sample. We will be able to report on the sensitivity and specificity of our risk prediction at a later timepoint.

Tab. 2: Comparison of changes in performance in the variables used to determine risk in the screening procedure at the two testing timepoints (N = number, M = mean, s = standard deviation) in the representative sample (R) and the risk sample (P)

| Screening task | Variable rated | Sample | Scores of changes in performance | | | | | t-Test | |
| | | | Testpoint 1 | | | Testpoint 2 | | | |
			N	M	s	M	s	t	p<
Recognition of rhyming word pairs	Correct decision	R	136	8.51	1.65	9.09	1.28	-4.91	0.001
		P	104	6.37	2.22	8.00	1.76	-7.36	0.001
Syllable segmentation	Correct pronunciation	R	133	8.02	2.40	8.21	2.19	-0.87	n.s.
		P	103	6.15	3.14	6.97	2.76	-2.43	0.05
Phoneme-word matching (initial phoneme)	Correct decision	R	133	7.98	2.04	9.02	1.53	-6.94	0.001
		P	102	5.97	2.06	7.47	2.06	-6.41	0.001
Phoneme blending (with picture)	Decision with same vowel	R	136	9.04	1.26	9.04	1.46	0.00	n.s.
		P	104	7.84	1.81	8.75	1.28	-4.47	0.001
Repeating pseudowords	Correct repetition	R	136	6.17	2.06	6.76	1.94	-3.73	0.001
		P	104	4.72	2.40	5.94	2.34	-6.63	0.001
Word matching	75-100% identical alternative	R	136	10.31	1.94	10.76	2.02	-2.35	0.05
		P	104	7.95	2.37	9.13	2.29	-4.90	0.001
	Median processing time (averaged)	R	135	7.62	4.11	8.04	3.65	-1.05	n.s.
		P	103	5.51	3.28	6.22	3.40	-2.03	0.05
Rapid naming of the colors of objects	Naming time 1	R	134	49.10	17.50	41.40	13.53	6.63	0.001
		P	95	72.14	29.92	57.80	23.45	5.70	0.001
Rapid naming of the colors of color-incongruent objects	Naming time difference 2-1	R	130	28.82	20.57	20.64	14.19	4.33	0.001
		P	87	42.54	29.75	28.55	22.71	3.78	0.001
Knowledge of object colors	Correct naming	R	133	7.94	0.39	7.92	0.60	0.37	n.s.
		P	98	7.37	1.30	7.70	0.97	-3.02	0.01

The mean increments in performance when the screening battery was repeated with 136 representative and 104 risk children are presented in Tab. 2 split for the different performances on the screening variables used to determine risk at the two testing timepoints. It is first noticeable that the mortality rate of 20.5% in the representative group was much lower than in the risk group (38.5%). Appropriate mean and variance comparisons showed that this reduction had no effect on either the representativity of the representative sample or on the variance in the risk sample. Nevertheless, it was noticeable that the parents of non–German children in both subsamples particularly failed to return the necessary signed forms granting permission for their children's participation. It was no longer possible to perform a separate analysis of these subgroups as originally planned. This response could be due to the different modes of approach at the two testing timepoints (over kindergarten supervisors at the first postal request at the second timepoint).

According to Construction Principle 7 of the screening procedure, the scores and type of processing in the single tasks should also reflect developments over time. Tab. 3 shows the absolute frequencies of improvements or deteriorations in performance in the single test procedures. The differences in performance observed over a period of almost 6 months were significant except for a few variables that were only found in the representative group. As, apart from the familiarity with the test material, the long interval between testing, the different experimenters, and the lack of feedback during the test tend to indicate negligible retesting effects, it would appear that the differential changes in development can be portrayed with the screening battery. In the risk sample, these, indeed, all took the direction of a quantitative improvement in performance. However, when it is considered that the attribution of risk was made according to a random criterion in some tasks (cf. Tab. 1), in a large number of the children the shifts in performance in precisely these tasks could indicate qualitative changes (e.g., turning away from guessing strategies) compared to the strategy adopted in the first testing. As well as quantitative, qualitative changes in performance also appeared to have occured in the representative sample. The high percentage of children who performed worse is notable in the nonsignificant changes in performance in syllable segmentation and in a weaker form in phoneme blending.

Tab. 3: Frequency comparison across the numbers of children of the representative sample (R), and the risk sample (P) with worse (−), better (+), or equal (=) raw scores at Testpoint 2 compared to Testpoint 1. The number of children with maximum raw scores (M) at both testpoints is given in brackets (df = 2)

Screening task	Variable rated	Sample	Frequency and direction of changes (maximum at both testpoints)				Frequency comparison	
			−	=	+	(M)	chi²	p<
Recognition of rhyming word pairs	Correct decision	R	15	21	57	(43)	2.85	n.s.
		P	17	13	68	(6)		
Syllable segmentation	Correct pronounciation	R	48	8	45	(32)	2.24	n.s.
		P	34	8	50	(12)		
Phoneme-word matching (initial phoneme)	Correct decision	R	17	9	75	(32)	3.06	n.s.
		P	20	15	61	(6)		
Phoneme blending (with picture)	Decision with same vowel	R	29	20	36	(51)	4.04	n.s.
		P	22	19	54	(9)		
Repeating pseudowords	Correct repetition	R	40	26	68	(2)	5.10	n.s.
		P	18	22	64	(0)		
Word matching	75-100% identical alternative	R	30	8	60	(38)	2.94	n.s.
		P	22	14	63	(5)		
	Median processing time (averaged)	R	46	25	64	(0)	1.75	n.s.
		P	33	13	55	(2)		
Rapid naming of the colors of objects	Naming time 1	R	14	51	57	(14)	2.72	n.s.
		P	9	35	60	(0)		
Rapid naming of the colors of color-incongruent objects	Naming time difference 2-1	R	24	34	55	(17)	4.30	n.s.
		P	16	15	51	(5)		
Knowledge of object colors	Correct naming	R	3	0	3	(127)	--	--
		P	5	3	21	(69)		

Alongside special experimenter effects (no child had the same experimenter at both testing timepoints), a new orientation toward other characteristics could be responsible for this developmental change in the wrong direction. The worse performers could have recognized the limitations of the most obvious solutions (such as paying attention to vowels or imitation of the clapping rhythm) in the between-test interval and tested new or different solution alternatives. Whether this assumption is true or not remains to be tested. Ceiling effects could — as Tab. 3 clarifies — be drawn upon to explain the findings in the knowledge of object colors screening task.

Such differential effects in a representative and a risk sample that, after only half a year, have already led to both quantitative and qualitative changes in predictive power without any directed intervention clarify the importance of the testing timepoint (cf. Lichtenstein and Ireton, 1984) and above all repeated testing for an estimation and evaluation of the risk classification in addition to the selection and analysis of the tasks. Whereas this aspect remains ignored in many longitudinal studies, we are in a position to show individual developments in performance in the predictors and estimate their contribution to the precision of the prediction. The further testing and intervention timepoints that are planned within the framework of this longitudinal study will then provide information on whether and at what timepoint the use of the screening procedure is more suitable for the prediction of difficulties in reading and writing.

References

Ackerman, B.P. (1986): The relation between attention to the incidental context and memory for words in children and adults. Journal of Experimental Child Psychology, 41, 149–183

Angermaier, M. (1977): Legasthenie — Pro und Contra. Weinheim: Beltz

Baddeley, A.D. (1986): Working Memory. Oxford: Clarendon Press

Baddeley, A.D., Lewis, V.J., and Vallar, G. (1984): Exploring the articulatory loop. Quarterly Journal of Experimental Psychology, 36, 233–252

Baddeley, A.D., Thomson, N., and Buchanan, M. (1975): Word length and the structure of short term memory. Journal of Verbal Learning and Verbal Behavior, 14, 575–589

Badian, N.A. (1982): The prediction of good and poor reading before Kindergarten entry: A four-year follow-up. The Journal of Special Education, 16, 309–318

Badian, N.A. (1986): Improving the prediction of reading for the individual child: A four-year follow-up. Journal of Learning Disabilities, 19, 262–269

Blachman, B.A. (1984): Relationship of rapid naming ability and language analysis skills to Kindergarten and first-grade reading achievement. Journal of Educational Psychology, 76, 610–622

Bosch, B. (1937): Grundlagen des Erstleseunterrichts. Leipzig: Barth

Bradley, L., and Bryant, P.E. (1983): Categorizing sounds and learning to read – a causal connection. Nature, 301, 419–421

Bradley, L., and Bryant, P.E. (1985): Rhyme and Reason in Reading and Spelling. Ann Arbor: University of Michigan Press

Butler, S.R. (1979): Predictive antecedents of reading disability in the early years of schooling. British Columbia Journal of Special Education, 3, 263–274

Butler, S.R., Marsh, H.W., Sheppard, M.J., and Sheppard, J.L. (1985): Seven-year longitudinal study of the early prediction of reading achievement. Journal of Educational Psychology, 79, 349–361

Deutsche Forschungsgemeinschaft (1978): Zur Lage der Legasthenieforschung. Mitteilung/ Kommission für Erziehungswissenschaft; 1. Boppard: Boldt

Denckla, M.B., and Rudel, R.G. (1976): Rapid "automatized" naming (R.A.N.). Dyslexia differentiated from other learning disabilities. Neuropsychologia, 14, 471–479

Edler, M., Ostrau, R., and Schulze, K. (1977): Rechtschreibtraining mit Legasthenikern. Unpublished master's thesis, University of Bochum Ehri, L.C., and Wilce, L.S. (1987): Cipher versus cue reading: An experiment in decoding acquisition. Journal of Educational Psychology, 79, 3–13

Elkind, D., Larson, M., and Doorninck, W. (1965): Perceptual decentration learning and performance in slow and average readers. Journal of Educational Psychology, 56, 50–56

Frith, U. (1985): Beneath the surface of developmental dyslexia. In: Patterson, K.E., Marshall, J.L., and Coltheart, U. (Eds.): Surface dyslexia. London: Erlbaum, 301–330

Frostig, M. (1972): Programm zum Training der visuellen Wahrnehmung (Deutsche Bearbeitung von Reinartz). Dortmund

Kagan, J. (1965): Reflection-impulsivity and reading ability in primary grade children. Child Development, 36, 609–628

Kavanagh, J.F., and Mattingly, J.G. (1972): Language by ear and by eye – The relationship between speech and reading. Cambridge (Massachusetts), London: MIT Press

Kolers, P. (1970): Three stages of reading. In: Levin, H., and Williams, J. (Eds.): Basic studies in reading. New York: Basic Books, 90–118

Lichtenstein, R., and Ireton, H. (1984): Preschool screening identifying young children with developmental and educational problems. Orlando: Grune & Stratton

Lindgren, S.D. (1978): Finger localization and the prediction of reading disability. Cortex, 14, 87–101

Lundberg, I., Olofsson, A., and Wall, S. (1980): Reading and spelling skills in the first school year predicted from phonemic awareness skills in kindergarten. Scandinavian Journal of Psychology, 21, 159–173

Mann, V.A., Tobin, P., and Wilson, R. (1987): Measuring phonological awareness through the invented spelling of Kindergarten children. Merrill-Palmer Quarterly, 33, 365–391

Mannhaupt, G., and Jansen, H. (in press): Phonologische Bewußtheit: Aufgabenentwicklung und Leistungen im Vorschulalter. Heilpädagogische Forschung

Marx, H. (1985): Aufmerksamkeitsverhalten und Leseschwierigkeiten. Weinheim: VCH und Göttingen: Hogrefe

Mattingly, I.G. (1972): Reading, the linguistic process and linguistic awareness. In: Kavanagh, J., and Mattingly, I. (Eds.): Language by Ear and by Eye. Cambridge, Mass.: MIT Press, 133–147

Morais, J., Carey, L., Alegria, J., and Bertelson, P. (1979): Does awareness of speech as a sequence of phonemes arise spontaneously? Cognition, 7, 323–331

Morais, J., Alegria, J., and Content, A. (1987): The relationship between segmental analysis and alphabetic literacy: An interactive view. Cahiers de Psychologie Cognitive. European Bulletin of Cognitive Psychology 7, 415–438

Neumann, O. (1980): Informationsselektion und Handlungssteuerung. Untersuchungen zur Funktionsgrundlage des Stroop-Interferenzphänomens. Unpublished dissertation, University of Bochum

Norman, D.A., and Bobrow, D.G. (1975): On data limited and resource limited processes. Cognitive Psychology, 7, 44–64

Odom, R.D., Cunningham, J.G., and Astor-Stetson, E. (1977): The role of perceptual salience and type of instruction in children's recall of relevant and incidental dimensional values. Bulletin of Psychonomic Society, 9, 77–80

Perfetti, C., and McCutchen, D. (1982): Speech processes in reading. In: Lass, N. (Ed.): Speech and Language: Advances in Basic Research and Practice. New York: Academic Press, 237–269

Perfetti, C.A., Finger, E., and Hogaboam, T. (1978): Sources of vocalization latency differences between skilled and less skilled young readers. Journal of Educational Psychology, 70, 730–739

Reber, A.S., and Scarborough, D.L. (1977): Toward a psychology of reading. The proceedings of the CUNY Conferences. Hillsdale: Erlbaum

Rosenthal, R.H., and Allen, T.W. (1980): Intratask distractibility in hyperkinetic and non-hyperkinetic children. Journal of Abnormal Child Psychology, 8, 175–187

Rourke, B.P., and Orr, R.R. (1977): Prediction of the reading and spelling performances of normal and retarded readers: A four-year follow-up. Journal of Abnormal Child Psychology, 5, 9–20

Satz, P., and Friel, J. (1978): Predictive validity of an abbreviated screening battery. Journal of Learning Disabilities, 11, 20–24

Satz, P., Friel, J., and Goebel, R.A. (1975): Some predictive antecedents of specific reading disability: A three-year follow-up. Bulletin of the Orton Society, 25, 91–110

Share, D.L., Jorm, A.F., Maclean, R., and Matthews, R. (1984): Sources of individual differences in reading acquisition. Journal of Educational Psychology, 76, 1309–1324

Stanovich, K. (1981): Relationships between word decoding speed, general name retrieval ability, and reading progress in first-grade children. Journal of Educational Psychology, 73, 800–815

Stanovich, K., Feeman, D., and Cunningham, A. (1983): The development of the relation between letter naming speed and reading ability. Bulletin of the Psychonomic Society, 21, 199–202

Stroop, J.R. (1935): Studies of interference in serial verbal reactions. Journal of Experimental Psychology, 18, 643–661

Tiedemann, J., Faber, G., and Kahra, G. (1985): Ausgewählte Frühindikatoren schulischer Lernschwierigkeiten − Lernvoraussetzungen des Erstunterrichts. Psychologie in Erziehung und Unterricht, 32, 93–99

Treiman, R. (1987): On the relationship between phonological awareness and literacy. Cahiers de Psychologie Cognitive. European Bulletin of Cognitive Psychology, 7, 524–529

Vallar, G., and Baddeley, A.D. (1982): Short-term forgetting and the articulatory loop. Quarterly Journal of Experimental Psychology, 34, 53–60

Vellutino, F. (1979): Dyslexia: Theory and Research. Cambridge, Mass.: MIT Press

Vellutino, F.R., and Scanlon, D.M. (1987): Phonological coding, phonological awareness, and reading ability: Evidence from a longitudinal and experimental study. Merrill-Palmer Quarterly, 33, 321–363

Vernon, M.D. (1957): Backwardness in Reading. Cambridge: University Press

Wagner, I. (1976): Aufmerksamkeitstraining mit impulsiven Kindern. Stuttgart: Klett

Wagner, R.K., and Torgesen, J.K. (1987): The nature of phonological processing and its causal role in the acquisition of reading skills. Psychological Bulletin, 101, 192–212

Wagner, R., Balthazor, M., Hurley, S., Morgan, S., Rashotte, C., Shaner, R., Simmons, K., and Stage, S. (1987): The nature of prereaders' phonological processing abilities. Cognitive Development, 2, 355–373

Wendeler, J. (1986): Prognose der Lese-Rechtschreibschwäche. Psychologie in Erziehung und Unterricht, 33, 10–16

White, M., Batini, P., Satz, P., and Friel, J. (1979): Predictive validity of a screening battery for children "at risk" for reading failure. British Journal of Educational Psychology, 49, 132–137

Wolf, M. (1984): Naming, reading, and the dyslexias: A longitudinal overview. Analysis of dyslexia, 34, 87–115

Wolf, M. (1986): Rapid alternating stimulus naming in the developmental dyslexia. Brain and Language, 27, 360–379

Language Development and Delays and the Predictors of Later Reading Failure

Jim Stevenson

1. Introduction

The link between initial language acquisition and reading ability has been explored in a number of different ways. These include (1) the study of the current language skills of children with reading problems, (2) the retrospective study of the early development of children with reading difficulties, and (3) the follow–up study of the later educational progress of children with initially delayed language development. Each of these approaches will be considered, and the implications for the planning of preventive services for children will be drawn, concentrating on their significance for the screening for children at risk of later reading difficulties.

In exploring the links between the two, it is usually assumed that the development of language and the development of literacy will be closely associated. This may have a superficial attractiveness, since the two systems have the same linguistic base. However, of course the learning of reading requires the association of a visual stimulus with an existing language system. This makes different demands from the initial acquisition of the language system itself. So although strongly linked, learning to read is more than a simple re–rehearsal of a previously undertaken learning task. There will therefore be alternative sources of difficulty, and some children may well find one task more difficult than the other. Not all children who found initial language acquisition problematic will have difficulties in learning to read, nor will all children who find reading problematic have had earlier language delays.

Throughout this chapter, attention will be paid to children with language delays and not necessarily to those with speech problems. Of course these problems often coexist, and any one child might suffer from multicommunication handicaps, for example, a combination of disarrthria, phonological disorder, and syntactic immaturity are not uncommonly found together (Crystal et al., 1976).

However, it has been repeatedly found that when language rather than speech problems are present, the prognosis is worse; both for later language based skills, such as reading, and for a wider range of educationally related problems (Hall and Tomblin, 1978).

2. Current Language Skills of Children with Reading Problems

There has been considerable research interest in this topic over the past decade. In two recent review papers by Wagner (1986) and Wagner and Torgesen (1987), the case has been made that at root the language problems of reading-disabled children center on phonological processing abilities. Deficits have been found in their phonological awareness (e.g., on tasks requiring blending or segmenting phonemes, and rhymes), phonological recoding in lexical access (e.g., in reading pseudowords), and in phonetic recoding in working memory (e.g., memory span for phonemically confusable letter names − B,C,D,G). It is of interest to note that one of the mechanisms suggested by Tallal et al. (1980) for the link between early language delay and reading difficulties is continuing deficits in the use of phonemic categories.

Some theorists have made a strong case for reading–disabled children's language difficulties being accounted for by a single dimension of phonological processing efficiency (Bradley and Bryant, 1985). It is important to note that this is a relatively specific deficit not attributable to general intelligence (Wagner and Torgesen, 1987). If this single dimension accounts for the language–based difficulties of children with reading failure, it could provide a key for preventive intervention. For example, Bradley and Bryant (1985) found that the correlation between reading achievement at 7–8 years and sound categorisation at 4 years was about +0.55. When IQ, age, and general memory abilities were controlled, sound categorisation still accounted for a unique 10% of the variance in reading scores.

It might be supposed that if children were screened for phonological processing abilities in the preschool period this would identify a group of children for whom intervention would be most beneficial. However as Bryant (1985) has shown there are difficulties with this approach. He identified children with scores on a sound categorisation task that were more than one standard deviation away from the mean. Of those in the extreme group below the mean, only about 25% were significantly underachieving in reading some 4 years later. Bryant concluded that since prediction at the individual level was so poor (i.e., over 75% of the poor readers would not be showing phonological awareness difficulties at age 4 years), screening for an at-risk group was not appropriate. Instead, the universal adoption of sound categorization training to all preschoolers may be the most effective way to prevent later reading difficulties.

This suggestion is of course premised on the notion that such phonological skills are trainable. Bradley and Bryant (1985) have claimed some success in this respect, but Wagner (1986) is more cautious, suggesting that "it is too soon to draw conclusions about the effects of training phonological abilities especially for poor readers". Ingvar Lundberg (1987) has provided further evidence that such a training programme made available to all children before school can indeed improve reading and spelling in the first years of school. Lundberg has gone on to demonstrate that the number of children with reading problems is also reduced by phonological awareness training. This study reinforces the view that "training for all" is a feasible approach to the problem of preventing difficulties in early reading development.

3. The Retrosprective Analysis of the Early Language Development of Children with Reading Difficulties

This method of investigating the link between language development and reading relies upon obtaining data retrospectively on the early development of children found to have reading difficulties. Such data can be obtained by retrospective recall from parents or by "follow-back" searches through educational or clinical records. The most obvious weakness with this approach is the reliance in cross-sectional and follow-back studies on the retrospective measurement of language development. It is difficult enough to gain concurrent validity in language assessments without having to rely on existing records or parental report. The second major difficulty with such approaches is the accurate estimation of the false alarm rate, that is, how many of the children with a putative characteristic indicative of later reading difficulty actually never develop a literacy problem. This estimation is problematic for two reasons. Firstly, the base prevalence rate of such a characteristic is usually unknown and cannot be estimated from data on the reading disabled group alone. Secondly, where control comparison groups are used, such a group is usually too small to allow the accurate estimate of the risk of false alarms for infrequently occurring characteristics.

The weakness of retrospective studies is illustrated by one language–based measure that is often thought to be of possible value in predicting later reading difficulties, that is, Verbal–Performance IQ discrepancies. Cross–sectional and therefore retrospective studies have identified specific reading–disabled children as showing a V–P decrement; for example, Rutter, Tizard, and Whitmore (1970). Indeed such a result has been used to support the notion that specific reading retardation (in contrast to general reading backwardness) is primarily a language–based disability. However, a prospective study by Bishop and Butterworth (1980) showed that: (1) V–P discrepancies are not stable between the ages of 4 years 6 months and 8 years 6 months, that is, less than 50% of those with a large V–P discrepancy at 4 years showed such a discrepancy at 8 years and vice versa; (2) there is no tendency for those with significant V–P discrepancy at 4 years to develop reading problems at 8 years; and (3) V–P discrepancies at 8 years were related to reading problems at 8 years, though this later association depended on how reading problems were defined. These conclusions militate against the adoption of V–P decrement as a predictor of reading problems and also suggest a further important methodological issue that effects retrospective analysis. That is, it is possible that reading problems *lead* to language difficulties in some children rather than the other way round. Retrospective studies cannot be used to make any strong statements about the likely direction of causal effects.

4. The Outcome of Early Language Delay

There have been a number of studies that have followed–up children showing initial delays in language development. Children with early language delays are at risk of developing a wide range of later disorders. There are a number of studies that have followed samples of language delayed children that have been referred for remedial help or assessment (e.g., Griffiths, 1969; Garvey and

Gordan, 1973; Aram and Nation, 1980). For the purposes of prevention it is more valuable to have information on samples representative of the general population and obtained by screening children in the preschool period. The characteristics of such children when identified by screening were described by Richman and Stevenson (1977). They show a high level of behavior problems (see Tab. 1).

Tab. 1: The association between language delay and behavior problems (based on data from Richman, Stevenson and Graham, 1982)

Rate of behavior problems

in the population of 3 − year − olds	14%
in 3 − year − olds with language delay	59%

Rate of language delay

in the population of 3 − year − olds	3%
in 3 − year − olds with behavior problems	13%

Tab. 2: Characteristics of children with language delay (based on data from Richman and Stevenson, 1977)

	Language delay (n = 24)	Matched controls (n = 24)	P*
Mother depressed	50%	24%	< .05
3 or more siblings	41%	13%	< .001
3 or more stresses	41%	24%	< .05

* chi − square test

The results in Tab. 2 show that they are also subject to a wide range of social adversities and stresses. It is necessary to control for the association with behavior problems if the outcome of language delay itself is to be established and the implications for intervention are to be identified.

4.1   General risk problems in middle childhood

There have been three major longitudinal studies of children with language delay who were obtained by screening the total population (Silva et al., 1983; Stevenson and Graham, 1982; Fundudis et al., 1979). Despite studying populations in very different geographical areas, the prevalence rate for language delays was similar in the three studies: in Dunedin, New Zealand — 4.9%, in Newcastle, England — 3.0%, and in Waltham Forest, England — 3.1%. The degree of delay in language acquisition that these figures represent is approximately 9 months behind chronological age at 3 years. This is a somewhat arbitrary degree of delay, that is, other definitions could have been used and would have produced a different prevalence figure. However, this degree is not only of clinical significance at this age, it also has predictive validity, as will be seen below. In a review of these studies (Stevenson, 1984), it was concluded that from 50 to 75% of these children would be experiencing at least one of the following problems: low IQ (below 85), behaviour problems (as measured by the Rutter Teacher or Parent scales, Rutter, 1967; Rutter, Tizard and Whitmore, 1970), or reading problems at 8 years of age. In comparison with other groups of children identified in the preschool period, the language–delay group was singularly at risk for later difficulties. For example, children with behavior problems were at risk for continuing behavioral difficulties (Richman, Stevenson and Graham, 1982). However, even after controlling for the association between early language delays and behaviour problems (by selecting a control group matched for preschool behavior disturbance), there were still significantly more problems at age 8 in the language–delay children. Most recently, Silva, Williams and McGee (1987) have followed the Dunedin sample through to 11 years and have confirmed the increased risk of behavior problems and lowered reading ability at this later age.

A subsequent analysis of a larger group of 535 children followed from 3 to 8 years showed there to be a link between individual differences in language development and later problems (Stevenson, Richman and Graham, 1985). In this case a representative sample was simply divided into those with better or less well-developed syntactic ability at age 3 years. They were then compared on the rates of behavior disturbance at 8 years. It should be noted that the problems at 8 years were those identified by the teachers at *school*. There was a specific risk of later behavior problems associated with the presence of poor syntactic ability at each of the score ranges for the early behavior measure. Whatever the degree of early disturbance, the child with poor language development was more at risk of behavior disturbance some 5 years later.

It is clear then that early language delays are associated with a wide range of later, educationally significant problems. Rutter and Howlin (1987) have reviewed the link between language delays and aspects of development. Many other studies confirm the link between such delays and both educational and psychiatric disturbances.

The question then arises as to whether there are particular sub-groups within the language-delayed group who are more at risk than others. The general issue of the heterogeneity of language-delayed children has been reviewed by Bishop (Bishop, 1986; Bishop and Edmundson, 1987. She concludes that most language-delayed children can be seen to suffering from a more or less specific maturational lag. It is rare to find a child with a qualitatively deviant pattern of language development. Rather the nature of current difficulties and the prognosis for the child is mainly determined by the extent of their initial handicap. The rate of catch up in language functions is linearly related to the initial lag. If this study can be replicated, the implications are considerable. It means that the vast majority of children with language delay can be considered as a relatively homogeneous group, and presumably are likely to respond to similar remedial help. Bishop and Edmundson (1987) also indicate that once the child has caught up the initial lag, there is little residual difficulty. This finding is difficult to reconcile with the previously mentioned results on the long-term follow-up of children with initial language delays. One explanation that can resolve this apparent inconsistency is that Bishop and Edmondson only studied their children over a relatively short time during the preschool period, that is, up to 5 years 6 months. It may be that problems reemerge to distinguish these children when they are confronted by a novel language-based activity such as

reading later in their schooling. It may also be that the group was less socially
disadvantaged than the samples studied by Stevenson et al. (1977), Silva et al.
(1983), and by Fundudis et al. (1979). Continuities in these social disadvantages
may represent a possible mechanism linking early language difficulties and later
educational difficulties. This possibility will be returned to later.

4.2   Risk of Later Reading Difficulties

Continuing difficulties in language ability and reading have been reported for
language- and speech-delayed children referred for treatment (e.g., Griffiths,
1969; Aram and Nation, 1980). The follow-up studies of samples obtained by
screening have found a similar level of risk. Again, compared to a control
sample matched for degree of behavior disturbance at three years, it was found
that the rate of reading backwardness (RB) was three times greater in
language-delayed children; there was no corresponding association with specific
reading retardation. The distinction between these two groups is one that has
recently come under some criticism (Stevenson, 1988; van der Wissel and
Zegers, 1985). For the present purposes the distinction is possibly of less
relevance. Some work by Glenda Fredman and myself (Fredman and Stevenson, 1988) has failed to establish any difference in the nature of the reading
process underlying these two forms of reading problem once reading age had
been controlled. For the present distinctions between different types of reading
difficulty will not be central to considerations about the link between reading
and language. Undoubtedly, when considering the early stages of reading development, there will be different types of strategy that are part of normal development which could be used to describe the reading processing difficulties of
formerly language delayed children. However at this moment the most promising formulations such as that of Frith (1985), are not sufficiently well developed to have been applied to the problem of predicting reading failure from
children's early language development. The follow-up studies of samples of
language-delayed children have shown them to be highly at risk of a number of
educationally related problems in middle childhood. These include reading
problems, though there is no strong association with specific reading retardation.

5. Retrospective vs. Prospective Analysis

The follow-up studies of children with early language delay has shown them to be a group distinctly at risk of later reading and other problems. These longitudinal studies allow direct comparison between retrospective and prospective analysis of the link between language delay and later reading problems. As shown above, children with language delay are prospectively at risk for later reading difficulties. However, retrospective analysis from the Waltham Forest study gives a rather different impression (Richman, Stevenson, and Graham, 1982; see also Tab. 3).

Tab. 3:   The association between reading problems at 8 years and language delay at 3 and 4 years (based on data from Richman, Stevenson and Graham, 1982)

	Percentage of children at 8 years with delay at 3 or 4 years			
	Specific reading retardation ($n = 16$)	$P*$	Reading back-wardness ($n = 17$)	$P*$
At 3 years				
Specific language delay	31%	ns	59%	ns
General language delay	31%	ns	71%	.03
At 4 years				
Specific language delay	38%	ns	59%	.02
General language delay	31%	ns	71%	.01

* chi−square comparison with children without reading problems

This shows that although 60-70% of children with reading backwardness at age 8 show some form of language delay in the preschool period, less than one third of the children with specific reading retardation would be identified in this way. In part this is due to differences in prevalence rate. Language delays were found in 3% of the population, whereas the rates of specific reading retardation and reading backwardness were 6% and 5% respectively. Therefore even if high continuity in language related problems was found for these children, they could not account for more than one third of all later reading problems. Of course the definition of language delay could have been modified to produce a higher prevalence, but it is very likely that the continuities in language related problems for an enlarged group would not have been so high. The implication of this is that in terms of identifying later poor readers, the sensitivity of language screening is low. However, the specificity is high, that is, there are few children with language delay who will not show some form of education-ally related problem at 8 years (false alarms).

Tab. 4:   Screening for language delay and behavior problems in a hypothectical population of
          3 − year − olds and outcome at 8 years

	At 8 years	
	No problems	IQ< 85 or behavior problems or reading problems
At 3 years		
Language delay (*n* = 30)	6	24
No language delay (*n* = 970)	820	150
At 3 years		
Behavior problems (*n* = 150)	75	75
No behavior problem (*n* = 850)	723	127

The implication of this for screening is shown in Tab. 4. It is of interest to note the comparison with behavior problems here. With behavior problems, the sensitivity is higher with about 40% of problem children identified by the screen. However, the false alarm rate is higher in that 50% of children identified by the screen as at risk do not show a later problem. The impact of successfully identifying and treating language delay (if such treatment were available) on later prevalence is going to be modest. However, in terms of the efficient use of professional time, they represent a singularly worthwhile group for intervention.

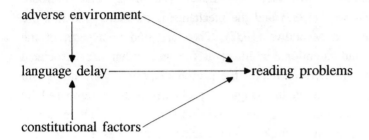

Fig. 1: Direct and indirect links between language delay and reading difficulties

It should be emphasized that even if successful treatment for their language difficulties were available, there may still be continuing environmental and biological influences acting on both early language delay and reading (see Fig. 1). A good illustration of such an environmental effect is maternal depression. This was one feature of the child's home environment at age 3 years that was strongly linked with specific reading retardation (Richman, Stevenson and Graham, 1982).

Tab. 5: The association between reading problems at 8 years and aspects of the family at 3 years of age (based on Richman, Stevenson and Graham, 1982)

	Specific reading retardation (n = 16)	P*	Reading backward-ness (n = 17)	P*
At 3 years				
Mother depressed	75%	.001	53%	ns
3 or more stresses	63%	ns	59%	ns
Poor marriage	31%	ns	44%	ns
Significant behavior problem	69%	ns	77%	.06

* chi square comparison with a mixed group of behavior problem children and controls

This association remained even when other factors were controlled, including language development at 3 years. The result has recently been independently replicated by McGlaughlin, Morrisey and Sever (in press) and Estrado, Arsenio, Hess and Holloway (1987) and the mechanisms mediating the link are being studied by Mills and Meadows (1987). They are finding aspects of the child's learning style and attentional abilities at 5.5 years that are associated with depression in their mothers earlier in the preschool period. An enthusiasm for early intervention centered on the language problem needs to tempered by taking into account the continuities in these environmental effects. There are of course constitutional factors that might be producing continuities in language-based problems. These include both genetic influences (Pennington and Smith, 1983; Stevenson et al., 1987) and developmental defects occurring during ontogeny.

Before leaving the issue of screening for language delayed children, mention must be made of the rather different conclusions reached by Stark et al. (1983). They argued that the prevalence of such problems was so much lower in the 7– to 8–year–old child that most children will grow out of their early language problems, and therefore it is inappropriate to screen before the age of 7. There are two problems with this argument. Firstly they used a much too high esti-mate for language delay in the preschool population. A figure of 25% was taken from Allen and Bliss (1979), which is way above the 4% figure given above for Britain and New Zealand. Secondly, they took no account of the language–delayed child being at risk for a wide range of educational handicaps.

6. Conclusions

The following conclusions can be made concerning the use of early language development as a predictor of later reading failure.

1. It is clear that language processing disabilities lie at the score of most chil-dren's reading problems.
2. There are preliminary indications that early training might help to improve some of the most important language skills, that is, phonological awareness.

3. Screening before school for such specific language deficits, that is, phonological awareness, is not going to be effective in identifying a significant proportion of later reading problems.

4. The screening for more general language delay might be justified since the false alarm rate is low.

5. Successful treatment of language delay alone will have only a modest impact on the prevalence of reading difficulties in middle childhood.

6. Combining screening with the universal provision of phonological training might prove to be a fruitful joint strategy. The work of Hewison and Tizard (1980) on paired reading for parent and child provides an excellent model for a program aimed at all children having a significant impact on reading problems.

7. Maximum benefit is only likely to occur if intervention with language-delayed children is designed to deal with some of the continuities in adverse environmental influences shared in common by language delay and reading failure.

These points need to be borne in mind by those concerned with planning future research programs in the early identification of children at risk for reading problems. They are also central to considerations about the strategy for developing services to prevent written language difficulties in school–age children.

References

Allen, D.V., and Bliss, L.S. (1979): Evaluation procedures for screening preschool children for signs of impaired language development. Second Interim Report, Contract NS6 2353, NINCDS, Bethesda, Md.: Dept. Health, Education and Welfare

Aram, D.M., and Nation, J.E. (1980): Preschool language disorders and subsequent language and academic difficulties. Journal of Communication Disorders, 13, 159–170

Bishop, D. (1987): The causes of specific developmental language disorder ("developmental dysphasia"). Journal of Child Psychology and Psychiatry, 28, 1–8

Bishop, D., and Butterworth, G. (1980): Verbal–performance discrepancies: relationship to birth risk and specific reading retardation. Cortex, 16, 355–389

Bishop, D. and Edmundson, A. (1987): Specific language impairment as a maturational lag: evidence from longitudinal data on language and motor development. Developmental Medicine and Child Neurology, 29, 442–459

Bradley, L., and Bryant, P. (1985): Rhyme and reason in reading and spelling. Ann Arbor: University of Michigan Press

Bryant, P. (1985): The question of prevention. In Snowling, M.J. (Ed.): Children's written language difficulties. Windsor: NFER–Nelson

Crystal, D., Fletcher, P., and Garman, M. (1976): The grammatical analysis of language disability. London: Edward Arnold

Estrada, P., Arsenio, W.F., Hess, R.D., and Holloway, S.D. (1987): Affective quality of the mother–child relationship: longitudinal consequences for children's school–relevant cognitive functioning. Developmental Psychology, 23, 210–215

Fredman, G., and Stevenson, J. (1988): Reading processes in specific reading retarded and reading backward 13 year olds. British Journal of Developmental Psychology, 6, 97–108

Frith, U. (1985): Beneath the surface of developmental dyslexia. In Patterson, K.E., Marshall, J.C., and Coltheart, M. (Eds.): Surface dyslexia: neuropsychological studies of phonological reading. London: Lawrence Erlbaum

Fundudis, T., Kolvin, I., and Garside, R. (1979): Speech retarded and deaf children: their psychological development. London: Academic Press

Garvey, M., and Gordon, N. (1973): A follow–up study of children with disorders of speech development. British Journal of Disorders of Communication, 8, 17–28

Griffiths, C.P.S. (1969): A follow–up study of children with disorders of speech. British Journal of Disorders of Communication, 4, 46–56

Hall, P.K., and Tomblin, J.B. (1978): A follow–up study of children with articulation and language disorders. Journal of Speech and Hearing Disorders, 43, 227–241

Hewison, J. and Tizard, J. (1980): Parental involvement and reading attainment. British Journal of Educational Psychology, 50, 209–215

Howlin, P., and Rutter, M. (1987): The consequences of language delay for other aspects of development. In Yule, W., and Rutter, M. (Eds.): Language development and disorders. Clinics in Developmental Medicine No. 101/102. Oxford: MacKeith Press/Blackwells

Lundberg, I. (1987): Two dimensions of decontextualization in reading acquisition. Unpublished manuscript, Umea University, Sweden

McGlaughlin, A., Morrisey, M., and Sever, J. (in press): Behaviour disturbances and educational attainments of 9 year olds. Infant Mental Health Journal

Mills, M. and Meadow, S. (1987): The impact of maternal depression on children – follow–up at age 5. Paper presented at the Annual Conference of the British Psychological Society Developmental Section, 11–14 September, University of York

Pennnington, B.F., and Smith, S.D. (1983): Genetic influences on learning disabilities and speech and language disorders. Child Development, 54, 369–387

Richman, N., and Stevenson, J. (1977): Language delay in 3 year olds: family and social factors. Acta Paediatrica Belgica, 30, 213–219

Richman, N., Stevenson, J., and Graham, P. (1982): Preschool to school: a behavioural study. London: Academic Press

Richman, N., Stevenson, J., and Graham, P. (1983): The relationship between language, development and behaviour. In Schmidt, M.H., and Remschmidt, H. (Eds.): Epidemiological approaches in child psychiatry II. New York: Thieme–Stratton

Rutter, M., Tizard, J., and Whitmore, K. (1970): Education, health and behaviour. London: Longmans

Silva, P.A. (1980): The prevalence, stability and significance of developmental language delay in preschool children. Developmental Medicine and Child Neurology, 22, 768–777

Silva, P.A., McGee, R., and Williams, S.M. (1983): Developmental language delay from three to seven years and its significance for low intelligence and reading difficulties at age seven. Developmental Medicine and Child Neurology, 25, 783–793

Silva, P.A., Williams, S., and McGee, R. (1987): A longitudinal study of children with developmental language delay at three years: Later intelligence, reading and behaviour problems. Developmental Medicine and Child Neurology, 29, 630–640

Stark, R.E., Mellits, E.D., and Tallal, P. (1983): Behavioural attributes of speech and language disorders. In Ludlow, C.L., and Cooper, J.A. (Eds.): Genetic aspects of speech and language disorders. New York: Academic Press

Stevenson, J. (1984): Predictive value of speech and language screening. Developmental Medicine and Child Neurology, 26, 528–538

Stevenson, J. (1988): Which aspects of reading ability show a "hump" in their distribution? Applied Cognitive Psychology, 2, 77–85

Stevenson, J., Fredman, G., McGloughlin, V., and Graham, P. (1987): A twin reading study of genetic influences on reading ability and disability. Journal of Child Psychology and Psychiatry, 28, 229–247

Stevenson, J. and Richman, N. (1976): The prevalence of language delay in a population of three year old children and its association with general retardation. Developmental Medicine and Child Neurology, 18, 431–441

Stevenson, J., Richman, N., and Graham, P. (1985): Behaviour problems and language abilities at three years and behavioural deviance at eight years. Journal of Child Psychology and Psychiatry, 26, 215–230

Tallal, P., Stark, R.E., Kallman, C., and Mellitis, D. (1980): Perceptual constancy for phonemic categories: a developmental study with normal and language–impaired children. Applied Psycholinguistics, 1, 49–64

van der Wissel, A., and Zegers, F.E. (1985): Reading retardation revisited. British Journal of Developmental Psychology, 3, 3–9

Wagner, R.K., and Torgesen, J.K. (1987): The nature of phonological processing and its causal role in the acquisition of reading skills. Psychological Bulletin, 101, 192–212

Wagner, R.K. (1986): Phonological processing abilities and reading: implications for disabled readers. Journal of Learning Disabilities, 19, 623–630

Part Three

Methodological Problems in Longitudinal Research

Problems of Longitudinal Studies with Children: Practical, Conceptual, and Methodological Issues

Wolfgang Schneider

1. The Need for Longitudinal Studies in the Field of Developmental Psychology

While there seems to be a broad consensus that developmental psychology should focus on changes occurring over time within the organism, the majority of research conducted in the field of developmental psychology has been based on a methodology inappropriate for the study of change (cf. McCall, 1977; Wohlwill, 1973, 1980). That is, most developmental studies cannot be considered truly developmental because they used cross–sectional designs. Consequently, they focused on developmental *differences* among various age groups and ignored developmental *changes* within individuals over age which can only be assessed via longitudinal approaches.

These criticisms represent serious challenges to the purpose of developmental psychology and the way its hypotheses are traditionally investigated and interpreted (cf. Appelbaum and McCall, 1983). Although these criticisms have been around for a while, their impact on current research methodology has been negligible. For example, a recent review on studies conducted in the field of memory development revealed that more than 99 % of these studies have been cross–sectional in nature (cf. Schneider and Weinert, in press).

Interestingly, this does not mean that researchers are still unaware of the problem: Calls for longitudinal studies are frequent in the developmental literature. Given the discrepancy between theory and practice, however, one conclusion could be that there are also various problems with longitudinal studies serious enough to keep off many developmental researchers. The critical analysis of potential problems and possible coping strategies will be a major goal of this chapter. When discussing problems of longitudinal studies, I will not restrict myself to the more general issues typical of most longitudinal investigations, but also refer to problems inherent in longitudinal studies with children.

Discussing problems of longitudinal studies is a complicated matter. First of all, it is difficult because we do not have a precise definition of what constitutes a longitudinal study. Actually, the term "longitudinal" does not describe a simple method but a broad variety of methods. As Baltes and Nesselroade (1979) pointed out, the spectrum ranges from single-case studies in time-series arrangements to broad-band panel designs including thousands of subjects. Moreover, available longitudinal studies range from repeated single-variable assessment completed within a couple of months to life-span multivariate investigations. The only common denominator of longitudinal research is variation of time and repeated observation of a given entity.

Given the broad variety of research designs subsumed under the label "longitudinal", it follows that the problems discussed in the remainder of this chapter may be relevant for many − so I assume − but not for all longitudinal studies conducted with young children. In my view, there has been considerable confusion about what has to be considered a "true", general, and uncurable problem of longitudinal investigations. It is one goal of the present chapter to illustrate the relativity of many problems and their dependence on research aims. More specifically, it is assumed that problems vary as a function of the respective rationale for longitudinal research. According to Baltes and Nesselroade (1979), there are three different rationales that relate to *description* of development: (1) direct identification of intraindividual change; (2) direct identification of interindividual differences in intraindividual change; and (3) the identification of interrelationships among classes of behavior during development. Two further rationales concern the *explanation* of development: (4) the analysis of causes of intraindividual change; and (5) the analysis of causes of interindividual differences in intraindividual change.

In the remainder of this chapter, general problems as well as problems specific to longitudinal research based on the above rationales will be discussed in more detail. Three classes of general problems will be considered: *Practical problems* concerning cost factors, the long-term recruitment of staff, data storage, and funding; *conceptual problems* referring to the fact that there seems to be no broad consensus among longitudinal researchers about how the concept of change should be defined (note that the solution of this conceptual problem is crucial for the realization of all five rationales for longitudinal research). Finally, general *methodological problems* will be addressed concerning the assessment of change and stability over time. The solution of these problems is equally important for all five research goals mentioned above. As will be shown below, related methodological problems, for example, the choice of adequate statistical tools, depend on the specific goal of longitudinal analysis. While those problems seem relevant to most longitudinal studies, their importance varies as a function of the type of longitudinal study under consideration.

In addition to these more general problems, longitudinal studies with young children have to cope with more specific problems that are primarily related to the data generation process. Examples from the Munich Longitudinal Study on the Genesis of Individual Competences (LOGIC; cf. Weinert and Schneider, 1986, 1987) will be used to illustrate problems of verbal assessments (e.g., interviews) with preschool and kindergarten children and their implications for stability of test scores.

2. General Problems of Longitudinal Studies

2.1 Practical Difficulties

Harway, Mednick, and Mednick (1984) summarize the most obvious practical problems of (long–term) longitudinal studies. Among those, the costs associated with conducting longitudinal studies over an extended period of time and difficulties with funding such costly projects are usually considered the major obstacles. According to Harway et al. (1984), this objection to longitudinal research has been typically overrated. In their view, the initial data collection phase is most costly in that staff has to be trained, tasks have to be developed and pretested, the samples have to be recruited, and the research design confined. Costs for subsequent follow–up assessment should be comparably low.

Given the variety of longitudinal designs mentioned above, however, it is difficult to evaluate the importance of the cost problem. Harway et al. (1984) judgment seems adequate for long–term longitudinal studies conducted with a single cohort and including only a few follow–ups or a rather restricted set of test instruments. The situation seems completely different, however, for a more complex longitudinal design. There is little doubt that the cost problem remains a serious practical difficulty for longitudinal studies operating with several cohorts, including a broad variety of test instruments and several measurement points. According to our own experience, costs are even likely to rise in later assessments if data collections in subsequent waves aim at the entire cohort — and do not limit themselves to subsamples, as Harway et al. suggest. The rise in costs experienced in the latter case is mainly due to mobility problems.

Researchers interested in keeping the attrition rate low have to spend additional (travel) money in order to keep mobile subjects in the sample.

Given the fact that long–term longitudinal studies are costly enterprises, obtaining and maintaining funding is not an easy task. Usually, a necessary (but not
sufficient) condition for obtaining funding is an elaborated research design
combined with a sophisticated developmental theory. It is most important to
convince reviewers that the planned study has to be longitudinal and cannot be
replaced by a series of related cross–sectional studies. As there is an obvious
lack of information on intraindividual changes in many developmental areas, the
task seems difficult but solvable in principle.

With regard to staffing, the likelihood that only a few staff members will stay
with a longitudinal study for the duration of the project is not a real problem.
Although shifts in personnel are often costly, periodic changes in personnel are
not necessarily unhealthy. The occasional addition of "fresh blood" does not
only minimize the risk of data bias due to frequent interactions among experimenters and subjects in a long–term longitudinal study, but also increases the
possibility that already existing data will be analyzed in ways not considered by
permanent staff members (cf. Harway et al., 1984).

Two other practical difficulties frequently mentioned by opponents of longitudinal research refer to the publication record of longitudinal investigators and
the timeliness of long–term longitudinal enterprises. In view of the "publish–or-
perish" principle guiding scientific careers, a longitudinal researcher may be in
a bad position because it usually takes several years before the first results are
available for publication. Even worse, the problem of timeliness of publication
arises in the case of long–term longitudinal studies in which it takes a long time
before the harvesting of data is possible. In those cases, publishing results could
be a difficult enterprise because the topic under investigation may be "out of
fashion"; a problem frequently encountered in various disciplines of social
sciences. However, there are solutions to both problems. More specifically, it is
of crucial importance to design longitudinal studies in a way that: (1) there
remains sufficient time for analyzing the data and writing up reports between
two adjacent measurement points, and (2) the design is flexible enough to allow
for the possibility of change. Accordingly, an extreme delay in publication can
be avoided if sufficient time is available for the different phases of a longitudinal study (i.e., data collection, data analysis, report writing). With regard to
flexibility, precautions should be taken to ensure that the study is not too
narrow in scope. That is, a broad–band investigation including several measures
from different domains copes with the problem of timeliness in that the data

might be reanalyzed at a later date and interpreted in the light of theoretical and technological advances (cf. Block and Block, 1980, 1984; Harway et al., 1984). All in all, there is no doubt that there are several practical difficulties with longitudinal studies. However, as there also seem to be practicable solutions to most of the problems discussed in this section, those problems should not be overestimated by researchers interested in conducting longitudinal research.

2.2 Conceptual Problems

All five rationales of longitudinal research listed above referred to the assessment of change. At first glance, there seems to be no problem with conceptualizing and studying developmental change. A closer look at the literature, however, reveals that conceptualizing human development is a complicated issue. As emphasized by Baumrind (1987), instability and discontinuity in human development can only be seen against a background of stability. The question of what stability can mean in the context of changing individuals (Wohlwill, 1980) has been answered differently by different researchers.

Given the space restrictions, I do not want to reiterate the discussion of conceptual discrepancies but summarize the existing consensus (cf. for a more detailed discussion Asendorpf, in press a; Kagan, 1980; Overton and Reese, 1981; Rutter, 1987; Wohlwill, 1973, 1980).

There is a general consensus that two types of longitudinal inquiry can be distinguished. One aspect of developmental inquiry concerns what Wohlwill (1973) called the developmental function, that is, the average value of a dependent variable plotted over age. Typical examples would be growth curves for physical height or weight based on a sample of individuals. The second realm of developmental inquiry concerns individual differences. More specifically, the question is whether individual subjects maintain approximately the same relative rank ordering within their group at one age as they do at another (cf. Appelbaum and McCall, 1983; McCall, 1977). McCall (1977) used the term *continuty/discontinuity* to refer to the developmental function, whereas *stability/instability* refers to the individual differences approach. Other researchers have further differentiated among various meanings of the stability concept: They make a distinction between the stability of a variable and the stability of an individual (Wohlwill, 1980), and further refer to ipsative stability as the persistence of a pattern of variables for an individual subject over time (cf. Asendorpf, in press a, 1987; Kagan, 1980; Rutter, 1987).

The important distinction to be emphasized here is between the continuity or discontinuity of a growth function for an attribute and the degree of stability or instability of individual differences in an attribute. Note that continuity/discontinuity in developmental function is *conceptually* independent from stability/instability in individual differences: The relationship between both concepts is an *empirical* question (cf. Appelbaum and McCall, 1983).

Longitudinal researchers have frequently overlooked the fact that developmental functions and individual differences represent two separate aspects of the same problem. Appelbaum and McCall (1983) provide examples for such confusions. One general problem of longitudinal research is the tendency to emphasize information on the stability of individual differences at the expense of data on developmental change. That is, most longitudinal researchers focused on predicting later differences in a given variable without considering the fact that this could not tell them anything about the developmental functions of that variable. McCall (1977) correctly stated that many longitudinal studies cannot be considered truly developmental because they ignored developmental change in individual differences over age.

In the present context, it is important to note that most longitudinal studies either focus on individual differences or the developmental function. Studies simultaneously combining these two aspects are rare. With regard to methodological problems, the conclusion is that only a few problems to be discussed below are representative of the two types of longitudinal studies. For example, the extensive literature on the problems of assessing individual changes over time only refers to those empirical studies dealing with data on the developmental function. The problem with measuring change has not been a relevant topic for the many longitudinal studies dealing with individual differences. The reader should keep in mind that many problems of longitudinal research to be discussed below are relative rather than general.

2.3   Methodological Problems of Longitudinal Research

Given the conceptual problems discussed above, it is not surprising that longitudinal research in the social sciences has been dominated by several fundamental misunderstandings and damaging myths (cf. Rogosa, 1988). Many problems are related to the use of inadequate designs or inappropriate statistical tools. Appelbaum and McCall (1983), for example, emphasize the fact that applied statistics has made considerable progress within the last few years, and that researchers engaged in longitudinal studies should become acquainted with more recent statistical developments useful for the study of change. Thus, narrowing the knowledge gap between statisticians and researchers is considered a pre-condition for improving longitudinal research. In the following, I will first refer to several well–established "myths" of longitudinal research and then go on to more serious problems related to the assessment of change.

2.3.1 Problems with Measuring Change

The debate about the measurement of change has a long tradition in the psy-chometric literature. Since the classical article by Cronbach and Furby (1970), longitudinal researchers have been warned repeatedly of the hazards of change scores. These warnings seem to have created the belief that change scores are unreliable, misleading, and unfair, and therefore should be avoided at all costs (cf. Maxwell and Howard, 1981). However, several methodologists have pro-vided evidence that it is high time to debunk this myth.

For example, Maxwell and Howard (1981) showed that the analysis of change scores is valid in randomized pretest–posttest designs. Social scientists familiar with the hazards of change scores may prefer a repeated measures ANOVA over an ANOVA on posttest–pretest change scores, assuming that any problem with change scores are avoided with the repeated measures ANOVA. They are obviously unaware of the fact that an ANOVA on posttest–pretest change scores yields exactly the same F value as obtained from the interaction test of the repeated measures design (cf. Maxwell and Howard, 1981; Nunnally, 1982). Accordingly, there is no problem with using change scores for *group* analyses.

However, what about the use of difference scores for the assessment of *indivi-dual* change? Again, there is strong evidence that problems have been overesti-mated. Proponents of difference scores emphasize the fact that they constitute the very heart of longitudinal investigations and represent unbiased estimates of true change (Nunally, 1982; Rogosa, 1988; Rogosa, Brandt, and Zimowski, 1982). Indeed, it can easily be shown that several objections (e.g., unreliability, unfairness, bias through regression toward the mean) do not generally hold.

For example, Rogosa et al. (1982) demonstrated that the reliability of difference scores is not generally low. The difference score will have low reliability as long as individual growth rates vary little across subjects. In this case, reliability indicates the accuracy with which subjects can be ranked on the growth rate function on the basis of their difference scores, whether the estimates of the growth rate function are precise or not. The important message is that low reliability does not necessarily imply lack of precision, that is, does not preclude meaningful assessment of individual change. Moreover, the reliability of the difference score is respectable when considerable individual differences in change are present (for illustrations see Rogosa and Willett, 1983).

Similarly, it has been shown that the importance of regression–toward–the–mean effects for the study of change has been overestimated in the social sciences literature (cf. Nesselroade, Stigler, and Baltes, 1982; Rogosa, 1988). While there is a lack of explicit descriptions of the phenomenon, the traditional meaning is that, on average, you are going to be closer to the mean at Time 2 than you were at Time 1. The crucial message provided by Nesselroade et al. (1982) is that regression toward the mean is not an ubiquitous phenomenon that has unalterable effects. On the contrary, Nesselroade et al. demonstrated that the often–held belief that measurement error necessarily produces a regression effect that makes it impossible or difficult to measure change properly is not correct, at least not with multiwave data.

It should be noted in this connection, that the popular assumption that residual change scores should be chosen instead of difference scores because they adjust for effects of individual differences in initital status is problematic. As Rogosa (1988; Rogosa et al., 1982) points out, there are logical problems with the residual change approach as well as statistical and psychometric shortcomings. Logically, the question "How much would individual p have changed on attribute x if all individuals had started out 'equal'" stimulates the subsequent question "Equal on what?". Does it mean equal on true initial status, observed initial status, initial status in combination with other background variables, or what? The correct answer is unknown. Obviously, addressing the question "How much did individual p change on attribute x?" is comparably simple (cf. Rogosa, in press). See Rogosa et al. (1982) as well as Rogosa and Willett (1985a) for a detailed treatment of statistical and psychometric shortcomings of residual change scores.

All in all, methodological papers written in defense of the difference score have accumulated over the past few years. The important message for the longitudinal researcher is that more effort should be invested into developing models of individual growth (cf. Bock, 1976; Bryk and Raudenbush, 1987; Rogosa et al., 1982) and constructing proper longitudinal designs. In general, two measurement points provide an inadequate basis for studying change. Data collected on multiple occasions are better suited to control for regression effects and estimate individual growth curves (cf. Nesselroade et al., 1980; Rogosa et al., 1982). To my knowledge, Bryk and Raudenbush's (1987) two–stage model of growth represents one of the most promising approaches to the study of change. It allows for studying the structure of individual growth, examining the reliability for measuring status and change, investigating correlates of status and change, and testing hypotheses concerning the effects of background variables. Given the impressive demonstrations presented by Bryk and Raudenbush, longitudinal researchers should be encouraged to adopt such a hierarchical linear modeling approach for their studies which seems broadly applicable to the study of change.

So far, our discussion has been restricted to change scores based on classical test theory. Note that probabilistic measurement models provide an alternative possibility to quantify individual change. Various versions of the linear logistic test model (Rasch model) exist that allow for unbiased estimation of item difficulty parameters and person ability parameters (cf. Fischer, 1976; Fischer and Formann, 1982). In these Rasch models, changes in either abilities or item difficulties over time can be simply assessed by analyzing the respective difference scores (see Schneider and Treiber, 1984, for an empirical example).

To summarize, there seem to be several possibilities of correctly assessing developmental change or the developmental function, mainly due to recent methodological advancements. Potential pitfalls have been definitively overrated by many researchers.

It should be noted, however, that this conclusion only holds if change scores are measured on a common scale. More specifically, the precondition for the analysis of change scores is that the same measurement instruments were used over time. It is obvious, then, that longitudinal studies with children run into serious problems whenever tests or questionnaires are designed for a restricted age range. While the same instrument can be used at all ages with certain measurements like height or weight, this is not true for the majority of measures designed to assess cognitive or personality development in children. Although Goldstein (1979) discusses the possibility of constructing a common scale for different instruments by using various transformation procedures, this only allows for the assessment of *relative* change, that is, for a comparison of subgroups of a given population. Consequently, while the use of different measurement instruments over time does not cause problems for the longitudinal analysis of individual differences, it definitively restricts the analysis of the developmental function.

But even when the same instrument is used on each occasion, the interpretations of it may differ (cf. Magnusson, 1981). As Baumrind (1987) emphasized, a variable or construct may appear to be the same at various ages when in fact it is not. An example referring to motor development may illustrate the case: There is no doubt that crawling has a different meaning for a 9–month–old child than it has for a 4–year–old child. Obviously, the neglect of *qualitative* change or discontinuity in the organization of individual behavior can lead to erroneous conclusions (see also Rutter, 1987). Block, Gjerde, and Block (1986) found considerable transformations in the psychological meaning of indicators of categorization breadth from age 4 to age 11. While the use of relatively broad categories in early childhood reflected an inability to organize experience effectively, the use of relatively broad categories in preadolescence reflected a rather creative ability (see Baumrind, 1987, for a similar empirical example). Baumrind (1987) and Block et al. (1986) recommend the use of multiple and diverse measures of behavioral constructs in order to examine whether continuity across time periods is given or not. Methodologically, this means that a cluster of variables defining a construct must load on second–order factors in the same way across time to have the same meaning and validity.

2.3.2   Problems of Longitudinal Studies Analyzing Individual Differences

As already mentioned above, longitudinal research focusing on individual differences is concerned with different definitions and types of stability. In most cases, correlation coefficients (e.g., Time 1 − Time 2 correlations) are used as measures of the consistency of individual differences. Further methods include repeated measures ANOVA, cross–lagged panel correlation analysis, path analysis regression, and structural equation models using latent variables.

Several myths or misunderstandings relate to the interpretation of the correlation coefficient. While there are several limitations with correlation coefficients and problems concerning their interpretation (cf. Rutter, 1987; Valsiner, 1986, one fundamental misunderstanding is that the correlation matrix for longitudinal data tells you whether or not you are measuring the same thing over time (Rogosa, 1988). Theoretically, it is possible that the rank ordering of individuals within a given group remains constant over time (indicated by a large correlation coefficient), although the theoretical construct under study changes its meaning for the subjects. Of course, the opposite could be also true. Consequently, more elaborated validation procedures (e.g., assessment of related reference variables) seem necessary to ensure that correlation coefficients are correctly interpreted.

A further misunderstanding concerning methods of the individual differences approach is that structural regression models tell us much about change, or that cross–lagged panel correlation procedures inform about reciprocal causal effects (cf. Rogosa, 1980, 1985, 1988). In the first case, the myth to be debunked is that structural parameters can be indicative of individual growth rates in observed or latent variables. As illustrated by Rogosa (1988), structural regression coefficients can actually badly mislead about exogeneous influences on growth. The message is that the analysis of correlations or covariance structures should not be undertaken to reach conclusions about individual growth. Rather, they should be used to investigate stability or consistency issues and be concerned with the prediction of events.

The myth concerning the potential of cross–lagged panel correlations seems even more popular. Roughly speaking, the research question is whether variable x causes y or vice versa. Thus studies of reciprocal effects investigate problems of causal predominance or causal ordering. In the two wave − two variable case typically used to illustrate the problems with the procedure, r_{x1y2} and r_{y1x2} represent the sample cross–lagged correlations of specific interest. The attribution of causal predominance is based on the difference between the two cross–lagged correlations. Usually, causal predominance is assumed when the null hypothesis of equal cross–lagged correlations is rejected. Rogosa (1980, 1985) has convincingly demonstrated serious methodological flaws of the procedure. Accordingly, cross–lagged panel correlations cannot be recommended in order to detect patterns of causal influences and should best be forgotten. Fortunately, several alternatives are available. In particular, structural equation modeling (SEM) procedures have been developed recently that can be used to systematically develop and test theories (cf. Bentler, 1980, 1985; Jöreskog and Sörbom, 1984; Lohmöller, 1984). SEM procedures using a latent variable approach like LISREL or EQS not only seem better suited for the analysis of reciprocal causal effects but are also appropriate for estimating and testing more complex causal models including intervening variables. While structural equation models can principally be applied to cross-sectional data, they seem promising when used with longitudinal data. In short, their major advantages − as compared to traditional regression analysis − are that: (1) a verbal theory has to be trans-lated into a mathematical model that can be estimated; (2) structural/causal relationships are estimated at the level of latent variables or theoretical con-structs and not on the basis of fallible observed variables; (3) the distinction between a measurement model describing the relationships among observed variables and latent factors and a structural model describing interrelations among theoretical constructs also allows for a separate estimation of measure-ment errors in the observables and specification errors in the structural part of the model: large specification errors usually indicate that the causal model is not completely specified, that is, important predictor variables are obviously missing; and (4) Several so−called goodness−of−fit tests exist that detect the degree of fit between the causal model and the data set to which it is applied. Causal models are said to be "confirmed" when the goodness−of−fit parameter indicates better−than−chance fit between the model and the data. (See the Spe-cial Section on Structural Equation Modeling in the first issue of *Child Devel-opment*, 1987, for a more detailed description of SEM procedures and for numerous applications drawn from different areas of developmental psycholo-gy.)

While SEM procedures generally operate on correlation or covariance matrices, mean structures can also be considered. For example, McArdle and Epstein (1987) illustrate the possibilities of a longitudinal model that includes correla-tions, variances, and means and is described as a latent growth curve model. The inclusion of mean structures makes this longitudinal model more similar to repeated−measures ANOVA and MANOVA traditions. As a consequence, this type of model may also be used to assess the developmental function, that is, group changes in the amount of a latent variable over time.

Although there is broad agreement that SEM procedures represent powerful general tools for the analysis of longitudinal data, they should not be conceived of as panaceas. Several potential problems with SEM procedures have been addressed in the literature (cf. Connell, 1987; Martin, 1987; Rogosa, 1988). First of all, the use of a multiple indicator approach based on an elegant statistical model cannot compensate for poor–quality data, careless operationalization of major constructs, and inappropriate designs (cf. Martin, 1987; Rudinger and Wood, 1987). It is the researcher who has to make sure that theoretical assumptions are justified, and that the longitudinal sampling of occasions and variables allows for the discrimination between interesting alternatives. Further, some SEM procedures (e.g., LISREL) require multivariate normality of data, a criterion rarely met in the case of longitudinal data (cf. Bentler, 1986, 1987). In addition, the effectiveness of most SEM procedures depends on the accessibility of large data sets (more than 100 subjects as a rule of thumb). Unfortunately, SEM procedures applicable to nonnormally distributed data (e.g., EQS) require even larger sample sizes (cf. Tanaka, 1987). As Tanaka puts it, the "cost" of making fewer distributional assumptions about data is the necessity of a large sample size. It should be noted, however, that this restriction does not apply to distribution–free, exploratory SEM procedures also known as soft-modeling procedures. For example, causal models with latent variables based on partial–least–squares (PLS) estimation procedures can be used as a starting point whenever theoretical knowledge is scarce and/or only small samples are available (cf. Lohmöller, 1984; Schneider, 1986).

One last problem to be mentioned concerns the adequate assessment of reciprocal causal effects discussed earlier in the paper. Traditionally, first–order autoregressive or simplex models have been argued to be optimal models for studying stability and change in developmental applications (cf. Rogosa, 1988). In these models, variables are represented as causes of themselves over two or more points in time. As it is well known that autoregressive models define changes over time to be independent of prior changes, they do not seem to be an optimal method for assessing change in many developmental applications. Note that the growth curve models introduced by McArdle and Epstein (1987) seem preferable in that they define changes over time to be dependent on the prior changes. Further, as Hertzog and Nesselroade (1987) illustrated, simplex models may be a particularly poor way of representing change and reciprocal causal relationships between state (nontrait) phenomena. Finally, there is also evidence that it is often too easy to fit autoregressive models (including cross-lagged regression models) to longitudinal data. For example, Rogosa and

Willet (1985b) demonstrated that a simplex model marvelously fit a covariance matrix from growth curves that were maximally "unsimplex".

All in all, the problems presented so far have illustrated that careful theoretical analyses are a prerequisite for an adequate model building process. Of course, the quality of data available for analyses further complicates the issue. Recent developments in SEM procedures, however, seem to minimize this problem. That is, long–linear path analysis models for discrete data or causal models with categorical/nonnormal dependent variables are now available for longitud-inal researchers who cannot rely on continuous variables (cf. Goldstein, 1979; Muthén, 1984, 1987). Altogether, the number of statistical techniques available for the analysis of discrete longitudinal data has considerably increased during the last decade (cf. for reviews Henning and Rudinger, 1985; Markus, 1979).

To summarize, there seem to be relatively few problems with analyzing longi-tudinal data focusing on individual differences and stability/instability issues. Due to recent methodological advancements, generally applicable and elegant statistical tools are available that can be used for elaborate model building. This is particularly true for the assessment of what Hertzog and Nesselroade (1987) call *mean* stability or *covariance* stability over time. Relatively little attention has been paid to *intraindividual* stability, that is, change within the given sampling unit (but see Asendorpf, in press a, b for the construction of a coeffi-cient assessing individual stability over time).

3. Specific Problems of Longitudinal Studies With Young Chil-dren: The Case of the Munich Longitudinal Study on the Gene-sis of Individual Competencies (LOGIC)

In the last section of this chapter, I will focus on problems typical of longitudi-nal studies with preschool and kindergarten children. Although these problems are well–known to most researchers working with young children, they are rarely mentioned in scientific reports. In particular, problems related to the test situation, to practice and experimenter effects will be discussed in more detail. Moreover, problems related to the instability of test scores and the implications for model building and prediction purposes will be addressed.

As already noted, empirical examples demonstrating some of the problems typical of longitudinal studies with young children will be taken from our

Munich longitudinal study on the genesis of individual competencies (LOGIC). In this study, a sample of about 220 four-year-old subjects was first tested immediately after the children had entered kindergarten. This was done to make sure that the subjects' experience with social groups was limited at the very beginning of the longitudinal study. As one of the major goals of LOGIC was the study of the effects of social group experiences on cognitive development, it seemed important to start at this particular point in time. Since 1984, children have been annually tested on a broad variety of variables, including measures of intelligence, memory and metamemory, social cognition, social competence, moral development, and achievement motivation. In order to identify important prerequisites and determinants of school (reading) achievement, a number of experimental tasks tapping different aspects of phonological processing (i.e., children's use of phonological information in processing oral or written language) were additionally included at the third measurement point, that is, at the end of the kindergarten period. The study is designed to be active until the end of elementary school (4th grade). The major methodological problems experienced during the kindergarten phase of the study are summarized below.

3.1   Problems Related to the Test Situation

It is well-known from cross-sectional studies that testing or interviewing young children is a complicated matter. Given the large number of experimental tasks, psychometric tests, and interview procedures included in LOGIC, it turned out to be an extremely difficult task to keep our subjects motivated and interested in the study. One problem repeatedly encountered during the first measurement point was that children felt insecure and uncomfortable in the test situation. It usually took a long warming-up phase before children were ready to participate in the various tasks and answer the numerous questions. In several cases, however, even extended interactions with the child before testing did not have the expected effects: A small number of 4-year-old children refused to answer any questions in several test situations, particularly in the more difficult and demanding interviews (e.g., the metamemory interviews). They also did not reproduce any items in several experimental tasks (e.g., recall of texts or word lists). How does one proceed with such "untestable" children? They surely cannot be treated like missing cases because they did not actually miss the test session. On the other hand, it seems obvious that their poor performance in the test situation represents a seriously biased estimate of their true competence. In other words, the problem of measurement error seems particularly serious in the case of "untestable" children.

A related problem concerns the experimenter or observer effect. Even if young children are willing to participate in an interview or test session, it may be that they only want to interact with certain experimenters. Methodologically, one "disadvantage" of an extended warming–up procedure is that young children get used to their adult partners. As a consequence, they do not want to be tested by other experimenters in subsequent sessions or measurement points. This phenomenon has been frequently observed in our study. The problem is that it is difficult if not impossible to control for experimenter or observer effects. Again, this means that there is systematic bias and additional noise in the data. Ways of coping with this problem will be described below.

3.2   Problems with Instability of Test Scores

An analysis of the LOGIC memory data (Schneider and Weinert, in press) revealed considerable test instability over time. That is, retest correlations for measures of word list recall, text recall, and memory span assessed at ages 4 and 6 were rather low with coefficients ranging between .22 (word span) and .36 (word list recall). This finding indicates that the subjects did not maintain their relative standing within their group, and that individual differences were not preserved between age 4 and age 6. These results are not in accord with those reported by Kunzinger (1985), who reported high across–age group stabilities for his sample of elementary school children between ages 7 and 9. Additional analyses concerning *individual* stability, that is, the amount of across–age variable shown in an individual's relative standing within the referent group, did not change the overall pattern of results. So–called "lability scores" (Kunzinger, 1985; Wohlwill, 1973), representing the across–age standard deviation of an individual's z scores, were computed for the various recall measures, and yielded considerably higher values (i.e., high lability) than those reported by Kunzinger (1985). This trend was not restricted to our memory data. When lability scores were computed to assess the across–age stability in text recall, verbal intelligence, and motor skills, we found them to be almost three times as high as those obtained by Kunzinger (1985). Interestingly, lability scores were comparable across the three tasks considered. It seems, then, that high levels of instability are not only typical of memory performance at that particular age, but can be generalized across different domains (Tab. 1).

Tab. 1:   Individual Across–Age Lability of Test Score for Selected Variables of the LOGIC Study, split for Sex (N = 208)

Variable	Boys	Girls	
General metamemory	.71	.55	s
Sorting in a sort–recall task	.79	.71	ns
Recall in a sort–recall task	.59	.64	ns
Text recall	.63	.66	ns
Memory span	.64	.61	ns
Verbal intelligence	.46	.50	ns
Nonverbal intelligence	.69	.74	ns
Motor skills	.52	.50	ns
Social competence	.87	.72	ns

Note: "s" indicates that sex differences were significant at the p = .05 level;
        "ns" indicates that no sex differences were found.

Given the high instability of test scores over time, an interesting question is whether this is due to high unreliability of measurement instruments or rather to the high fluctuation of the phenomenon under study. Note that low stability over time does not necessarily mean low reliability or low internal consistency of the measure in question: Hertzog and Nesselroade (1987) used SEM procedures to demonstrate that so–called state measures like anxiety or fatigue showing low stability over time can nevertheless be reliably and validly assessed.

Interestingly, in the case of young children, trait measures such as indicators of psychometric intelligence seem to "behave" like the state measures in the case of Hertzog and Nesselroade's (1987) study with older adults: Whereas their stability over time is rather low, their internal consistency is not.

The situation seems more complicated, however, when internal consistency of measures cannot be assessed, that is, whenever the measures of interest consist of only one of a few items. Unfortunately, this is true for many experimental tasks (e.g., measures assessing different aspects of memory). In those cases, short–term, test–related correlations should be obtained to make sure that the variables of interest are indeed measured reliably (cf. also Asendorpf, in press a).

Problems with low stability of test scores obtained from young children are not restricted to longitudinal assessment. We found similarly low intraindividual consistency across related tasks in cross–sectional settings. For example, only weak to moderate intercorrelations were obtained when memory tasks tapping similar skills were compared for one point in time.

Young children's low intraindividual consistency across similar measures re-presents a serious problem when the researcher's goal is to predict future performance. In the LOGIC study, for example, the Bielefeld Screening Test developed by Marx and Skowronek (this volume) was used in the last period of kindergarten to identify children at risk, particularly with regard to reading and spelling. The screening procedure consisted of nine different tests assessing various aspects of phonological processing (e.g., rhyming, syllable segmenta-tion, visual word matching, or sound blending). Although intertask correlations were moderate to high, there were only a few children scoring consistently low on most measures. Tab. 2 illustrates the degree of inconsistency observed for the screening test measures. We checked the number of times each child be-longed to the bottom 10% of the distribution in the nine subtests of the screen-ing test. As can be seen from Tab. 2, there were only 8 out of 208 subjects who belonged to the bottom 10% in more than five out of nine subtests. Given the low intraindividual consistency across measures, it seems that the early prediction of school achievement is a difficult task.

Tab. 2:   Number of Times a Subject Belonged to the Bottom 10% in the Various Subtests of
          the Bielefeld Screening Test (N = 208)

N of times	N of subjects	Percent
0	99	47.6
1	60	28.8
2	21	10.1
3	11	5.3
4	9	4.3
5	4	1.9
6	2	1.0
7	2	1.0

3.3   Possible Coping Strategies

How can we cope with all the problems related to longitudinal studies with
young children? It seems that the risk of working with measures swamped by
error is particularly high in studies using preschoolers and kindergarteners as
subjects. To enhance the reliability and validity of test scores, several measures
can be taken (cf. Block and Block, 1980; Block et al., 1986). First, the use of
multiple kinds of data seems advantageous. If test data, observational data,
self–report, and questionnaire data are available that all refer to the same theoretical concept, the chances of getting closer to the "true" score increase.
Similarly, multiple measurement within each kind of data seems suited to
reduce error variance. Block et al. (1986) refer to the psychometric truism that
the proportion of concept–related variance in a given measure can be improved
by basing that measure on an average or composite of a number of concept–related items, each of which may contain only a small proportion of concept–related variance. Moreover, the use of multiple measures also allows for more
sophisticated model building and theory testing via SEM procedures.
In addition, it seems important to draw independent cross–sectional samples to
check generalizability of findings and to assess possible practice effects.
Furthermore, this measure could be useful for identifying cohort effects. How-

ever, while controlling for cohort effects seems a very important problem of life–span longitudinal studies (see Baltes, Cornelius, and Nesselroade, 1979, for a detailed treatment of this point), they do not seem equally relevant in longitudinal studies with young children conducted within a comparably restricted time interval. Nonetheless, the recruitment of independent samples in studies with young children may well be informative in that the existence of age–group–related influence patterns can be examined.

4. Concluding Remarks

All in all, the discussion of selected practical, conceptual, and methodological problems of longitudinal studies with children revealed that the importance of different kinds of difficulties has been overrated in the literature. This is particularly true of methodological problems: As has been shown above, several myths concerning the problems of change scores or the analysis of cross–lagged panel data still exist and need to be debunked. Recent developments in applied statistics have made it possible to effectively deal with change scores and also provide several possibilities for the analysis of reciprocal causal effects. Thus the message is that most methodological problems of longitudinal studies can be successfully handled, regardless of whether the focus is on the developmental function or individual differences.

On the other hand, the overview of the literature also revealed that longitudinal studies have to be planned carefully in order to be successful in the long run. For example, many practical problems reported in the literature seem related to poor planning efforts; for example, insufficient time lags between data assessment and data analysis. Other studies suffered from the problem that their long–term goals were never precisely defined. That is, it remained unclear in those cases whether the focus was on developmental changes or on individual differences. As mentioned above, this decision should be made early in the planning process because it definitively affects the choice of measurement instruments. For example, the selection of conceptually related but different measures does not cause major problems in studies dealing with individual differences, but seems disadvantageous in studies focusing on the developmental function. In fact, one of the few serious problems discussed in this chapter concerns the question of how to build up a common scale for different measures tapping the same underlying construct.

Taken together, however, it seems that numerous coping strategies are available that can deal effectively with potential problems of longitudinal work. Given the unique importance of longitudinal data for our proper understanding of child development, we can only hope that the powerful tool of longitudinal analysis will be more frequently used in future developmental studies than it is today.

References

Appelbaum, M.I., and McCall, R.B. (1983): Design and analysis in developmental psychology. In P.H. Mussen (Ed.), *Handbook of child psychology* (Vol. 1, pp. 415–476). New York: Wiley

Asendorpf, J. (in press a): Individual, differential, and aggregate stability of social competence. In B.H. Schneider, G. Attili, J. Nadel, and R. Weissberg (Eds.): *Social competence in developmental perspective.* Dordrecht: Kluwer

Asendorpf, J. (in press b): Coefficients of individual and differential stability. *Methodika*

Baltes, P.B., Cornelius, S.W., and Nesselroade, J.R. (1979): Cohort effects in developmental psychology. In J.R. Nesselroade, and P.B. Baltes (Eds.), *Longitudinal research in the study of behavior and development.* New York: Academic Press

Baltes, P.B., and Nesselroade, J.R. (1979): History and rationale of longitudinal research. In J.R. Nesselroade, and P.B. Baltes (Eds.): *Longitudinal research in the study of behavior and development.* New York: Academic Press

Baumrind, D. (1987): *The permanence of change and the impermanence of stability.* Paper presented at the biennial meetings of the Society for Research in Child Development, Baltimore

Bentler, P.M. (1980): Multivariate analysis with latent variables. Causal modeling. *Annual Review of Psychology, 31,* 419–456

Bentler, P.M. (1985): *Theory and implementation of EQS: A structural equations program.* Los Angeles: BMDP Statistical Software Corp.

Bentler, P.M. (1986): EQS — Ein Ansatz zur Analyse von Strukturgleichungsmodellen für normal- bzw. nichtnormal verteilte quantitative Variablen. In C. Möbus and W. Schneider (Eds.), *Strukturmodelle für Längsschnittdaten und Zeitreihen.* Bern: Huber–Verlag

Bentler, P.M. (1987): Drug use and personality in adolescence and young adulthood. Structural models with nonnormal variables. *Child Development, 58,* 65–79

Block, J., Gjerde, P.F., and Block, J.H. (1986): Continuity and transformation in the psychological meaning of categorization breadth. *Developmental Psychology, 22,* 832–840

Block, J.H., and Block, J. (1980): The role of ego–control and ego–resiliency in the organization of behavior. In W.A. Collins (Ed.): *Minnesota Symposia on Child Psychology* (Vol. 13). Hillsdale, NJ: Erlbaum

Block, J.H., and Block, J. (1984): A longitudinal study of personality and cognitive development. In S.A. Mednick, M. Harway, and K.M. Finello (Eds.): *Handbook of longitudinal research, Vol. 1: Birth and childhood cohorts* (pp. 329–352). New York: Praeger

Bock, R.D. (1976): Basic issues in the measurement of change. In D.N.M. de Gruijter, and L.J.T. van der Kamp (Eds.): *Advances in psychological and educational measurement.* New York: Wiley

Bryk, A.S., and Raudenbush, S.W. (1987): Application of hierarchical linear models to assessing change. *Psychological Bulletin, 101,* No. 1, 147–158

Connell, J.P. (1987): Structural equation modeling and the study of child development: A question of goodness of fit. *Child Development, 58,* 167–175

Cronbach, L.J., and Furby, L. (1970): How should we measure "change" — or should we? *Psychological Bulletin, 74,* 68–80.

Fischer, G.H. (1976): Some probalistic models for measuring change. In D. De Gruijter, and L. Van der Kamp (Eds.): *Advances in psychological and educational measurement.* New York: Wiley

Fischer, G.H., and Forman, A.K. (1982): Veränderungsmessung mittels linear–logistischer Modelle. *Zeitschrift für Differentielle und Diagnostische Psychologie, 3,* 75–99

Goldstein, H. (1979): *The design and analysis of longitudinal studies.* London: Academic Press

Harway, M., Mednick, S.A., and Mednick, B. (1984): Research strategies: Methodological and practical problems. In S.A. Mednick, M. Harway, and K.M. Finello (Eds.): *Handbook of longitudinal research, Vol. 1, Birth and childhood cohorts.* New York: Praeger

Henning, H.J., and Rudinger, G. (1985): Analysis of qualitative data in developmental psychology. In J.R. Nesselroade, and A. von Eye (Eds.), *Individual development and social change: Explanatory analysis.* Orlando: Academic Press

Hertzog, C., and Nesselroade, J.R. (1987): Beyond autoregressive models: Some implications of the trait-state distinction for the structural modeling of developmental change. *Child Development, 58,* 93–109

Jöreskog, K.G., and Sörbom, D. (1984): *LISREL VI — Analysis of linear structural relationships by maximum likelihood instrumental variables, and last squares methods. (Users Guide).* Mooresville: Scientific Software

Kagan, J. (1980): Perspectives on continuity. In O.G. Brim, Jr., and J. Kagan (Eds.): *Constancy and change in human development* (pp. 26–74), Cambridge, MA: Harvard University Press

Kunzinger, E.L. (1985): A short-term longitudinal study of memorial development during early grade school. *Developmental Psychology, 21,* 642–646

Lohmöller, J.B. (1984): *LVPLS program manual.* Köln: Zentralarchiv für Empirische Sozialforschung

Magnusson, D. (1981): Some methodology and strategy problems in longitudinal research. In F. Schulsinger, S.A. Mednick, and J. Knop (Eds.): *Longitudinal research — Method and uses in behavioral science.* Boston: Martinus Nijhoff Publishing

Markus, G.B. (1979): *Analyzing panel data.* Beverly Hills: Sage Publications

Martin, J.A. (1987): Structural equation modeling: A guide for the perplexed. *Child Development, 58,* 33–37

Maxwell, S.E., and Howard, G.S. (1981): Change scores — necessarily anathema? *Educational and Psychological Measurement, 41,* 747–756

McArdle, J.J., and Epstein, D. (1987): Latent growth curves within developmental structural equation models. *Child Development, 58,* 110–133

McCall, R.B. (1977): Challenges to a science of developmental psychology. *Child Development, 48,* 333–344

Muthén, B.O. (1984): A general structural equation model with dichotomous, ordered categorial, and continuous latent variable indicators. *Psychometrika, 49,* 115–132

Muthén, B.O. (1987): *LISCOMP — Analysis of linear structural equations using a comprehensive measurement model.* Mooresville, In Scientific Software, Inc.

Nesselroade, J.R., Stigler, S.M., and Baltes, P.B. (1980): Regression toward the mean and the study of change. *Psychological Bulletin, 88*, 622–637

Nunnally, J.C. (1982): The study of human change: Measurement, research strategies, and methods of analysis. In B.B. Wolman (Ed.), *Handbook of Developmental Psychology.* Englewood Cliffs, NJ: Prentice Hall

Overton, W.F., and Reese, H.W. (1981): Conceptual prerequisites for an understanding of stability–change and continuity–discontinuity. *International Journal of Behavioral Development, 4*, 99–123

Rogosa, D. (1980): A critique of cross–lagged correlation. *Psychological Bulletin, 88*, 245–258

Rogosa, D. (1985): Analysis of reciprocal effects. In T. Husen, and N. Postlethwaite (Eds.): *International Encyclopedia of Education.* London: Pergamon Press.

Rogosa, D. (1988): Myths about longitudinal research. In K.W. Schaie, R.T. Campbell, W.M. Meredith, and C.E. Rawlings (Eds.), *Methodological problems in aging research.* New York: Springer

Rogosa, D., Brandt, D., and Zimowski, M. (1982): A growth curve approach to the measurement of change. *Psychological Bulletin, 90*, 726–748

Rogosa, D., and Willett, J.B. (1983): Demonstrating the reliability of difference scores in the measurement of change. *Journal of Educational Measurement, 20*, 333–343

Rogosa, D., and Willett, J.B. (1985a): Understanding correlates of change by modeling individual differences in growth. *Psychometrika, 50*, 203–228

Rogosa, D., and Willett, J.B. (1985b): Satisfying a simplex structure is simpler than it should be. *Journal of Educational Statistics,* 10

Rudinger, G., and Wood, P.K. (1987): N's, times and number of variables in *longitudinal research.* Paper presented at the European Science Foundation workshop on methodological issues in longitudinal research. Rönneberga, Stockholm, Schweden

Rutter, M. (1987): Continuities and discontinuitites from infancy. In J.D. Osofsky (Ed.), *Handbook of infant development (Vol. 2).* New York: Wiley

Schneider, W. (1986): Strukturgleichungsmodelle der zweiten Generation: eine Einführung. In C. Möbus, and W. Schneider (Eds.): *Strukturmodelle für Längsschnittdaten und Zeitreihen.* Bern: Huber

Schneider, W., and Treiber, B. (1984): Classroom differences in the determination of achievement changes. *American Educational Research Journal, 21*, 195–211

Schneider, W. and Weinert, F.E. (in press): Memory development: Universal changes and individual differences. In A. de Ribaupierre (Ed.): *Transitional mechanisms in cognitive–emotional child development.* New York: Cambridge University Press

Tanaka, J.S. (1987): "How big is big enough?": Sample size and goodness of fit in structural equation models with latent variables. *Child Development, 58*, 134–146

Valsiner, J. (1986): Between groups and individuals. Psychologists' and laypersons' interpretations of correlational findings. In J. Valsiner (Ed.): *The individual subject and scientific psychology.* New York: Plenum Press

Weinert, F.E., and Schneider, W. (1986): *First report on the Munich Longitudinal Study on the Genesis of Individual Competencies (LOGIC).* Munich: Max Planck Institute for Psychological Research

Weinert, F.E., and Schneider, W. (1987): *LOGIC-Report No. 2: Documentation of assessment procedures used in waves one to three (Technical Report).* Munich: Max Planck Institute for Psychological Research

Wohlwill, J.F. (1973): *The study of behavioral development.* New York: Academic Press

Wohlwill, J.F. (1980): Cognitive development in childhood. In O.G. Brim, Jr., and J. Kagan (Eds.): *Constancy and change in human development.* Cambridge, Mass.: Harvard University Press.

Zero–Missing Non Existing Data: Missing Data Problems in Longitudinal Research and Categorical Data Solutions*

Alexander von Eye

1. Introduction

Many data sets in social science research contain missing data. That is, some of the values in the data matrix are not observed. Examples include a respondent participating in a mail survey who fails to complete a questionnaire because of an extended out–of–country trip or, some recall rates in a memory experiment are not recorded because the computer breaks down or, in a decision experiment, a subject leaves a question blank because he/she does not have a clear opinion or he/she is not aware of the alternatives.

There are at least three reasons for missing data. As with the first two examples, in many instances it is meaningful to assume that there are values existing in principle, albeit not available to the researcher. This is the usual case of missing data. For these cases it seems natural to apply techniques to replace the missing values with estimated ones that meet certain optimality criteria. Most of the literature on missing data is devoted to these techniques (cf. Little and Rubin, 1987; Lösel and Wüstendörfer, 1974; Rovine, Petersen, and Delaney, in press), and many of these techniques have made their way into statistical software packages (cf. Dixon, 1983), even though in most instances cases with missing data are simply deleted.

The third example covers two cases. In the first, the subject has not made up his/her mind. Therefore, a missing value does not indicate that there is an underlying true value that could have been observed with better data collecting

---

* I would like to thank Constance Jones for helpful comments on an earlier version of this paper

techniques. Rather, it indicates that it would have been better if the researchers had included a category for "do not know" or "unable to come up with a decision." This problem typically is considered to be either a validity problem for the scale or − wrongly − an ordinary missing data problem.

The second problem covered by the third example leads us to the topic central to the present paper. The example shows that data may be missing not because researchers failed to collect them or because of lack of validity of the scales used, but rather because they *do not exist*. In the example the subject does not know the alternatives and, therefore, it would be meaningless to force a decision or to note "did not make up his/her mind". Another example is a subject who solves a problem in an experiment in fewer trials than other subjects and, therefore, does not provide values for the later trials.

The problem of non existing data is most prevalent in developmental, longitudinal research. It is generally treated under the labels of attrition or experimental mortality (cf. Baltes, Reese, and Nesselroade, 1977). For example, a student may fail to show up for a wave of data collection because he/she is sick; another student might be in the process of deciding what track to select and, therefore, be unable to communicate a decision; an elderly individual might have died between two observation points. Only the last example shows a case of non existing data.

Methods for treating missing data can be classified using the following taxonomy (Little and Rubin, 1987). All of these techniques assume that the data are a random sample and that the missing values are also random in nature.

1. *Deletion of incomplete records.* A standard procedure in early versions of many statistical software packages is the casewise deletion of incomplete records (cf. Nie et al., 1975). This procedure leads to the analysis of complete data sets. It heavily relies on the assumption of randomly distributed missing values. Therefore, it is most inappropriate in longitudinal research when one has to assume that attrition is a selective process. Under such circumstances casewise delection can lead to serious biases.

2. *Imputation of missing values.* Imputation is the replacement of missing values. Examples of imputation procedures include substitution of means and estimates based on predictions made using regression.

3. *Weighting procedures.* These procedures estimate parameters using design weights which allow one to adjust for missing values. The weights typically reflect the probability of missing values.

The present paper discusses the problem of non existing data. In particular, the handling of non existing data in categorical data analysis will be covered. A data example from experimental research on problem solving will be given.

2. Description of the Problem

For the sake of simplicity, suppose a researcher conducts a longitudinal study observing only one variable. Then, the equation relating observation values to observation points is:

$$y_i = x_0 b_0 + x_i b_1 + e_i \tag{1}$$

that is, the score of subject i depends on some scaling factor and the point in time at which the person was observed. If a sample containing n subjects was observed, Equation 1 can be expressed as:

$$y = Xb + e \tag{2}$$

Suppose, for example, two subjects are observed on two occasions. Then, one obtains the matrix:

$$\begin{bmatrix} y_{11} \\ y_{12} \\ y_{21} \\ y_{22} \end{bmatrix} = \begin{bmatrix} 1 & x_1 \\ 1 & x_2 \\ 1 & x_1 \\ 1 & x_2 \end{bmatrix} \begin{bmatrix} b_0 \\ b_1 \end{bmatrix} + \begin{bmatrix} e_{11} \\ e_{12} \\ e_{21} \\ e_{22} \end{bmatrix}$$

Solutions for (2) are well known:

For instance, the **Least Squares** criterion is:

$$(y - Xb)^T (y - Xb) \overset{!}{=} \min$$

and the solution is:

$$b = (X^T X)^{-1} y^T X$$

Using this solution, the expected outcome vector is:

$$\hat{y} = Xb \tag{3}$$

A **Maximum Likelihood Solution** is:

$$\hat{y}_{ij} = \frac{(\pi_i y_{ij}) \ (\pi_j y_{ij})}{n} \tag{4}$$

Suppose, in an experiment, the first subject solves the experimental problem in the first trial, whereas the second subject needs two trials. This is an example of non existing data. Then, the data matrix given above looks like:

$$\begin{bmatrix} y_{11} \\ - \\ y_{21} \\ y_{22} \end{bmatrix} = \begin{bmatrix} 1 & 1 \\ 1 & 2 \\ 1 & 1 \\ 1 & 2 \end{bmatrix} \begin{bmatrix} b_0 \\ b_1 \end{bmatrix} + \begin{bmatrix} e_{11} \\ - \\ e_{21} \\ e_{22} \end{bmatrix}$$

Obviously, the solutions for the estimation of expected values given in (3) and (4) do not allow one to consider the case of missing values. Application of (3) only leads to $\hat{y}_{ij} = 0$ if the inner product $Xb = 0$, and application of (4) only yields $\hat{y}_{ij} = 0$ if the first, the second, or both factors in the numerator are zero. Typically, missing data procedures provide maximum likelihood estimates for missing values. These estimates are consistent, that is, they converge toward the expected value if the sample size increases, they are efficient, that is, they have the smallest variance, and they are normally distributed. However, when one applies these procedures to non existing data, the resulting estimates are meaningless.

Substantively oriented researchers often apply one of the following strategies for dealing with attrition or experimental mortality. The first is to eliminate those cases that dropped out during the investigation (see casewise deletion, above). The second is to compare the available data of those who later dropped out with those who remained in the sample. These comparisons often suggest that attrition is a nonrandom process. That is, in most instances there are significant differences between these two groups (Schaie, Labouvie, and Barrett, 1973). Therefore, results obtained with only those cases that remained in the sample can in most instances be considered biased.

Again, the problem with the second strategy is that within the group of dropouts there may be two or more reasons for missing values: ordinary missing data or non existing data. Another problem with this strategy is that the stratification breaks the sample apart. This might be counter to the intentions of the researcher and, in addition, may cause problems with the sample size in either subgroup. Therefore, the following sections will present an approach to handle the non existing data problem in such a way that the original sample is conserved as a unit.

3. Non Existing Data in the Analysis of Categorical Variables in Longitudinal Research

The present section describes a solution of the non existing data problem that meets the following two criteria:

1. The original sample is conserved as a unit; therefore, data from those subjects who do not provide data after a given point in time must be analyzed simultaneously with the data from those subjects who provide complete data;

2. the timing of non existing data for each subject, an important variable in its own right, is conserved for statistical analysis.

One first solution to this problem has been discussed by Lienert and von Eye (1986). These authors analyzed data collected in a learning experiment during which subjects went through trials until they had reached either a learning criterion or the maximum number of trials. The resulting data set consisted of learning curves of different lengths. The authors defined the following three criteria for the evaluation of the learning curves:

1. *Monotonous Trend Criterion.* This criterion requires weak monotony, that is, $x_{i+1} \geq x_i$ for all $i = 1, ..., t-1$, in which t denotes the number of observation points. If there is at least one pair of adjacent measures for which this criterion is violated, the respective learning curve is treated as nonmonotonic. This criterion requires a minimum of two values.

2. *Early Success Criterion.* If a subject reached the learning criterion before the maximum number of trials allotted, the Early Success Criterion is considered met. This criterion requires a minimum of one value.

3. *Mistake Avoidance Criterion.* This criterion was considered fulfilled if the number of items incorrectly recalled by a subject lies below the grand median of incorrectly recalled items in the entire sample. This criterion, too, requires a minimum of one value.

The approach discussed by Lienert and von Eye (1986) has several advantages over casewise deletion or splitting the sample in subgroups. First, it allows one to analyze subjects with learning curves of different lengths simultaneously. Second, it allows one to consider both formal characteristics of learning curves such as trend parameters, and substantive characteristics such as mistake avoidance.

The present paper will adopt an approach that differs from Lienert and von Eye's approach in two respects. First, there is no need to transform the raw data into categories reflecting characteristics of the time series. Rather, one can operate with raw data. Second, the exact point from which a subject no longer provides data is considered.

One possible solution to the problem of non existing data in the analysis of repeatedly observed categorical variables can be seen in the introduction of an ordinal variable that describes the point in time at which a subject participated for the last time in an investigation. This variable can be crossed with the observables to form a contingency table which may be analyzed using, for instance, log–linear modeling, prediction analysis, or configural frequency analysis. However, there are several problems connected with this solution:

1. The number of cells in the table increases exponentially. Therefore, the sample size must be increased accordingly to enable the researcher to perform statistical data analysis.

2. The number of sampling zeros can become very large. In particular, at the beginning of the series of observations, the number of subjects who do provide data can be expected to be high.

3. Because of the second problem, estimation of expected frequencies and, even more so, the application of the usual fit tests such as the Pearson or the likelihood ratio Chi–Square tests can become problematic. The likelihood ratio test statistic is not defined for observed zero frequencies; the term X^2 = o log (o/e) is undefined because log (0) is undefined, where o denotes the observed and e the expected frequencies. The adjustment of the df to the number of sampling zeros can be problematic because it may limit the complexity of the models fitted. Pearson's $X^2 = (o-e)^2/e$ is defined even if $o = 0$. One obtains X^2 = e. However, because of the distributional characteristics of this ordinal variable, expected frequencies can become smaller than the lowest acceptable value of $e = 0.5$ for which Pearson's test statistic is considered valid (Larntz, 1978).

4. Because of (2) and (3), one is either unable to properly perform standard data analysis or is tempted to declare many cells structural zeros that, in principle, cannot contain any cases.

5. The researcher will have to perform transformations as discussed by Lienert and von Eye (1986). Thus, simultaneous analysis of raw data is not possible.

Because of these problems, the present paper adopts another solution. For the sake of simplicity this solution will be described for a design in which one dichotomous variable is observed three times. For multivariate designs or designs with more observation points, this solution applies accordingly. In terms of the equations given above, Equation 2 takes the following form for the present example:

$$
\begin{bmatrix} y_{11} \\ y_{12} \\ y_{13} \\ \cdot \\ \cdot \\ \cdot \\ y_{n1} \\ y_{n2} \\ y_{n3} \end{bmatrix}
=
\begin{bmatrix} 1 & x_1 \\ 1 & x_2 \\ 1 & x_3 \\ & \cdot \\ & \cdot \\ & \cdot \\ 1 & x_1 \\ 1 & x_2 \\ 1 & x_3 \end{bmatrix}
\begin{bmatrix} b_0 \\ b_1 \end{bmatrix}
+
\begin{bmatrix} e_{11} \\ e_{12} \\ e_{13} \\ \cdot \\ \cdot \\ \cdot \\ e_{n1} \\ e_{n2} \\ e_{n3} \end{bmatrix}
$$

This form is equivalent to an ordinary regression equation that views the observables as dependent only on the observation points. Suitable coding variables can be introduced that analyze, for instance, contrasts. Suppose non existing data occur for the first time at the second observation. Then, if we assume Subject 1 drops out, the equation becomes:

$$
\begin{bmatrix} y_{11} \\ - \\ - \\ \cdot \\ \cdot \\ \cdot \\ y_{n1} \\ y_{n2} \\ y_{n3} \end{bmatrix}
=
\begin{bmatrix} 1 & x_1 \\ 1 & x_2 \\ 1 & x_3 \\ & \cdot \\ & \cdot \\ & \cdot \\ 1 & x_1 \\ 1 & x_2 \\ 1 & x_3 \end{bmatrix}
\begin{bmatrix} b_0 \\ b_1 \end{bmatrix}
+
\begin{bmatrix} e_{11} \\ - \\ - \\ \cdot \\ \cdot \\ \cdot \\ e_{n1} \\ e_{n2} \\ e_{n3} \end{bmatrix}
$$

When crossed, the dichotomous values from the three observation points form a Time 1 x Time 2 x Time 3, that is, a 2x2x2 contingency table. The cells of this table are given in the left–hand column of Tab. 1.

Suppose, again, non existing data occur, beginning with the second observation. Then, the strategy proposed in the present paper is to add a category to each variable from the observation point on at which the first subjects dropped out. For instance, a dichotomous variable becomes from this moment on a variable with three categories, where the third category denotes "dropped out." As a result, in the present example, the 2x2x2 table is transformed into a 2x3x3 table. The cells of this table are listed in the right-hand column of Tab. 1.

Tab. 1:   Cells of a Contingency Table for One Dichotomous Variable, Observed Three Times
          with Non Existing Data following the Second Timepoint

Cells without non existing data	Cells with non existing data following a second timepoint
111	111
112	112
121	113
122	121
211	122
212	123
221	**131**
222	**132**
	133
	211
	212
	213
	221
	222
	223
	231
	232
	233

Note: Cells printed in bold face are structural zeros

The present approach has several important characteristics. First, the data from the entire sample can be analyzed simultaneously. It is not necessary to divide the sample into two or more groups and, thus, adopt a differential perspective. Thus, this approach meets the first criterion set above. Second, the point in time at which subjects drop out of the sample is part of the analysis. It is obvious from the design shown in Tab. 1 which cases dropped out at any given observation point. The pattern of values of cases that drop out later is also obvious from Tab. 1. From this characteristic, we may conclude that the present approach allows one to perform data analysis at a more refined level than the approach presented by Lienert and von Eye (1986).

Tab. 1 shows that there are certain cells that cannot contain any cases. These are cells that would contain cases that dropped out at an earlier point in time in the sense of non existing data, and joined the sample again at a later point in time. Examples of such cases include the subject who solved a problem in the second trial and provides a value for time needed to solve the problem in the sixth trial. Because the definition of non existing data excludes such cases, the frequencies in cells that would contain these cases must be declared structural zeros. In the present example, Cells 131, 132, 231, and 232 are structural zeros. A subject in, for example, Cell 231 would display Behavior Category 1 at the first observation, drop out for good before the second, and come back and display Behavior Category 1 at the third.

4. Estimation of Expected Frequencies in Designs With Non Existing Data

One of the major advantages the present approach shares with Lienert and von Eye's approach (1986) is that the estimation of expected frequencies can be performed with standard methods from log–linear modeling (Bishop, Fienberg, and Holland, 1975). The following gives an example of an estimation procedure, the maximum likelihood estimation obtained by the iterative algorithm described by Darroch and Ratcliff (1972); (cf. Bishop et al., 1975). The algorithm is given for three–dimensional problems. An example of such a problem is given in Tab. 1.

To start the iteration one sets the parameter:

$$d_{ijk} = \begin{cases} 1 \text{ for cells that can contain Ss} \\ 0 \text{ otherwise} \end{cases}$$

The model under which the expected frequencies are estimated is a **quasi-in-dependence model** which assumes that there are no interactions among the variables at all. For the example given above, in which one variable was observed three times, the model of quasi-independence can be expressed by:

$$\log f_{ijk} = u + u_i + u_j + u_k \qquad \text{for cells with } d = 1$$

In other words, quasi-independence is given if:

$$f_{ijk} = \begin{cases} \dfrac{\sum\limits_{i} f_{i..} \cdot \sum\limits_{j} f_{.j.} \cdot \sum\limits_{k} f_{..k}}{n^2} & \text{for cells with } d = 1 \\[2ex] 0 \text{ otherwise} \end{cases}$$

As starting values one sets:

$$e_{ijk}^{(0)} = d_{ijk}$$

At the mth cycle of the iteration ($m > 0$) the following steps are performed:

$$e_{ijk}^{(3m-2)} = \frac{e_{ijk}^{(3m-3)} \cdot f_{i..}}{e_{i..}^{(3m-3)}}$$

$$e_{ijk}^{(3m-1)} = \frac{e_{ijk}^{(3m-2)} \cdot f_{.j.}}{e_{.j.}^{(3m-2)}}$$

$$e_{ijk}^{(3m)} = \frac{e_{ijk}^{(3m-1)} \cdot f_{..k}}{e_{..k}^{(3m-1)}}$$

After estimating expected cell frequencies, statistical analysis can be performed as usual. In the present context, two approaches will be discussed. The first approach asks whether the variables that form the table are independent of each other. A goodness–of–fit test will be performed to answer this question. If the frequencies expected under the log–linear model of quasi–independence do not differ substantially from the observed frequencies, the repeated observations can be viewed as not autocorrelated. If the model fit is not acceptably good, one may ask what kind of relations among the variables exist.

The second approach asks what kind of relations exist in a data set. To answer this question, prediction analysis of cross–classifications will be applied (Hildebrand, Laing, and Rosenthal, 1977; von Eye and Brandtstädter, 1988). This method is suitable if there are explicit hypotheses about local relationships in a given data set. Prediction analysis requires the researcher to specify exactly those cells that are supposed to contain high or low frequencies. The pattern of cells specified reflects the assumed local relationships among the variables.

Consider, for example, the two dichotomous variables diligence and grades in school. Then, an example of a hypothesis in prediction analysis is: High diligence (1) leads to good grades (1), and lack of diligence (2) leads to poor grades (2). If put in the format of a contingency table, this hypothesis refers to Cells 11 and 22 of a fourfold table:

11 = **high diligence, good grades**
12 = high diligence, poor grades

21 = lack of diligence, good grades
22 = **lack of diligence, poor grades**

To test whether or not this relation exists, the postulated frequency distribution is compared with an expected one in which the assumed relation is not present. More specifically, prediction analysis compares the observed frequency distribution in those cells that contain subjects who meet the prediction with the expected frequency distribution in which independence of predictors and criteria is assumed. The result can be expressed as the percentage to which more subjects who confirm the hypothesis are found in the observed rather than in the expected frequency distribution. This approach to data analysis will be illustrated in the next section.

5. A Numerical Example: Response Times in a Longitudinal Experiment on Problem Solving

In a longitudinal study on the development of information processing (Hussy, 1987) subjects between the ages of 6 and 60 were presented with the master mind game. They played the game with a personal computer (PC). The PC computed measures as amount of information exhausted in each step, and recorded the subjects' response times. The maximum number of trials per subject was restricted to eight. However, some subjects were able to solve the problem before the eighth step. Thus, if one looks at the response time series provided by the subjects one faces the problem of non existing data: Because a certain number of subjects solved the problem before the eighth trial, they did not provide information on response times for the remaining trials. It is obvious that estimating response times for these subjects would lead to highly artificial results and, most likely, to distorted pictures of the relations in the data set under study.

In the present context, for illustrative purposes only a small subset of the entire data set will be analyzed. The response times provided by 118 3-, 5- and 7-grade students in the sixth, seventh, and eighth trials will be analyzed. The data will be approached first by casewise deletion of those subjects who solved the given problem before the eighth trial. In this case, 20 subjects or almost 20% of the entire sample are omitted. The data will then be analyzed including the information provided by the master minds, that is those subjects who solved the problem before the maximum number of trials.

Tab. 2: Analysis of Response Times in Three Trials of a Master Mind Problem

Response Time		In Trial 8					
		1		2		3	
In Trial 6	In Trial 7	Obs.	Exp.	Obs.	Exp.	Obs.	Exp.
	1	18	7.63	4	6.06	0	8.31
1	2	0	1.04	1	0.83	2	1.13
	3	1	1.39	0	1.10	3	1.51
	1	0	3.47	4	2.76	6	3.78
2	2	3	6.59	3	5.23	13	7.17
	3	6	7.98	6	6.34	11	8.68
	1	4	2.08	1	1.65	1	2.27
3	2	1	1.73	4	1.38	0	1.89
	3	1	2.08	4	1.65	1	2.27

Model: [6,7] [8]; $df = 16$; Chi-square $= 56.14823$; $p <$ alpha

Proportionate increase in hits (PIH) $= 23.88\%$
z(PIH) $= 2.1877$, $p(z) = 0.0144$

Tab. 2 gives the observed frequency distribution and the expected frequencies estimated under the assumption that the problem solving time in the final, eighth trial is independent from the problem solving times in Trials 6 and 7. The problem solving times in the sixth and seventh trials were allowed to be correlated.

In the construction of this table, the time needed for each decision had to be discretized. Three categories were set:

1:          $0 < X \leq 10$ sec
2:          $11 \leq X \leq 20$ sec
3:          $21 \leq X$ sec.

The frequencies of the combinations of problem-solving times are given in Tab. 2. In the first step of the analysis, it was asked whether or not the log–linear model of quasi–independence of variables six and seven (treated as a group) from eight would provide a sufficient explanation of the empirical frequency distribution. For $df = 16$, the result was Chi–square $= 56.14823$. This value is above the critical Chi–square $(16;0.05) = 26.3$. It can be concluded that there are relations in this data set that go beyond the autocorrelation between the problem solving times in the sixth and the seventh trial.

To identify these relations it was assumed that there is stability in the response times such that transitions between response times occur only between adjacent categories. Following this assumption, a subject responding quickly in one trial is not expected to display very long response times in the next trial, and a subject taking his or her time in one trial is not expected to respond very quickly in the following trial. Cells containing subjects displaying response times as predicted are underlined in Tab. 2.

If this hypothesis holds true, the cells underlined in Tab. 2 should contain more subjects than expected if this relation does not prevail. Application of prediction analysis to test this relation shows that there is empirical evidence in favor of the hypothesis. In the empirical frequency distribution there are 23.88% more subjects in the critical cells than in the expected frequency distribution. This difference is significant ($z = 2.1877$, $p = 0.014346$).

To illustrate the methodology presented in this paper, the response times in Trials 7 and 8 were given an additional category for those subjects who had solved the master mind problem in previous trials. The resulting cross classification is given in Tab. 3.

Tab. 3:   Analysis of Response Times in Three Trials of a Master Mind Problem Including
the Subjects who Solved the Problem

Response Time		In Trial 8							
		1		2		3		4	
In Trial 6	In Trial 7	Obs.	Exp.	Obs.	Exp.	Obs.	Exp.	Obs.	Exp.
	1	18	7.02	4	5.58	0	7.64	1	2.76
1	2	0	1.48	1	1.18	2	1.61	2	0.74
	3	1	1.18	0	0.94	3	1.29	0	0.59
	4	–	–	–	–	–	–	2	2.00
	1	0	3.36	4	2.67	6	3.66	1	1.32
2	2	3	6.41	3	5.09	13	6.98	2	2.52
	3	6	8.24	6	6.55	11	8.97	4	3.24
	4	–	–	–	–	–	–	2	2.00
	1	4	1.78	1	1.41	1	1.93	0	0.88
3	2	1	1.78	4	1.41	0	1.93	1	0.88
	3	1	2.75	4	2.18	1	2.99	3	1.08
	4	–	–	–	–	–	–	2	2.00

Model: [6,7] [8]; $df = 24$; Chi–square $= 67.50535$; $p <$ alpha

Proportionate increase in hits (PIH) $= 13.24\%$
z(PIH) $= 2.0313$, $p(z) = 0.0211$

The expected frequencies in Tab. 3 were estimated under the same assumptions as in Tab. 2. That is, there may be an autocorrelation between the
response times in Trials 6 and 7, and there is independence between the
response times in these two trials combined and the response time in Trial 8. In
addition, structural zeros were taken into account. Those cells that would describe the transitions from problem solved to problem solution attempted in
later trials would contain structural zeros. Structural zero cells in Tab. 3 do
not contain observed nor expected frequencies.

In this statistical analysis, the log–linear model of quasi–independence does not fit. The empirical Chi–square = 67.50536 is greater than the critical Chisquare (24;0.05) = 36.4.

Prediction analysis was applied to Tab. 3 under the same assumption as before. In addition, it has to be assumed that subjects who are in the "problem solved before" cell remain there. In Tab. 3, cells that contain subjects confirming the hypothesis are underlined.

Application of prediction analysis reveals that in the critical cells there are 13.24% more subjects than was expected under the assumption of the quasi–independence model. With a z–value of $z = 2.031335$ ($p = 0.02111$, onesided), this difference is significant.

Up to this point the difference between the two approaches can be described by stating that the hypothesis is a little more obviously confirmed when the subjects who have dropped out are left aside than when they are analyzed simultaneously with the subjects remaining in the experimental trials. However, a closer look at the results shows that there are indeed differences.

To compare the results of the two analyses in detail, the prediction of success measures can be decomposed in such a way that an indicator of success can be determined for each proposition in the hypothesis to be tested. To do this, Tab. 4 was set up. For each hypothesis the expected cell frequencies, the observed frequencies, and two measures of prediction success are given. The first measure refers only to the proposition under study, the second measure shows the effect of each proposition on the global measure of prediction success. The middle panel of Tab. 4 gives the results for the analysis without the cases that dropped out, while the right hand panel gives the results for the complete sample.

Tab. 4: Comparison of Two Analyses of Response Times at the Level of Propositions in Prediction Analysis

Proposition number	Frequencies Obs.	Approach 1			Approach2		
		Exp.	PIH$_j$	PIH$_{cum}$	Exp.	PIH$_j$	PIH$_{cum}$
1	22	13.69	0.61	0.185	12.60	0.75	0.120
2	3	3.00	0.00	0.185	4.27	-0.30	0.103
3	3	2.61	0.15	0.194	2.23	0.35	0.113
4	2				2.00	0.00	0.113
5	4	6.13	-0.35	0.146	6.03	-0.34	0.087
6	19	19.00	0.00	0.146	18.48	0.03	0.094
7	17	15.02	0.13	0.189	15.52	0.10	0.113
8	2				2.00	0.00	0.113
9	5	3.73	0.34	0.218	3.19	0.57	0.136
10	5	5.00	0.00	0.218	5.12	-0.02	0.135
11	5	3.92	0.28	0.239	5.17	-0.03	0.132
12	2				2.00	0.00	0.132

Tab. 4 shows that in both approaches the first proposition is the most successful. In both cases, more than 75% of the entire prediction success is covered by this proposition. Tab. 4 also shows that in the second approach, the propositions concerning the cells that contain the subjects who solved the problem before the sixth trial do not contribute anything to the prediction success.

Major differences between the two approaches can be seen where the signs of the prediction success measures differ. This is the case, for instance, in Proposition 11. Whereas in the first approach this proposition favors the hypothesis with the partial prediction success 28%, in the second approach evidence speaks against the hypothesis. In the cells that are targeted by this proposition there are 3% fewer subjects than expected by chance. It can be concluded that the differences between the two approaches may increase with the number of subjects dropping out.

6. Discussion

The present paper attempts to distinguish between the well-known missing data problem and the problem of non existing data. While the problem of non existing data is known as an empirical problem, it has rarely been treated as a methodological problem. Rather, it typically led to a switch from a general to a differential perspective.

A solution for categorical data analysis was introduced that enables the researcher to simultaneously analyze data from those subjects who, for natural reasons, do not provide data from a given point in time on with data from subjects who still remain in the sample. This solution is achieved by defining a category that provides information on the configuration under which a subject dropped out, and the point in time at which this happened.

This solution has the following characteristics:

1. The sample as unit is maintained. While there is no need to adopt a differential perspective, this perspective is possible.
2. The solution can be applied to both uni– and multivariate approaches.
3. The methodology to estimate expected frequencies exists. Many of the widely distributed program packages provide suitable programs (e.g., SYSTAT for PCs, and SPSSX for mainframe computers).

Alternative solutions were considered. In addition, one might be interested in a solution for the analysis of continuous variables. Such a solution can be sketched out as follows:

1. Describe the time series of observed values using orthogonal polynomials.
2. Introduce a variable that provides information on the exact point in time after which a subject no longer provided information.
3. Analyze both kinds of variables simultaneously using, for instance, methods from the general linear model.

Another way to generalize focuses on the period of time for which subjects do not provide data in the non existing data sense. In certain instances, data may not be available because a subject cannot provide information at the beginning of an investigation. Examples include subjects who are not married and participate in a longitudinal cohort comparison study that asks questions on marital satisfaction, and subjects who enter a study late because their legal status did not make them eligible for participation. In other instances, subjects may not be able to provide information because they only change status for a transient period of time. For instance, investigations including only civilians will have to exclude those individuals who serve in the military for a limited amount of time.

References

Baltes, P.B., Reese, H.W., and Nesselroade, J.R. (1977): Life−span developmental psychology: Introduction to research methods. Monterey (Cal.): Brooks/Cole.

Bishop, Y.M.M., Fienberg, S.E., and Holland, P.W. (1975): Discrete multivariate analysis. Cambridge, Ma.: The MIT Press.

Darroch, J.N., and Ratcliff, D. (1972): Generalized iterative scaling for log−linear models. Annals of Mathematical Statistics, 43, 1470−1480.

Dixon, W.J. (Ed.) (1983): BMDP statistical software. Berkeley, Ca.: University of California Press.

Hildebrand, D.K., Laing, J.D., and Rosenthal, H. (1977): Prediction analysis of cross−classifications. New York: Wiley.

Hussy, W. (1987): Zusammenfassender Bericht zu den bisherigen Ergebnissen im EIS−Projekt. Unpublished manuscript.

Larntz, K. (1978): Small sample comparisons of exact levels for chi−squared goodness−of−fit statistics. Journal of the American Statistical Association, 73, 253−263.

Lienert, G.A., and von Eye, A. (1986): Nonparametric two−sample CFA of incomplete learning curves. In F. Klix, and H. Hagendorf (Eds.): Human memory and cognitive capabilities, (pp. 123−138). New York: Elsevier.

Little, R.J.A., and Rubin, D.B. (1987): Statistical analysis with missing data. New York: Wiley.

Lösel, F., and Wüstendörfer, W. (1974): Zum Problem unvollständiger Datenmatrizen in der empirischen Sozialforschung. Kölner Zeitschrift für Soziologie und Sozialpsychologie, 26, 342−357.

Rovine, M.J., Petersen, A.C., and Delaney, M. (in press). Missing data in longitudinal research. In A. von Eye (Ed.): New statistical methods in longitudinal research. New York: Academic Press.

Schaie, K.W. (Ed.) (1983): Longitudinal studies of adult psychological development. New York: The Guilford Press.

Schaie, K.W., Labouvie, G., and Barret, T.J. (1973): Selective attrition effects in a fourteen−year study of adult intelligence. Journal of Gerontology, 33, 848−857.

von Eye, A. (Ed.) (in prep.): New statistical methods in longitudinal research. New York: Academic Press.

von Eye, A., and Brandtstädter, J. (1988): Formulating and testing developmental hypotheses using statement calculus and non−parametric statistics. In P.B. Baltes, D. Featherman, and R.M. Lerner (Eds.): Life−span developmental psychology (Vol. 8, pp. 61−97), Hillsdale, NJ: Erlbaum.

Identifying and Separating Types of Behavior Problems by Latent Class Analysis: Results of a Prospective Study on Pregnancy Course and Child Development

Theodor Ehlers and Herbert Remer

1. Introduction

The origin of problem behavior in children is often obscure, and therefore appropriate treatment is a problem. Many symptoms that are regarded as signs of brain dysfunction might also be considered as main symptoms of primary neurotic or emotional disorder. This difficulty is often caused by the way in which empirical data are analyzed, especially if the model of linear regression is used.

In our longitudinal study, we found a correlation of about .25 (N ≈ 600) between the amount of problem behavior at the age of ten and the sum of risk factors during pregnancy and birth; which means a highly significant correlation. However, this correlation is far too low to infer that these problems are the results of constitutional factors caused by hazards during pregnancy and birth in an individual case with many risks and behavior problems. We also found a correlation of .25 between the respective behavior problems and an environmental variable that defined the emotional pressure on the child during upbringing. In this case the correlation was also significant but too low to decide in a single case that the problems are only produced by environmental pressure.

Under these conditions, a discrimination between constitutional and environmental influences on observed symptoms will only then be possible if further information about the development or the environment of the child are considered. But this consideration of additional variables has often a surprisingly small effect. This is partly a methodological problem. Common and most frequently used models for combining several variables are *LISREL* and factor analysis. These models only make use of linear relations between the variables, and, in addition, their results show a great sample bias (Kalveram, 1968).

2. Method

We therefore used another qualitative method to find efficiently discriminating combinations of several variables. This model is called latent class analysis (LCA) and was developed by P. Lazarsfeld in the early 1950s. Formann (1976) proposed a method (and a computer program) that avoided the initial problems of parameter estimation.

The idea of LCA is to explain the relation of variables by dividing the sample into homogeneous subgroups called latent classes. In each class the variables are considered to have local stochastic independence. The classes differ from each other by the probabilities of the variable levels; these are called the variable latent probabilities. So each class is described by a configuration of the variable latent probabilities called a class structure. These class structures allow − as will be shown − an interpretation of the psychological particularity of different groups in the sense of types.

The parameters of the LCA-model are estimated by an iterative procedure (Formann, 1976). The parameters are (1) class−sizes and (2) class−specific probabilities of the variable levels. These probabilities are specifically objective and therefore should be stable in different samples. This means that the class structure of an LCA model should be equal for boys and girls, younger and older children, and so forth. Now we will present the results of the LCA model based on our data. For this analysis we took four characteristics of the children and two characteristics of their environment into consideration.

Tab. 1:   Selected Variables and Their Definitions for the "Latent Class Analysis"*

	Test (Variable)	
Age: 6 years	10 years	code for level > Mdn

Variables of Development

(1) Intelligence
CFT 1, HAWIVA–Block Design (Wechsler), Draw–a–Man Test (sum of z–scores) — CFT 20, HAWIK–Block Design, HAWIK–Vocabulary, KFT–Test of Cognitive Abilities: Verbal Tests (sum of z–scores) — 1

(2) Sensorimotor development
GFT–Sensorimotor Development Test (mistakes) — 0

(3) Motor Development
KTK–Motor Development Test — Rostock Oseretzky–Motor Development Scale — 1

(4) Behavior Problems
Marburg Questionnaire for Problem Behavior; Childrearing problems, Mothers checklist of child disorders, Teachers checklist; AFS–Manifest Anxiety; AFS–Test Anxiety (sum of z–scores) — 1

Variables of the environment

(1) Expectations of early independent behavior (Questionnaire) — 1
(2) Emotional pressure in child–rearing through guilt and fear (Questionnaire) — 1

*   An exact description of the variables is given by Ehlers et al. (1979, 1981, 1983)

The characteristics of the children were:

— intelligence,
— sensomotor development,
— motor development, and
— behavior problems.

The two characteristics of the environment were:

— expectations of early independent behavior, and
— emotional pressure in child–rearing through guilt and fear.

The six variables were defined by standardized tests. For the analysis, each variable was divided by a median split.

3. Results and Discussion

The best model fit was achieved by accepting a solution with 4 classes (x^2-Goodness–of–fit test: 50.75, $df=36$, $p>0.05$). The result is presented in Fig. 1. It shows the probabilities of the above–median levels for each variable and class.

The first class contained 20% of the children. The variable latent probabilities pointed out that these were children with a cognitive and motor development that was well above the average, and who did not have any behavior problems. In this case there was no emotional pressure elicited by the parents, whose expectations with regard to early independent behavior had been normal.

Class II contained the largest portion of the whole sample: 45%. The variables showed a normal developmental status and a normal environment. Generally the variable latent probabilities were about $p=0.5$.

Class III contained children who showed a normal cognitive and motor development, but this was accompanied by behavior problems. The probability that a child who belongs to Class III had behavior problems was well above the average. At the same time, the parents of these children often acted with emotional pressure.

Class IV with 14% was the smallest one. The children in this group showed poor cognitive and motor development. Like the children in Class III, they often had behavior problems. The parents showed some emotional pressure on their children during upbringing, and their expectations for early independent behavior from their children were rather low.

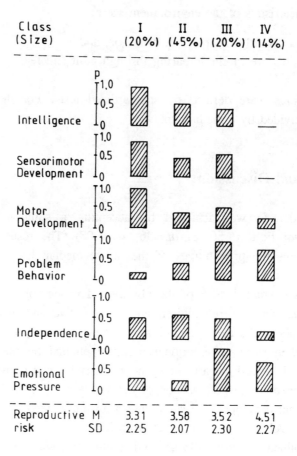

Fig. 1: Results of Latent Class Analysis for 6– and 10–year–old Children combined (N = 674). Latent probabilities of variable levels > median

To study our question about the origin of behavior problems, we have to compare Classes III and IV. Both groups included children with behavior problems. But in both cases we found different class structures, that is, different profiles with regard to the other variables. In Class III the class structure was defined by problem behavior and frequent environmental stress. The cognitive development of the children was normal. Consequently, the assumption can be made that in Class III the problem behavior was mainly influenced by the environmental variable.

In Class IV we found a configuration of problem behavior, poor mental and motor development, and low expectations of the parents concerning independent behavior. Class IV also differed from the other classes in pre- and perinatal risk factors. The mean frequency of these reproductive risks per class and the standard deviations are shown in the last rows of Fig. 1. The difference between Class IV and the other groups was statistically significant ($p > 0.001$).

This result may indicate that the behavior problems of Class IV could be mainly caused by constitutional variables.

What kind of differences in problem behavior can be found between Classes III and IV? A screening procedure based on all items yielded the following results: The behavior problems of the children in Group IV were mainly reported by their teachers and by the research psychologists who administered the tests. The symptoms indicated were suggestibility, tiredness, daydreaming, shyness, and poor performance stability. In the *self-ratings*, the children in Class IV showed higher test anxiety than those in Class III. The problem behavior of the children in Class III was more closely related to their family situation and was mainly reported by their parents. The main symptoms were aggressive behavior and hyperactivity.

This observed interdependency between class and kind of problems supports the notion that problem behavior in Class III was the expression of an underlying neurotic process, whereas in Class IV it was mainly the expression of disorders caused by cognitive deficiencies. As a result we can state that the LCA model described or defined two classes of children with behavior problems, whereby the causes of the problems were obviously different. If we put this finding into practice, we have to choose different treatments for both groups in order to provide a successful psychological intervention. Such solutions of LCA provide us with a classification procedure for the single case. On the basis of the class-specific probabilities of the variables, it is possible to infer which latent class the child belongs to.

One of the above-mentioned advantages of the LCA is that the class structures (not the class sizes!) are valid for several samples. To demonstrate this characteristic, we divided our cohorts into subsamples. For each subsample, we recomputed the proportions of the four classes. The eight subgroups were:

(1) boys versus (2) girls, (3) 6-year-old children versus (4) 10-year-old children, (5) children with high-SES homes versus (6) children with low-SES

homes, (7) children with many pre– and perinatal risks versus (8) children with few risks.

Naturally, these eight groups showed differences with regard to the size of the four classes. This is demonstrated in the following table:

Tab. 2:   Sizes of Latent Classes (%) in Different Samples*

			Class		
Sample	N	I	II	III	IV
Age: 6	(221)	19	42	20	19
Age: 10	(453)	17	45	24	14
Boys	(347)	12	46	26	16
Girls	(327)	24	42	19	15
Parental ≤MD	(347)	10	38	29	23
level of edu–					
cation*) >MD	(322)	27	50	16	7
Pre– and ≤MD	(349)	21	44	25	10
perinatal					
risks >MD	(313)	15	44	20	22

* defined by the sum of the SES–scales I and II (Ehlers, 1981)

It can be seen that the portion of girls in the first class was higher than that of boys. This difference was the result of the accelerated development of girls during school age. Other differences between subsamples in the first class can be seen concerning family status and risks during pregnancy and birth. Although there were differences between the subsamples with regard to the size of the latent classes, there was only very little variation of class structure. This is shown in Tab. 3.

The class–specific probabilities of the variables of each latent class always had quite a small range, particulary the cognitive variables in Class I or Class IV, the variable "problem behavior" in Class III or IV, or the variable "emotional pressure" in Class III. In all subsamples we found comparable structures in each of the four classes.

Tab. 3:   Range of the Class–Specific Probabilities of Variable Level >Median Based on eight Subgroups (Compare Tab. 2)

Variables	I	II	III	IV
Intelligence sensomotor	.89 — 1.00	.45 — .55	.36 — .64	0
development motor	.83 — 1.00	.37 — .47	.49 — .76	0
development problem	.94 — 1.00	.30 — .44	.40 — .56	.23 — .41
behavior	.12 — .18	.21 — .39	.91 — 1.00	.74 — .83
independence	.48 — .63	.46 — .73	.35 — .80	0 — .21
emotional pressure	.16 — .34	.16 — .32	1.00	.59 — .79

Our first attempt was to show that the LCA may be helpful in developing classification procedures in situations with complex relationships between variables. The presented analysis yields a classification system which enables us to find the right explanation and subsequently the right treatment for behavior problems in particular cases.

References

Ehlers, T. (1981): Fragebogen zur Beschreibung der Umwelt und der Verhaltensbesonderheiten von Kindern durch die Eltern. Berichte aus dem Fachbereich Psychologie der Philipps-Universität, Nr. 79, Marburg.

Ehlers, T., Hanel, E., Kalveram, H., and Merz, F. (1979): Psychologische Längsschnittuntersuchungen an Kindern aus dem Schwerpunktprogramm "Schwangerschaftsverlauf und Kindesentwicklung". Zwischenbericht über das erste Projektjahr. Philipps-Universität, Fachbereich Psychologie, Marburg.

Ehlers, T., and Merz, F. (1983): Psychologische Längsschnittuntersuchungen an Kindern aus dem Schwerpunktprogramm "Schwangerschaftsverlauf und Kindesentwicklung". Zwischenbericht über das vierte Projektjahr und die erste Hälfte des fünften Projektjahres. Marburg: Mauersberger.

Formann, A.K. (1976): Schätzung der Parameter in Lazarfelds Latent-Class-Analysis. Research Bulletin, 18.

Kalveram, K.T. (1968): Faktorenanalyse und Selektion. Marburg: Mauersberger.

Part Four

Issues in Prevention, Intervention, and Rehabilitation

Prevention of Psychopathology and Maladjustment in Children of Divorce*

Gerald Caplan

1. A Model of Prevention

Twentyfour years ago when I wrote my book, Principles of Preventive Psychiatry (1964), the main goal of our model building was to adapt traditional
public health theories and practices for use in the mental health field. We
focused in those days on two issues: (1) developing a list of past biopsychosocial stressful events and processes that were thought to increase the risk of
future mental disorder in an exposed population; and (2) studying so–called life
crises, namely, limited time periods of upset in the psychosocial functioning of
individuals, precipitated by current exposure to environmental stressors, which
appeared to be turning points in the development of mental disorder. Methods
of primary prevention were directed toward influencing decision makers to
change conditions of community life so as to reduce the occurrence or intensity
of biopsychosocial hazards; toward modifying health, education, and welfare
services so that community caregivers would intervene preventively during life
crisis provoked by stress; and toward developing and disseminating techniques
of preventive intervention for use with individuals in crisis and their families.
Much of this ciris intervention was directed at helping target individuals and
their families reduce the intensity and incapacitating effects of their crisis–in-
duced emotional upset and at offering them guidance and material help in
grappling with their predicaments.

---

*) Based on Chapter IX of Population–Oriented Psychiatry, Gerald Caplan (1989): Human
Sciences Press, New York. This book is due to appear in March 1989.

Another goal was to develop viable roles for mental health specialists as ener-
gizers of primary prevention programs that would be implemented mainly by
community decision makers and caregiving professionals. Our approach was to
use the limited number of mental health specialists as consultants and educators
to the network of community key workers, who in turn would influence high-
risk groups on a widespread scale in the population they served. In my second
book on preventive psychiatry, Theory and Practice of Mental Health Consultation (1970), I described the techniques we had worked out over the previous
decade to accomplish this goal.

During the past ten years the two elements of the original model have been
supplemented by postulating: (1) *competence* as an internal constitutional and
acquired quality of individuals that enables them to withstand the harmful
effects of hazardous circumstances; and (2) *social supports* as an external
mechanism that protects individuals against the damage that might be caused by
environmental stressors.

Tab. 1 summarizes how these elements articulate and reverberate with each
other in the manner of the themes of a musical composition. For example, the
hazardous circumstances of past risk factors reappear as the current stressor
that precipitates a crisis; the elements of competence that enable an individual to
master both a past hazard and a current stress recur in a modified form in the
outcome of the individual's reaction to current stress as changed vulnerability to
mental disorder that may predispose eventually to actual psychopathology; and
adequate social supports not only buffer reaction to current stress but also were
probably a crucial element in determining whether a past risk factor led to a
current unhealthy outcome, as well as being a central element in the mediated
learning process whereby children acquire self–efficacy and problem–solving
skills that form the core of competence. Because of these reverberations, I have
given to the overall conceptual structure the name of the Recurring Themes
Model of Primary Prevention. Tab. 1 provides a summary of present–day
conceptualizations of the field, and I believe that it shows how crisis intervention and the promotion of support systems articulate with the other elements in
a comprehensive primary prevention program.

Tab. 1: Recurrent Themes Model of Primary Prevention*

Past risk factors			Intermediate variables		Outcome
Bio-psycho-social hazard (episodes or continuing)	Teaching of competence	Competence (constitutional and acquired)	Reaction to recent or current stress (crisis)	Social supports	
Examples Genetic defects Pregnancy problems Birth trauma Prematurity Congenital anomaly Developmental problems Accidents Illness Hospitalization Poverty Cultural deprivation School failure Family discord Family disruption Parental mental or physical illness Sibling illness	Parents and teachers provide opportunities for child to learn self-efficacy and problem-solving skills. Exposure to increasing stress while providing guidance, emotional support, and teaching skills.	Self-efficacy Quality of self-image and identity. Expect mastery by self and support by others. Tolerance of frustration and confusion. Problem-solving skills Social and material.	Bio-psycho-social hazard Bodily damage. Current or recent life change events: loss, threat, or challenge. Adaptation by *Active Mastery* versus *Passive Surrender*. Hopeful perseverance despite cognitive erosion and fatigue. Containment of feelings. Enlisting support.	Cognitive, emotional, and material Supplement ego strength in problem solving. Validate identity. Maintain hope. Help with tasks. Contain feelings. Counteract fatigue.	Sense of wellbeing. Capacity to study, work, love, and play. Enhanced or eroded competence. Actual psychopathology (D.S.M. III)

Types of intervention

Social action in health, education, welfare, and legal services Consultation collaboration, and education for professionals	Education of parents and child-care professionals	Education of children and parents	Crisis intervention by anticipatory guidance and preventive intervention	Promote supports Convene network. Convene mutual-help couple. Help mutual-help organizations. Support the supporters.	

Preventive intervention to target populations (highest risk groups)

* Caplan, G. (1986): Recent developments in crisis intervention and in the promotion of support services. In Kessler, M., and Goldston, S.E. (Eds.): A decade of progress in primary prevention. Hanover: University Press of New England, 240

2. Utilizing the Model for Children of Divorce

In this paper I will describe how I have made use of this model in organizing a program of primary prevention of psychopathology and maladjustment for children whose parents are contemplating divorce or who have already divorced.

The following are the steps in organizing such a program:

1. Identify and define a target population at risk.
2. Specify the dimensions of the problem: possible pathological effects and their incidence.
3. Plan services to serve total target population and prepare ground for eventual evaluation; articulate with community caregivers and caregiving systems.
4. Identify pathogenic factors that should be reduced and psychosocial supports that should be increased.
5. Clarify ethical, political, and legal aspects of such intervention.
6. Develop procedures for case–finding and case–recruitment. Ensure easy access and flexible fee schedule. Promote wide range of professional referrals and direct contact by self–referral.
7. Develop comprehensive list of intervention services that can be tailored to different individual needs of heterogeneous population at risk.
8. Develop and precisely describe intervention methods so that they can be replicated and evaluated.
9. Evaluate results of different methods in terms of reducing incidence of pathological sequelae.

My clinical practice as a child psychiatrist has over the last few years convinced me of the increasing significance of parental divorce as the major threat to the mental health of today's children. Because of this I helped to establish in 1985 the Jerusalem Family Center, an ambulatory service that seeks to prevent child psychopathology and maladjustment by intervening in families at the time of divorce and afterwards. The frequency of divorce is lower in Israel than in many Western countries: Only one marriage in five ends in divorce compared, for example, with one in three in Britain and one in two in the United States. But divorce is still a major problem with us.

Tab. 2: Statistical Report 9.7.87 – 182 Cases

Lawyers	Order Beth Din[1]	Beth–Din Letter[2]	District Court Order	School	Welfare Worker	Psychologist	Self	Former Client	Physician	Friend
16	35	7	31	7	35	8	24	10	4	4

Living together: 69
Living apart: 114

Jerusalem Cases: 152
Outside Jerusalem: 30

Initiation of Separation
Mother: 92
Father: 31   Both: 2

Total Children: 406   0–6 : 151   7–8 : 163   9–13 : 110   14–18 : 82

With Whom Do Children Live After Separation?
Mother: 82 Cases   Father: 8 Cases   Split[3]: 12 Cases   Joint[4]: 12 Cases   Other Relative: 1 Case

Interval Between Separation and Intake

Under 6 months	1/2–1 Year	1–2 Years	2–3 Years	3–4 Years	Over 5 Years
21	22	17	12	22	15

Length of Marriage Before Separation

| Never Married: 3 Cases | 5 Years or Less: 38 Cases | 6–10 Years: 35 Cases | Over 15 Years: 50 Cases |

Tab. 2/continued

Couples in Which at least One Parent has Psychopathology:

Psychosis	Antisocial Personality	Narcissistic Personality	Paranoid Personality	Borderline Personality	Schizoid Personality
11 = 6.0%	5 = 2.7%	6 = 3.3%	16 = 8.8%	4 = 2.2%	2 = 1.1%

Type of Intervention

Conciliation Regarding Divorce Agreement	Report to Court or Beth Din on Custody or Visitation	Counseling Re Child Care and Child Adjustment after Divorce	Marriage Counseling and Child Care Counseling
70 Cases	43 Cases	47 Cases	35 Cases

Child Psychopathology: 20 Cases = 11%   Child Partisan[5]: 13 Cases = 7.1%

Notes:

1) *Beth – Din* – The rabbinical court that handles the process of divorce.
2) *Beth – Din Letter* – Circular letter inviting all divorcing parents to a voluntary guidance session.
3) *Split* – Children divided between homes of father and mother.
4) *Joint* – All children live together part of the time with each parent alternately.
5) *Child Partisan* – Cases in which a child actively sides with one parent against the other.

During my first two years' experience in the Family Center, I personally counselled 182 parental couples and their 406 children under 18. I worked collaboratively on these cases with lawyers, welfare workers, and school personnel; and I made recommendations on custody and visiting of children to our rabbinical and civil courts.

This experience has been the most fascinating in my entire career: The intensity of emotional arousal in parents and children and the victimization of children caught up in the parental battles aroused in me a profound empathic involvement. It was particularly exciting to participate in the unfolding of dramatic events of obvious significance for the future well-being of the children. I was also able in certain cases to intervene actively in their tumultuous family drama to modify the current balance of forces, and so to fulfil my basic mission of primary prevention.

This work has taught me to study and treat each case in accordance with its own complicated indiosyncratic elements, and to beware of premature generalizations that may oversimplify. But some regularities of pattern across cases are beginning to emerge in my mind.

3. Harmful Sequelae of Parental Divorce

Kalter (1977) reviewed the records of 400 children seen in 1974–75 in the Department of Psychiatry at the University of Michigan. He found that children of divorced parents appeared in the outpatient clinic at double their rate in the general population: 32.6% as compared with 16%. He reported that the children of divorce suffered principally from symptoms associated with poor control over aggression. In the younger children the hostility was directed inside the home against parents and siblings. In the older children and adolescents the aggressive behavior took the form of antisocial acts and delinquency, as well as alcoholism, drug addiction, and in girls, sexual promiscuity.

Kalter and Rembar (1981) repeated the study with a new sample of 500 cases seen in the University of Michigan psychiatric outpatient clinic in the period 1976–77, and obtained much the same results.

McDermott (1970) has emphasized the importance of depression in the clinical picture of children whose parents were divorced at least 2.5 years earlier. He found moderate or severe depression in 34.3% of his sample of 116 child psychiatry outpatient clinic cases whose parents had been divorced.

Wadsworth, Pekham, and Taylor (1985), reporting on a long-term follow-up study of a national sample of 5,362 children born during one week in Britain in 1946, found that 36.5% of men whose families had been disrupted by parental divorce, separation, or death before they reached age 5, suffered from psychopathology or social maladjustment (hospitalization before age 26 for affective psychiatric illness or for stomach ulcers or colitis, or delinquency by 21 years) compared with 17.9% of men from intact families. They also found that 23.3% of women whose families were disrupted by parental divorce, separation, or death before age 5 suffered from psychopathology or social maladjustment (hospitalized by 26 years for affective psychiatric illness or for stomach ulcers or colitis, delinquency by 21 years, divorce or separation by 26 years, or illegitimate children by 26 years) compared with 9.6% of women from intact families.

Wadsworth (1979) tabulates other findings of the 1946 longitudinal cohort study that permit the following recalculation: 29% of men whose families were disrupted by parental divorce, separation, or death before the children reached 16 suffered by age 26 from psychopathology or social maladjustment (hospitalization for affective psychiatric illness, delinquency, or divorce and separation) compared with 18% of men from intact families. Twenty–one percent of women whose families were disrupted by parental divorce, separation, or death before the children reached age 16 suffered by age 26 from psychopathology or social maladjustment (hospitalization for affective psychiatric illness, delinquency, illegitimate children, or divorce and separation) compared with 10.1% of women from intact families.

The British risk figures of 29% for men and 21% for women can be compared with the findings of Wallerstein and Kelly (1980) in the United States that 35% of the sons and daughters of divorced parents they studied suffered from psychopathology or delinquency.

Wadsworth and Maclean (1986) analysed other data from the 1946 longitudinal cohort study. They found that men from manual social class families had significantly lower income at age 26 if their parents had divorced or separated before they were 16 compared with men from intact families. They also found that children of both sexes of divorced or separated parents had significantly lower educational qualifications, such as matriculation or attending university, by the age of 26 years than children of intact families. By comparison, parental death had very little impact on a child's later educational achievements and may even have increased the chance of children of manual social class going to university. These findings indicate that parental divorce or separation has a considerable harmful impact on the lives of children that is expressed not only in psychopathology or social maladjustment but also in lower educational attainment in both sexes and lower socioeconomic achievements in males.

4. Psychosocial Hazards

In order to understand why parental divorce is associated with an increased likelihood that the children will develop psychopathology or social maladjustment during childhood or in later adult life, it seems advisable to focus on the following factors:

1. Parental Quarreling

Most divorces are preceded by months or even years of quarreling. These quarrels often go through three phases:

— Phase I is linked with disappointments and frustrations in the expectations of each other that motivated their marriage, with incompatibilities of temperament that became salient between them, or in a minority of cases with manifestations of psychopathology in one or both spouses. Mutual provocations typically lead to escalation of hostility and to episodes of irrational shouting, screaming, and verbal or physical abuse. The children may be involved as bystanders. The younger children are frightened by these scenes, and, whatever their age, the children are burdened and upset by the breakdown of rational control in their parents. Most children, however, do not appear to be drawn in to take sides in these conflicts at this stage.

— Phase II begins with one or both parents' decision to start the process of divorce. They begin an adversarial process to wrest from each other an optimal share of their joint property and to safeguard their links with their children. Often, their hostility intensifies, they inflict on each other mental or physical wounds; in consequence, especially if this phase is protracted, they may become increasingly bitter and vengeful. Often, they actively try to recruit their children to side with them by maligning the other parent and by inciting the children against him or her.

— Phase III begins when the parents separate or divorce. In many cases the separation of the combatants leads to a period of relative tranquility, and since a contract has been signed or the case has been adjudicated, the immediate conflict of interests has been terminated. Previous animosities become a fading memory of past pains, and the former spouses begin to adjust to the burdens of reestablishing their homes and dealing with the adaptive problems of their children.

Often, however, the hatred and bitterness stimulated by the narcissistic wounds inflicted in the previous phase, or in certain cases by the image of the former spouse having been introjected to play an enduring part in the individual's psychopathological inner world, lead to long-term vengeful hostility. In these cases the plight of the children may well become worse than before the divorce. They are more likely to be recruited as protagonists in the fight, particularly as the bone of contention is often disagreements between the parents about implementing the terms of the divorce contract in regard to custody and visitation. The other major factor is that the separated parents can no longer give direct vent to their hatred through face-to-face contact or even through the medium of a telephone conversation, and therefore they send their hostile messages through their children.

2. Conflict of Interests Between Parents and Children

Spouses who continually quarrel with each other may well feel that they should cut their losses and end their marriage. Their children, however, will rarely be in favor of divorce. In my experience, although most children of quarreling parents feel burdened by the rows, very few accept divorce as a solution, because they feel that the splitting of their home and their separation from one of their parents will involve them in worse burdens. Even in cases of physical violence, many children say they prefer the present painful reality to their becoming involved in an unknown and frightening future after divorce. For instance, Gideon aged nine, told me, "It is often pretty bad at home, especially when Dad comes home drunk and starts beating us up. But I still love him, and I don't want my mother to throw him out of the house for good".

Many children feel that their interests were ignored by their parents, and that they were passive victims of adult decisions about adult issues. Shimon, aged 14, said, "Our parents have decided to divorce. We feel angry that they didn't pay any attention to what this will mean to us children. They never even talked to us about it till after they had decided". Existentially the children may be right. This is not to say that if their parents had been fully aware of the needs and views of their children they would have changed their decision to divorce. However, they might have found ways of reducing the feelings of passivity and helplessness of the children, which impose a major additional burden on them.

3. Communication Issues

Feelings of passive victimization of children are often exacerbated by the parents not preparing them ahead of time and not explaining to them what is happening during and after the divorce, which would give the children the opportunity at least to gain cognitive mastery over their predicament. This is particularly the case with preschoolers and young school children (James, 1897). For instance, Ester, aged 5, told me, "Three months ago I woke up one morning and found that Daddy had disappeared. Mummy told me he had gone off to do his army reserve duty; but this can't be true because he always comes back from army service at the end of a month. She won't tell me where he has gone!"

This absence of authentic communication often leads to the child developing fearful fantasies that the departing parent no longer loves him and has left home because of the child's badness. Ester said, "I think he has left us because I used to make so much noise and he couldn't stand it".

Another and more serious hazard, particularly for older children, is their being used by parents as message carriers between them. These messages are usually heavily loaded with hatred and disparagement. Even for children who have not been recruited to take sides, the conveying of such hostile messages is most disturbing.

This hazard becomes exaggerated, when, as often happens, a child rebels against his feeling of passivity by choosing to play an active role in the parental conflict. He will then modify the messages he carries between them. Sometimes he tones down the hostile elements in order to reduce the animosity between the parents. Often he distorts the messages, as well as the stories he himself tells each parent about the other, in an effort to stir up further trouble. In either case, the child's manipulations give him the feeling that he is exercising some active mastery over the situation. Haviv, aged 14, said, "I can't bear to see how much it hurts mother when I give her father's messages; so I change them; that makes everyone happier. I wish my parents wouldn't behave so childishly so that I have to quiet them down".

4. Partisanship of Children

A child may begin to hate one of the parents because he has been brainwashed and incited by the other. He may take sides because of his own interpretation of the relative merits of the adversaries, particularly if one parent was repeatedly violent, or was the one the child felt caused the family breakup. For instance, Talia, aged 11, told me, "Mother suddenly changed. She began to make hysterical scenes and to call the police to stop father hitting her; but it was she who attacked him, and she also scratched my brother's arm. She shamed us in front of the neighbors — I began to hate her. She was the cause of all the trouble in the home". The child is likely to develop a stereotyped view of one parent as ideally *all-good* and the other as *all-bad*. Perceptions and expectations of the bad parent usually become colored by fantasy elements that increase the child's rejection and fear. Typically, this leads to the child's trying to cut down his interactions with the bad parent; and in provocative behavior when meetings do take place, which often stimulates hostile reactions in the parent that reinforce the child's prejudices. Talia said, "Mother takes it out on me because she knows I am on father's side". Her mother told me, "She is impossible; she continually attacks me and behaves like a rebellious brat!" Such behavior leads to an escalation of animosity that results in the child, and often the parent, cutting links with the other. In effect, the child divorces that parent or is abandoned by him or her.

Courts have limited power to force a recalcitrant child, even as young as 8 or 9, to visit a rejected parent. Rifka, aged 10, told me, "I absolutely refuse to visit that man. He is no longer my father. Even if you send police to take me by force I won't go; I will jump off the balcony and kill myself. If you invite me to your office and I know he is coming I will not come to you".

The net result is most unfortunate. Absence of contact allows the child's fantasies about the satanic evils of his parent to flourish without an opportunity for the child to modify his stereotypes by real experience. This promotes the continuation in the child of splitting of ambivalence — he may perceive not only his parents as divided into an all-good one and an all-bad one but also everyone else in the world, himself included. And he may introject the evil image as a rejected part of his own psychic structure, inherited from his bad parent. Rifka, who is a deeply religious girl, genteel, shy, and fastidious, said, "A couple of years ago when I used sometimes to visit him, he and the whore he lives with used to lie together half naked on the living room couch and behave in a disgusting manner. They also used to have competitions as to who could make the loudest noise by expelling gases". Later, she said, "He is an absolute monster. He once tried to strangle my mother when she was weak after an illness". In fact her father is an uncouth, insensitive, and brutal man, but he is eager to renew links with his children, although he does not know how to behave with them.

Since the internalized bad object is likely to be highly colored by hostile and sexually aggressive elements linked with actual or imaginary aspects of the conflicts between his parents, the situation is conducive to the development of antisocial violence, substance abuse, and sexual promiscuity in adolescence, when the child's psychic equilibrium becomes upset, and his previously rejected impulses become dominant.

5. Abandonment

In several of my cases a noncustodial parent deserted the children. In one case, a mother, without prior warning, ran off to Australia with her lover, leaving behind three small children with her husband, whom she subsequently divorced. In several cases, a divorced father refused to see his children because they had chosen to live with their mother. In other cases, the father took revenge on his former wife by severing his links with their children, on the grounds that she was living in sin with another man. In some cases the father stopped visiting the children because he claimed the mother had turned them against him and had put obstacles in the way of his visits. In other cases, the father visited only at irregular, long intervals in contravention of the divorce agreement that he had signed.

In all these cases the children suffered greatly. David, aged 6, told me, "Daddy has gone off and left us. It makes me very, very sad. I can't fall asleep at nights and I have bad dreams. In school I think about him the whole time instead of doing my lessons. I long for him and I cry a lot".

Myriam, aged 4, said, "Daddy doesn't live with us anymore. I don't know what I have done to drive him away. Sometimes he telephones and I beg him to visit us. He promises to come, but he never keeps his promises".

Many of these deserting parents are psychiatrically disturbed, usually suffering from major personality disorders, paranoid, narcissistic, or borderline; and before they deserted they behaved cruelly to their children, linked with their lack of capacity to love. Although I believe that ideally children should be given the opportunity to recognize the reality of their parents as human beings, I feel that these children might sometimes be worse off if I were to engineer contact between them and a sick parent. For instance, Leah, aged 14, told me, "I went to see Daddy last week. I had thought that after not seeing me for a year he would be nicer than in the past. But he spent the whole visit shouting and screaming. He told me that he had evidence that mother was having affairs with several different men, and that she has brainwashed me to become his enemy. He demanded that I leave her at once and come to live with him, because otherwise I will become a whore like her. He says that if I don't come to him he will no longer accept me as his daughter, and as far as he is concerned I will be dead". Her father suffers from a borderline personality disorder with paranoid features.

In such cases I have learned not to be doctrinaire about fostering contact between children and a sick parent, but to weigh the evidence very carefully before intervening, lest I make a bad situation worse.

6. Loss of a Parent: The One-Parent Home

Children of divorce usually suffer from a significant reduction in regular contact with one of their parents. Intermittent contact of a few hours a week with a nonresidential parent does not effectively make up for interruption of parenting. Adequate parenting requires that on a continuing basis the father or mother, nurtures, controls, guides, and supports the child by active involvement in the details of the child's daily life. A child needs two parents, who play complementary roles in child care and education, who support each other in supporting the child in mastering the expectable stresses of growing up, and who provide him with two differentiated sexual role models on which to base the identifications that form the core of his identity. Weiss (1975) has reported on the findings of research at our Harvard Laboratory of Community Psychiatry which documented the expectable burdens of the one-parent home for both the parent and the children. It is important to emphasize that divorce leads not to "one-parent-families" but to split two-parent families and to one-parent-homes. If the divorced parents live close to each other, communicate freely with each other, and are able to collaborate well in joint parenting, some of these burdens on their children may be reduced by joint-custody arrangements which involve children in living part of every week with each parent. When it succeeds, this pattern allows the children to relate in a more healthy way to both parents, and allows each parent more fully to play his or her child-rearing role; but when animosities and disorders of communication continue between the parents after the divorce, this arrangement can be particularly burdensome to the children.

Divorcing parents not infrequently try to solve conflicts over child custody by dividing up their children. This does not solve the children's problem of losing daily contact with their nonresidential parent. It also reduces the support the children get from being part of a stable sibling group, and often leads to the children being burdened by unsatisfied longings for absent siblings as well as for the absent parent.

Many children after parental divorce lose their conviction that until they grow up they will be nurtured and protected by their parents. The breakup of their home and the fact that they feel they have lost one parent often arouses the fear that they may also lose the other. This fear may be strengthened if the residential parent, usually the mother, has to absent herself during the day from the home to go out to work, and if she comes home tired out because of this, as well as suffering from depression as a reaction to the failure of her marriage and to the practical burdens of running a one–parent home. The child may then feel that he has lost or will lose both his parents; and this leads to a feeling of being alone and unsupported that will render him less resilient in facing and mastering situations of adversity (Rutter, 1985).

7. Loss of Income

Two homes cost more than one. Almost all families are economically worse off after divorce, despite the efforts of the mother, who is usually the parent with whom the children live, to increase her earnings and thus make up the deficit, and despite governmental family welfare allowances in some Western countries to reduce the financial deprivation. Wadsworth and Maclean (1986) have recently confirmed the findings of a study by Fogelman (1983) that family income is almost certain to be reduced after divorce, and that this is likely to lead to downward social mobility and to a socioeconomically disadvantaged status for children that is in turn associated with lower educational achievements and reduced future earning power in their adult life.

8. Moving

A child, especially a young child, derives a significant part of his feelings of basic security from the stability of his familiar home and neighborhood, and from his continuing relationships with his neighborhood friends and the children and adults he meets daily in his kindergarten or school classroom. Divorce often results in the children and the parent with whom they live being forced to move house. Not infrequently, the mother has to take her children to live for a while with relatives. Often, the downwardly mobile family is forced to move repeatedly so that the mother can find accessible work, or so they can locate a home they can afford. Often these moves have to take place in the middle of the school year. Each move is likely to interrupt schooling and to separate the children from their neighborhood friends. Each move is likely to face them with the burdens of adjustment to new classrooms and new teachers and with the task of making new friends. These frequent moves still further erode the sense of security of the children.

9. Stigma

The rapidly increasing incidence of divorce is related to, and results in, a reduction of the social and religious stigma that used to be associated with it even a generation ago. And yet, apart from places like California, where two out of three children will probably soon be children of divorce, this status is generally not the norm. And school children are particularly sensitive to being regarded as different and hence inferior; they are apt to suffer by being stigmatised by their peers.

10. Sex

Marital conflicts that lead to divorce not infrequently focus on sexual dissatisfactions. Frequently, angry accusations of sexual infidelity or misconduct are recurring features of verbal battles between parents. The children also often overhear a parent complaining bitterly to a friend about the sexual misconduct of the spouse. A small child may not at first understand the meaning of these complaints, but will fill out the story from his own fantasies. His sexual curiosity is likely to be much stimulated by these passionate complaints, as portrayed so well by Henry James (1897).

After divorce, parents not infrequently engage in a flurry of sexual overactivity to counteract feelings of inferiority about not having succeeded in marriage. Eventually, each parent may initiate exploratory dating with a succession of prospective sexual partners with a view to remarriage.

These situations are likely to stimulate precocious development of sexual curiosity in the children, and to their taking upon themselves the unnatural role of critic or intervener in the sex life of their parents. Especially during adolescence, when parents normally have a sensitive role to play in helping their children grapple in a socially acceptable way with the complications of their tumultuous sexual awakening, a loss of respect by the children for the sexual maturity of their parents erodes an important source of support and control inside the family.

5. Adjustment Reactions

Children typically react to these psychosocial burdens and to reductions in parental support by signs of strain that persist for several weeks or months after divorce. These symptoms vary somewhat with age and developmental level. Younger children are confused, frightened, and clinging. Older children are angry, irritable, and restless; they have difficulty concentrating in school because of the intrusion of worries about the parental battles and the breakup of their home. Many children of all ages have difficulty falling asleep, and their sleep is disturbed by frightening dreams. After divorce many children become sad and depressed. Most children are aggressive with their siblings and with peers at school and in the neighborhood. Adolescents have difficulty with impulse control and tend to be more rebellious than the norm.

In my Jerusalem caseload, these immediate adjustment reactions have generally cleared up by the end of the first year; but in 11% of cases they have been succeeded by signs of psychopathology described earlier in this chapter. I expect that a follow-up study would show that possibly another 15–20% of my cases will develop signs of similar psychiatric illness in the future; but on the basis of their present clinical picture and pattern of adjustment I do not feel able to predict which these will be. Such predictions must await the results of further research. Until then, the acute adjustment reactions should be regarded as normal signs of strain and should not be interpreted to the prodromata of eventual psychopathology, which some of them will by hindsight eventually be determined to have been.

6. Ethical and Political Aspects of Preventive Interaction

Primary prevention of psychopathology and maladjustment in the children of divorce requires *proactive* intervention to modify the conditions of life of the children; namely, reaching out by caregivers who seek to initiate change processes in the family, without having received a prior invitation by the parents to intervene. Our goal is to identify harmful factors and to modify them, or to introduce supportive factors before many parents will be aware of the risks to their children; particularly as these parents are likely to be preoccupied with their own conflicts and the complications of the divorce process, and will be less motivated and able than usual to focus attention on the needs of their children. This raises significant ethical and political questions.

In democratic societies the care and protection of children is largely left to their parents within their private domain. Representatives of society are only permitted to penetrate the boundaries of this domain if there is convincing evidence that a parent is causing major damage to a child by maltreatment or battering or by gross neglect and deprivation. This philosophy is justified, because the vast majority of ordinary parents do care adequately for their children on their own or with help that they themselves seek from others. And in most societies the rights of the parents to privacy in regard to how they fulfil their responsibilities to their children are protected by law and by public opinion; and are defended politically against governmental or professional encroachment by advocates of civil liberty.

This situation is, however, altered in the case of divorce. By voluntarily approaching the courts to dissolve their marriage, parents explicitly open up their private domain to public scrutiny and intervention. Their request for divorce is a formal statement that their marriage has broken down and constitutes an invitation to the representatives of society to assess the consequences for themselves and their children. And indeed, most laws governing the procedure of divorce make explicit provision for the protection of the interests of the children, which are felt to be endangered by the upheavals of the divorce and its aftermath.

Moreover, I have already cited evidence that the very fact of divorce implies that the children are in significantly greater danger than children in intact families. Divorce must therefore be seen as a marker indicating the need for societal intervention to protect these children from expectable damage, which cannot be left entirely in the private domain of their parents. This is a special case, and we must avoid being persuaded by the arguments of zealous political advocates of civil liberty to romanticize the competence of all parents, including those who have failed to maintain a stable marriage and have thus involved their children in this major extra risk to their mental health.

On the other hand, although authoritarian adjudication by the courts may be essential in determining the pattern of child care following divorce, the details of how children will be cared for in their family throughout their years of dependency after the divorce cannot be completely determined by court prescriptions; they must sooner or later be once more returned to the field of responsibility of their parents within the reconstituted boundaries of their private domain. Intervention by agents of society must necessarily be temporary. My own feeling is that it should be as short as possible, and that the invoking of authoritarian coercion, or its threat, should be minimal, lest it have a counterproductive effect when the care of the children inevitably will be returned to their parents.

Although it may sometimes be necessary to force divorcing parents to modify their behavior for the benefit of their children at the time of court proceedings during divorce, or during subsequent court action to change custody or access, I believe that a more stable long–term pattern of child care will generally be achieved if the parents are educated, guided, and enabled through mediation to work out plans which they feel meet their own idiosyncratic needs and which they voluntarily decide to accept. In my experience, many parental divorce agreements about their patterns of future child care are not implemented because eventually the parents do what they want and not what they feel they were forced to agree to do.

Other things being equal, and in the absence of major psychopathology, the likelihood of implementation is greater in proportion to the degree of freedom of choice of the parties in designing the contract. But I do not agree with those who idealize a pure mediation approach, namely that an intercessor at the time of divorce should restrict himself to merely enabling the parents voluntarily to work out a plan for their children with which they can personally feel comfortable. On the contrary, I believe that if the intercessor is a specialist in child development he should add information to the planning discussions that increases the knowledge and understanding of parents about the needs and development of children and about child care, as well as about the special problems commonly encountered by children of divorce. And although the intercessor should surely avoid imposing his own plan, he should not hide from the parents his opinion about the relative merits for their children of some of the options one or other parent may propose.

Even though I advocate the initiation of intercession without waiting for divorcing parents to ask for it, I believe that once contact has been made, the first task of the intercessor must be to arouse the motivation of both parents to invite him to continue his work with them in helping them plan how to terminate their marriage with minimal harm to their children. I advocate this approach irrespective of the auspices of the intercession, whether in a voluntary agency outside the courts or within the actual framework of the court, for example, in a court clinic or welfare unit. All such interventions connected with divorce are likely to be felt by the parents to be formally or informally linked with the court process. Parents will therefore usually feel obliged to choose arrangements for their children that they believe will be in conformity with the terms of the eventual court adjudication (Mnookin, 1978).

7. Planning a Preventive Program

In the light of the foregoing, I propose that a comprehensive preventive program should provide a range of services to intervene successively, as relevant, in the lives of a very large heterogeneous population that will mainly be composed of normal parents and their children, but will include a substantial minority of parents with psychiatric disorders. The program will center on the courts, through which all divorcing couples must pass, and will extend out into the community to units that provide services in response to voluntary requests. These services may operate within a variety of administrative auspices, which may or may not be under the control of the courts, and which may or may not have a formal link with each other. No service should, however, operate in isolation; it should articulate voluntarily with other units and with community professionals and nonprofessional caregivers, and should see its own role as part of the overall long–term community mission of reducing the risk of psychopathology and maladjustment throughout childhood in the entire population of children whose parents divorce.

The service elements of such a comprehensive program should include:

1. Education
Services to disseminate information about the significance for children of parental divorce and about expectable reactions of children and how they may be handled. This information may be disseminated to the general population through the mass media. It might be focused on the population of parents contemplating divorce by brochures provided by the courts. It should be made available through in–service training programs and case consultation to relevant caregiving professionals such as judges, lawyers, family doctors, nurses, welfare workers, educational personnel, rabbis, and clergymen.

2. Guidance
Similar information should be provided to all parents who initiate divorce proceedings, through face–to–face meetings on an individual or group basis, in which there may be discussion of problematic issues that are geared to the idiosyncratic needs and capacities of the individual cases.

3. Reconciliation
Marriage counseling should be provided in cases of marital disharmony to enable some parents to avoid divorce, possibly influenced by gaining a better understanding of the significance for their children of the different options.

4. Conciliation
Mediation by intercessors, who may or may not have expertise in child devel-

opment, to enable divorcing parents to work out on a voluntary basis a mutually acceptable contract that will determine custody of children, access to parents, and other aspects of child care, and the division of parental responsibilities for children after divorce.

5. Reports to Divorce Court
Specialist appraisal of family relationships on which may be based recommendations to the court on such issues as child custody and contacts between children and parents after divorce.

6. Adjudication of Divorce Court
This basic obligatory procedure should include judicial appraisal of the effectiveness of child-care provisions in the divorce contract in safeguarding the rights of the children. The judges should be able to order additional specialist consultation in cases of doubt or continued conflict.

7. Postdivorce Surveillance
Services should be available in questionable cases of court-ordered, obligatory, long-term surveillance to ensure that provisions of the divorce contract are actually being implemented and are indeed benefiting the children. In other cases, follow-up monitoring on a voluntary basis should be available to be organized systematically at intervals or at the request of one of the parties.

8. Postdivorce Crisis Intervention
A service should be available, to be invoked at the request of one of the parents or by a community professional, for intermittent short interventions, when new conflicts arise between the parents about the implementation of the plan for child care, or when the plan does not appear to be serving the developing needs of the children. Such intervention should have the goal of preventing escalation of hostility between the parents and offering them guidance on care of the children and on how best the parents should collaborate in providing such care.

8. Methods and Techniques

Constraints of space prevent me from providing details of all the methods and techniques that we have so far developed in Jerusalem to achieve our preventive goals. The following summarized samples of our work give some indication of how we have operated within the framework of our model: The first two samples are taken from handouts we prepared in our program to educate family doctors and parents, and the third summarizes the principles of our approach to conciliation.

8.1   Family Doctor's Role as a Counselor

The doctor should aim to influence the current behavior of the parents by offering guidance, and he should not concern himself about underlying reasons why they might have behaved differently if he had not intervened. He realizes that he may be tipping the balance of a complicated set of psychological forces by exerting his influence on the final outcome in the "here and now". The following are among the issues he may wish to emphasize during the course of his many contacts with the parents:

a) He should foster open communication between the parents about the children. They should avoid making use of the child as a communication channel between them. Children tend to distort messages because of intrusion of their fantasies. Parents should take their children's stories about each other with a large grain of salt. The child often tries to curry favor by telling each parent what he imagines he or she wants to hear about the other; he may take sides or may aggravate existing tensions to give himself a feeling of mastery in order to counteract his feelings of helplessness and insecurity because of the parental conflicts.

b) The doctor should foster maximum access of the children to the nondomiciliary parent. He should emphasize the importance of each parent, counteracting partisanship by the child in order to avoid the psychological damage this will cause the child.

c) He should urge both parents to talk well of each other to the children despite their antagonism to each other.

d) He should continually focus the attention of parents on the current needs of their children, which he should observe and communicate to them.

e) The doctor should support the parents in catering to the emotional neediness, especially of younger children; for instance, the mother should take the child into her bed at night if he wakes frightened and insecure. But the doctor should warn her against using the child unduly to comfort herself or as a replacement for her absent spouse when she feels cold and lonely in bed.

f) The doctor should assure the parents that the sadness, anger, and regressive behavior of their children is temporary in nature; a reaction to their upset feelings because of the breakup of their home. He should emphasize that such a reaction is normal; but he should himself monitor the behavior of the children, and if he identifies prolonged holdups in their psychological development he should refer the children for investigation by a child psychiatrist or psychologist.

g) Although the primary mission of the general practitioner is to safeguard the mental health of the children, he should also be concerned about parents' feelings of sadness, emptiness, and loneliness, which occur not uncommonly, even after divorce from a hated spouse that perhaps was expected to usher in an era of happiness and freedom from care. He should be particularly alert to the occurence of depression or related deterioration in physical health due to loss of interest in a domiciliary parent who did not initiate the divorce proceedings; he should counteract the underlying sense of failure and the loss of self-esteem, and he should mobilize psychosocial support by family and friends, and mutual help by divorced persons in the neighborhood who have succeeded in mastering a similar predicament.

h) Eventually, the doctor may advise the parents about balancing the satisfaction of their own needs against focusing only on the needs of the children. He should offer them guidance on how to deal tactfully and discreetly with their children in regard to the latters' heightened curiosity about the sex life of their parents. The children must not be allowed to dictate how the parents should lead their lives. On the other hand, the doctor should try to counteract any tendency of newly divorced parents to embark on a frenzy of sexual overactivity as an escape from sadness and mourning for a terminated relationship, or as a denial of lowered self-esteem because of the conjugal failure.

8.2   Role of Parents

Parents intending to divorce should discuss the issues with their children before the separation, in order to prepare the children for what is about to happen in words and at a time that is geared to the age and developmental level of the children. With preschool children this discussion should take place about a week or two before the family breakup; with 5–8 year olds the discussion should be a month or two beforehand; older children should be given longer notice. If possible, parents should talk jointly to their children to demonstrate that they agree on their message. They should expect that after this first discussion there will be the need to continue talking about the issues with the children as a group or individually in response to the reactions of the children and the questions they will raise. The initial discussion should cover the following points:

a) The parents intend to end their marriage, to live in separate homes, and no longer to be husband and wife, because they have stopped loving each other and cannot live peacefully with each other; *this divorce has not been caused by anything the children have done.*

b) The couple intend to continue as parents of their children, to love them, and to care for them throughout childhood. They promise this without regard to what may happen in future years, when one or other of the parents may possibly remarry and have additional children.

c) The children will live in the home of one parent and will visit the other parent at regular intervals. Both parents know that a child needs continuing contact with his two parents as a basis for healthy growth and development, and both want the child to maintain close links with each parent.

d) The divorce will be permanent. If the parents stop quarreling after the separation and if they become friendly, as once they used to be, this will not mean that they will again live together.

e) The parents realize that the children will probably oppose the divorce because it breaks up their home, but the children cannot alter the situation and should not try to do so. The decision has been made by adults because of their adult problems.

f) The parents know that the children may feel angry, upset, and insecure. The parents have taken these understandable reactions into account and are sorry about them. They will help the children master these feelings; most children succeed in accomplishing this over a period of a few months.

g) Divorce is very common: Every second (third) marriage ends in this way. So the children should not feel so different from others; they should not feel ashamed because their parents have divorced. Like other family matters this is private and not for public consumption; but the children should feel free to talk about it to their close friends and to their teachers. It often helps to share such matters with others who can provide support in times of difficulty. If, for a few weeks, thoughts about the family troubles interfere with the capacity to concentrate in the classroom or in homework, it would be good that the teacher should know what is happening and help the child overcome the temporary difficulties.

h) The children should stay out of the quarrels between the parents. *They should definitely not take sides.* Even though the parents have stopped loving each other, they continue to love their children, and will always do so. They each *want the children to love the other parent.* They will do their best not to say bad things about the other parent to the children; if because of anger they do not always succeed in this, the children should forgive them.

i) The parents do not wish the children to carry messages from one to the other, and promise to try not to send messages through the children. They do not wish the children to tell them what the other parent has been doing.

j) The parents jointly or individually will talk to the children about these matters from time to time before and after the divorce. The parents know that it will be hard for the children to understand and to come to terms with what is happening, and that it will take a long time for them to adjust to the division of their family unit into two separate homes. The children should express their feelings in any way that is comfortable to them and should feel free to ask questions, which the parents will try to answer.

8.3   Conciliation

a) Build relationship of trust in each parent that the conciliator is sensitive to his or her needs and problems and is eager to help find the best way of safe-guarding the welfare of the children during and after the divorce.

b) In short series of joint interviews, support each parent in expressing his or her point of view and help them overcome emotional blocks that distort their communicating with, and hearing, the other parent.

c) Prevent each from being undermined and bullied, through the conciliator interrupting coercive behavior on either side and equalizing power.

d) Exercise a firm chairman's control to ensure focus of discussions on current issues of planning a divorce contract for welfare of children.

e) Allow only limited expression of negative feelings. Interrupt overt or covert attacks on each other.

f) Accept that the two parents have conflicting points of view. Do not seek "objective truth" or try to adjudicate between right and wrong.

g) Clarify and reformulate those statements of each that seem productive options. Ensure that these are heard and understood by the other. If "noise" is too great, meet with each separately and report back to the other by "shuttling" between them.

h) Conciliation is a step–by–step process. Start with points of agreement and progress gradually to resolve disagreements.

i) Investigate attitudes and needs of children and feed these into parental discussions. Occasionally invite children to participate personally.

j) Conciliator should oppose parental plans that infringe on rights of the children but should not dictate his own plan.

k) Prevent premature closure, and ensure opportunity for "working through" by examining implications of various aspects of the plan.

l) Divorce plan should include a clause to facilitate future mediation and counseling regarding postdivorce problems of caring for the children.

9. Summary of Jerusalem Program

The following Tab. provides an overview of our caseflow and the characteristics of our clientele and of our types of intervention. It will be noticed that we draw our cases from a wide range of sources, implying a low intake threshold that is a necessary feature of any serious preventive program, and also that a significant proportion of our clients come for help years after marital separation or divorce, which is consonant with our thesis that important pathogenic factors for the children emerge from the long–term continuing sequelae of divorce and are not just time–limited to the period of the crisis of the divorce process and its immediate aftermath. The fact that in only 11% of our cases did we diagnose current psychopathology in the children validates the preventive character of our program.

This Tab. also demonstrates the skewed nature of our sample. Because of my local reputation as a specialist in psychopathology, judges, lawyers, doctors, educators, and social workers refer to our center their most problematic cases, and particularly those they suspect of emotional disturbance. Of course, it would not be valid to extrapolate from the finding that in 24% of our sample at least one parent suffers from manifest severe psychopathology to an estimate that there is a similar prevalence of psychiatric disturbance in the total population of Jerusalem parents who divorce. But at least our findings do imply that a substantial minority of divorcing couples are burdened in this way. It remains for a future study to determine the size of this minority, and to elucidate the implications of this for our preventive program. For instance, it has already become clear to me that our usual verbal techniques of mediation and counseling do not succeed if one of the parents is significantly disturbed and perseveres in a campaign of hatred and vengeance that endangers the children because of projective identification or other deep psychopathological mechanisms that are not amenable to modification by rational discussion and verbal persuasion. In such cases only the authority of the courts as an arbitrating mechanism and a clear system of imposed constraints can be expected to modify the potentially damaging behavior.

References

Caplan, G. (1964): Principles of preventive psychiatry. New York: Basic Books.

Caplan, G. (1970): Theory and practice of mental health consultation. New York: Basic Books.

Fogelman, K. (1983): Growing up in Great Britain. London: Macmillan.

James, H. (1897): What Maisie knew. London: The Bodley Head.

Kalter, N. (1977): Children of divorce in an outpatient psychiatric population. American Journal of Orthopsychiatry, 47, 40–51.

Kalter, N., and Rembar, J. (1981): The significance of a child's age at the time of parental divorce. American Journal of Orthopsychiatry, 51, 85–100.

McDermott, J.F. (1970): Divorce and its psychiatric sequelae in children. Archives of General Psychiatry, 23, 421–427.

Mnookin, R. (1978): Bargaining in the shadow of the law. Oxford University: Centre for Sociolegal Studies.

Rutter, M. (1985): Resilience in the face of adversity. British Journal of Psychiatry, 147, 598–611.

Wadsworth, M.E.J. (1979): Roots of delinquency. New York: Barnes and Noble.

Wadsworth, M.E.J., and Maclean, M. (1986): Parents' divorce and children's life chances. Children and Youth Service Review, in press.

Wadsworth, M.E.J., Pekham, C.S., and Taylor, B. (1985): The role of national longitudinal studies in prediction of health, development, and behavior. In: Walker, D.B., and Harvard, Richmond J.B. (Eds.): In monitoring child health in the United States. Cambridge, Mass.: University Press, 63–83.
Wallerstein, J.S., and Kelly, J.B. (1980): Surviving the breakup. New York: Basic Books.
Weiss, R.S. (1975): Marital Separation. New York: Basic Books.

The Concept of Social–Pediatric Developmental Rehabilitation

Theodor Hellbrügge

1. Introduction

Among the various social–pediatric tasks, which include primary prevention with preventive measures for healthy patients and secondary prevention with early detection of existing or developing disorders by screening methods, developmental rehabilitation has become a new focal point for tertiary prevention (Hellbrügge, 1981).

According to its definition, developmental rehabilitation utilizes the unique chances of early development in order to help children with inherent or early acquired defects in such a way that they do not become handicapped.

2. Ethological Pediatrics — Social Development as a Basis

Developmental rehabilitation is less based on classical elements of medicine, that is, morphology and physiology. Instead, it is based more on ethology, as ethological criteria are mainly used for the basic elements of developmental rehabilitation. These basic elements are early diagnosis, early therapy, and early social integration.

Developmental rehabilitation builds upon the social development of young infants, that is, the development of independence and sociability. Its impulse came from scientific findings of research in maternal deprivation (Hellbrügge, 1966; Pechstein, 1974) which showed that even healthy children suffer retardations in their speech and social development if they are cared for in institutionalized groups of children of the same age. Therefore, the decisive therapeutic basis of developmental rehabilitation is the family, and, if the child does not have one, a foster or adoptive family.

3. Early Diagnosis by Screening Methods

Screening by parents. Parental observation is a very important diagnostical instrument for early detection of developmental disorders. For this purpose, a parents' book was developed which illustrates in pictures the most important developmental steps in functional areas in such a way that parents can follow the development of their infant at monthly intervals (Hellbrügge and von Wimpffen, 1976). The functional areas include crawling, sitting, walking, grasping, perception, speech, language comprehension, and social development. Meanwhile, this book has been published in 14 languages (German, English, French, Spanish, Italian, Dutch, Flemish, Serbo–Croatian, Greek, Turkish, Finnish, Japanese, Korean, Indonesian), which points out that development in the first year of life is almost identical internationally.

It is important to note that the typical behavior patterns in this parents' book show 90% values. Therefore, most parents observe a faster development of their child when comparing it to the pictures in the book. If, on the other hand, parents observe a retardation of any function, they should consult a pediatrician a soon as possible.

Children's medical check-ups. Any suspicion parents may have can be confirmed by a system of medical check-ups for children which was introduced into the Federal Republic of Germany in 1970 and which guarantees 8 medical check-ups for each child free of charge (for details see Hellbrügge, 1985). These medical check-ups take place immediately after birth, between 3 and 10 days of age, at 4 to 6 weeks of age, at 3 to 4 months, at 6 to 7 months, at 10 to 12 months, at 21 to 24 months, and between 3 1/2 and 4 years of age.

On the day of birth, the mother of each child receives a booklet in which the pediatrician marks his findings. A copy is sent for statistical purposes to the central institute for physicians participating in the German health insurance plan (Zentralinstitut für die kassenärztliche Vereinigung in der Bundesrepublik).

These medical check-ups for children are constructed as a screening method. It is no problem to uncover metabolic diseases during infancy. The detection of psychomotor, hearing, and visual disorders, however, still needs to be improved. There is a lack of effective screening tests, for example, a newborn screening for hearing disorders, a developmental screening method, and so forth. The Denver-test is insufficient since it hardly considers neuromotor disorders.

4. Special Diagnostic Methods

Developmental diagnosis. As a basis for an early developmental therapy of young infants, the "Munich Functional Developmental Diagnostic System — First to Third Year of Life" (Hellbrügge, 1978; Köhler and Egelkraut, 1984) has proved to be very effective. It is the equivalent of the parents' screening, and measures the same functional areas in monthly steps. For diagnostics, the following criteria are considered: crawling age, sitting age, walking age, grasping age, handskill age, perception age, speech age, language comprehension age, social age, and independence age.

Contrary to other internationally used developmental tests (Bayley Scales, Griffith, Uzgiris et al., Brunet-Lézine, etc.), the "Munich Functional Developmental Diagnostic System" avoids a developmental quotient. The developmental quotient, similar to an intelligence quotient, contains the basic danger of labelling children negatively without giving concrete hints for therapeutic consequences.

Neurokinesiological diagnostics. The kinesiological diagnostics based on postural reactions according to Vojta have proved to be an excellent method of early detection of neuromotor disorders. This method is based on well-known pediatric reactions to sudden postural changes (e.g., Traction reaction, Landau-reaction, Axillary suspension reaction, Side-tilt-reaction according to Vojta, Horizontal side-suspension reaction according to Collis, Vertical suspension reaction according to Peiper-Isbert, Vertical suspension reaction according to Collis). These reactions, observed in connection with the testing of certain primitive reflexes in young infants, allow the determination of neurological age, which is identical with chronological age in healthy children, even without knowledge of the date of birth. Neurokinesiological diagnosis can, for example, detect an impending cerebral palsy before the first symptoms appear. It is also the preferred system used in diagnosing all other neuromotor disorders.

Early detection of hearing disorders. Even in medically well-provided countries like the Federal Republic of Germany, the early detection of hearing disorders is not at all ensured. On the average, it still takes 3 years until a hearing disorder is diagnosed and speech therapy, along with the fitting of a hearing aid, is started.

Screening at the age of 7 to 8 months is possible with the Ewing-test used in Great Britain, Israel, and the Netherlands as well as the BOEL-test in Scandinavia. From the point of view of developmental rehabilitation, the application of these tests will improve the situation, but effective help can only be derived from a newborn screening that still needs to be developed.

5. Programs of Early Therapy

Concrete programs have been developed in the "Kinderzentrum München" for early therapy of infants with multiple and variable disorders or with impending handicaps. On the basis of a multidimensional diagnosis, the programs are prepared for each child individually and for a certain period of time. They are then shown to the parents in such a way that the therapy can be integrated in the daily routine of the child. The individual program for a certain child is combined by respective specialists (i.e., pediatrician, child psychologist, and therapists such as physiotherapists, occupational therapists, speech therapists, music therapists, etc.). Under the coordination of the pediatrician, the parents receive a comprehensible exercise which they can then carry out at home.

Developmental therapy Developmental therapy based on the "Munich Functional Developmental Diagnostic System" is begun as early as possible, especially for infants suffering from maternal deprivation — that is, children who are impaired in their social development - for infants with hearing disorders as a basis for an early speech intervention; and finally, for mentally retarded children, for example, Down syndrome. All possibilities of optical and acoustical stimulation, and especially social interactions, are used to their full potentials in developmental therapy with young infants. Schamberger (1978), in comparing studies of Down syndrome children treated early with those of Down children who did not receive an early treatment, showed that the treated children were superior in all measured functional areas. Nine years later, the success of treatment could still be recognized.

A *stimulating oral therapy* (according to Castillo–Morales) improves orofacial pathologies of children with Down syndrome as early as possible. Oral plates with a cone designed to induce the tongue to a special activity are implanted. This again not only strengthens the tongue muscles, but also improves the well-known symptomatology of the open mouth, hypersalivation, protruding tongue, and so forth, in a way that changes the physiognomy of the children decisively (Avalle et al., 1985; Fischer–Brandies, 1986).

Kinesiological therapy. The kinesiological therapy according to Vojta has proved to be very efficient. Compared to Bobath–therapy, this therapy is much more successful when applied to motor disorders. In a comparative study of both methods, the advantage of Vojta–therapy was so obvious that Bobath–therapy is now only occasionally applied in the "Kinderzentrum München". Vojta–therapy stimulates central functions of the nervous system starting from the periphery.

Indications for Vojta–therapy. In addition to impending cerebral palsies and fixed cerebral palsies, indications for Vojta–therapy apply especially to the treatment of meningomyelocele, including obvious improvements of hydrocephalus; the therapy of peripheric birth paralysis (e.g., Erb and Klumpke); and finally, scoliosis.
A mentally normal child with an impending cerebral palsy has a 95% chance of normal motor development. The therapy is all the more successful if it is started early. Therefore, it should begin immediately after birth with children at risk and, at the latest, at 4 months of age.

Orff music therapy. Orff music therapy, developed by Gertrud Orff in her work with handicapped children at the Kinderzentrum München, is an active form of music therapy which has its roots in the Orff–Schulwerk. Basis principles of Orff–Schulwerk — the unity of movement, speech, singing, and playing and the idea of creative, spontaneous improvisation — also exist in Orff music therapy. However, in Orff music therapy these principles are implemented in a nondirective manner to achieve a nonmusical goal — reaching the handicapped, especially the severely handicapped child, in order to further him in his development. In addition to the Orff instrumentarium, other instruments and objects, for example, whistles, balls, rings, are available for use by the children in activities involving the auditive, visual, tactile, and kinesthetic modalities. These activities can lead to the development of perceptual motor skills, that is, the integration of sensory perception and motor skills, which are necessary in all areas of learning.

Early speech therapy. For early speech intervention of mentally handicapped or deaf children, the close interplay of sensorimotor, social, and communicative developmental processes are utilized for the conception of learning programs. An important goal of early therapy for deaf children is the construction of a natural phonetic speech without gestures, a method supported by Van Uden (1982) and Horsch (1982).

Early treatment of speech retardations of different causes demands exact knowledge of normal child development as well as a special imagination for the constructing of various logopedic promotional strategies. Parents and speech therapists cooperate closely and continually in all speech programs. With mentally retarded children, behavior patterns based on learning psychology receive special attention.

6. Early Social Integration — Montessori Medical Pedagogy

The decisive goal of developmental rehabilitation is the social integration of disturbed, disabled, and thus more or less handicapped children. This goal is contrary to the wide-spread efforts of special education which has created special institutions for specific disorders or handicaps, resulting in the segregation of the children affected.

Montessori medical pedagogy (Aurin, 1978; Hellbrügge, 1977; Hellbrügge and Montessori, 1978) has proved to be an excellent method of integration. It has been developed in the "Kinderzentrum München" on the basis of the most important elements of the internationally known Montessori education.

This type of education considers the neurophysiological elements of learning, with emphasis on the use of the sense organs. It is an active and not a reactive way of learning which induces the child to work with the autodidactic Montessori material according to the principle of trial and error. The furtherance of the child with integrated education not only includes

— activities of practical life,
— furtherance of the senses through sensory material, and
— furtherance through didactic material,

but especially the social development of the child.

Integration into the family. The first step of social integration is integrating the child into the family. After their shock at the birth of a child who is not normally developed, parents are in need of special psychological help. In many cases psychotherapy for parents is necessary. According to our experience, most parents wish a clear counseling about what to do with their child. Family therapy as practiced in some children's centers may be advantageous for some families. However, it often hinders controlled therapy for and furtherance of the child, because the main goal of this psychotherapy is parental treatment.

In Montessori individual therapy, parents receive clear therapeutic instructions. The smallest learning steps in the already mentioned activities of practical life, of sensory material, and of didactic material are to be transfered from the therapeutic to the home situation.

The purpose of Montessori small–group therapy is to further the social development of the child and to promote the communication of disordered or handicapped children in the presence of their parents, so that the children become capable of functioning within a group. Here, the goal is also to show parents in small steps how to improve the integration of their affected child into their immediate environment (neighborhood).

Adoption and foster care of handicapped children. Care within a family is especially important for disordered or handicapped children. Therefore, with the help of social workers, we search for adoptive and/or foster parents if the child lives in a broken home.

In the period from January 1981 to February 1984, with the additional help of social workers, 48 children could be reintegrated into their own families after thorough parental therapy was completed.

41 children were mediated into foster homes, including
13 mentally retarded children,
 9 physically handicapped children,
18 children with learning disabilities or behavior disorders, and
 1 blind child.

32 children could be mediated into adoptive homes, including
 1 mentally retarded child,
 5 physically handicapped children, and
26 children with learning disabilities or behavior disorders.

These procedures are only possible under great expenditure of time and personnel. The preparation time for foster or adoptive care is about 4 months, the intensive follow-up treatment about half a year, and the average long-term treatment several years.

Integration into kindergarten. The Montessori method has also proved to be very successful in integrating multiply and variously handicapped children into a normal kindergarten. Since this method is a child-centered method of education, it is possible to further highly intelligent, healthy children in their cognitive learning processes as well as children with physical handicaps (cerebral palsy, meningomyelocele) or blind, deaf, and mentally retarded children without difficulty. There are 20 to 25 children in a kindergarten group, including up to 6 children with various disorders. Such a group composition induces the children to help each other, which, in turn, furthers the development of independence. This also applies to the handicapped children when, for example, a mentally retarded child proudly pushes the wheelchair of a paralysed child.

Integration into school. The Montessori method is also an ideal educational instrument for the integration of children with multiple and variable disorders into school. According to the experiences of the "Kinderzentrum München", children with high intelligence quotients as well as children with mental retardations profit from this kind of education. As the Montessori method does not divide into age groups, the social learning processes of experienced and non-experienced children are of central importance. This decisively furthers social development, that is, the development of independence and the capability of communicating with others.

The integration of handicapped children reinforces these social learning processes in all children, through which their cognitive learning is increased. The results of integrated education thus affect nonhandicapped children (unproblematic transfer to secondary schools) as well as handicapped children (some "mentally retarded" children manage to complete intermediate school education). Additional methods like motology, Orff music, and so forth, have helped to improve integration in school.

7. German Academy for Developmental Rehabilitation

For the various programs of developmental rehabilitation, the German Academy for Developmental Rehabilitation organises courses and seminars in the "Kinderzentrum München". These include, among others:

"Munich Functional Developmental Diagnostic System" and
"Developmental Therapy",

"Kinesiological diagnostics according to Vojta" and
"Kinesiological Therapy",

"Montessori Medical Pedagogy",
"Orff Music Therapy",
"Neuro–linguistics" (e.g., speech procurement according to Schmid–Giovannini),

"Motopedagogy",
"Orofacial therapy according to Castillo–Morales",
"Psychotherapy of MCD–children according to Naville", and so forth.

These courses are in the German language. If interested, please contact the Congress Bureau of the German Academy for Developmental Rehabilitation, Heiglhofstrasse 63, D–8000 München 70, Phone: (089) 71009–239.

References

Aurin, M. (1978): Das erste Montessori-Kinderhaus mit integrierter Erziehung in München. Erfahrungen bei den Kindern. In: Th. Hellbrügge (Ed.): Die Montessori-Pädagogik und das behinderte Kind. München: Kindler-Verlag.

Avalle, C., Fischer-Brandies, H., Schmid, R.G. (1985): Zur Mundtherapie bei Zerebralparese. Erste Erfahrungen bei der Behandlung von neuromotorischen Störungen im Mundbereich bei Kindern mit zerebraler Parese nach der Konzeption von Castillo-Morales. Sozialpädiatrie in Praxis und Klinik 7, 116–121.

Fischer-Brandies, H. (1986): Entwicklungsmerkmale des Schädels und der Kiefer bei Morbus Down unter Berücksichtigung der funktionellen kieferorthopädischen Behandlung der orofozialen Fehlfunktionen nach Castillo-Morales bei Säuglingen und Kleinkindern. Habilitationsschrift zur Erlangung des Grades eines habilitierten Doktors der Medizin an der Ludwig-Maximilians-Universität München.

Hellbrügge, T. (1966): Zur Problematik der Säuglings- und Kleinkinderfürsorge in Anstalten – Hospitalismus und Deprivation. In H. Opitz, and F. Schmid (Hrsg.): Handbuch der Kinderheilkunde Bd.3, Soziale Pädiatrie. Berlin-Heidelberg-New York: Springer Verlag, 384–404.

Hellbrügge, T. (1977): Unser Montessori-Modell. München: Kindler-Verlag.

Hellbrügge, T. (Ed.) (1978): Münchener Funktionelle Entwicklungsdiagnostik erstes Lebensjahr. Bd.4, Fortschritte der Sozialpädiatrie. München-Wien-Baltimore: Urban & Schwarzenberg.

Hellbrügge, T. (Ed.) (1981): Klinische Sozialpädiatrie. Ein Lehrbuch der Entwicklungs-Rehabilitation im Kindesalter. Berlin-Heidelberg-New York: Springer.

Hellbrügge, T. (Ed.) (1985): Screening und Vorsorgeuntersuchungen im Kindesalter, Bd. 8 Fortschritte der Sozialpädiatrie. Lübeck: Hansisches Verlagskontor.

Hellbrügge, T., von Wimpffen, J.H. (Eds.) (1976): Die ersten 365 Tage im Leben eines Kindes. 4th edition. München: TR-Verlagsunion. English edition: Bombay 1980.

Hellbrügge, T., Montessori, M. (1978): Die Montessori-Pädagogik und das behinderte Kind. München: Kindler-Verlag.

Horsch, U. (1982): Kommunikative Erziehung zur Früherziehung Behinderter –erörtert am Beispiel hörgeschädigter Kinder. Heidelberg: Julius Groos-Verlag.

Köhler, G., Egelkraut, H. (1984): Münchener Funktionelle Entwicklungsdiagnostik für das zweite und dritte Lebensjahr. Handanweisung. Durchführungs-, Beurteilungs- und Interprätationshinweise. Eigenverlag der Aktion Sonnenschein, Hilfe für das mehrfachbehinderte Kind e.V. München.

Pechstein, J. (1974): Umweltabhängigkeit der frühkindlichen zentralnervösen Entwicklung. Schriftenreihe aus dem Gebiete des öffentlichen Gesundheitswesens, 34.
Stuttgart: Georg-Thieme.

Schamberger, R. (1978): Frühtherapie bei gesitig behinderten Säuglingen und Kleinkindern. Untersuchungen bei Kindern mit Down-Syndrom. Weinheim-Basel: Beltz.

Van Uden, A. (1982): Das gehörlose Kind – Fragen seiner Entwicklung und Förderung. Heidelberg: Julius-Groos-Verlag.

Prevention and Intervention From the Perspective of Child Psychiatry

Friedrich Specht

1. Introduction

From my perspective as a child psychiatrist, I can only attempt to present an overview of certain problems of intervention and prevention here. Some questions have to remain open, and answers frequently remain hypothetical. I shall focus on three rather complex questions:

— To what extent do the concepts of prevention and intervention refer to different directions and forms of action?
— What relationships exist between prevention, self-help, counseling, and treatment, and which persons or groups of persons are reached through prevention and intervention?
— To what extent can preventive measures be justified, and what should be their orientation?

2. To What Extent Do the Concepts of Prevention and Intervention Refer to Different Directions and Forms of Action?

This problem field can be viewed from two sides: One involves the preventive effectiveness of *interventions*, and the other is concerned with the fact that some forms of prevention clearly differ from interventions. For this reason, intervention is also often defined as a therapeutic *or* preventive measure (e.g., in the Rothe–Lexikon Medizin). In any case, all forms of planned, and mostly therefore professional, interference can be regarded as intervention. Interventions among children and adolescents are mostly triggered when the adults concerned are confronted with problems that they can no longer cope with by themselves, or they at least believe to be beyond their capabilities. The procedures involved range from problem–centered counseling within the child's or adolescent's environment to more long–term, methodologically structured therapeutic contact with the child, adolescent, or its family. I also include justified nonintervention as a measure of intervention. Although this may appear to be paradoxical, a justified nonintervention requires a previous clarification of the problem. As a result, further interventions — for example, an extended therapy — may be unsuitable and unjustified.

Interventions have a *preventive* effect when the extent of intervention brings about changes of perception, attitudes, and behavior in the persons involved. It is not just the members of the family who are involved in a crisis or problem, but also other persons who deal with a child or adolescent, such as teachers.

For more than 10 years, I have been counseling teachers at regular intervals in a comprehensive secondary school. The direct cause for this counseling is generally a student whose behaviors or learning difficulties are a cause of concern, by whom the teachers have found that little can be achieved with educational methods. The goal of this joint counseling is to find insights into the relationships as well as explanations and action plans that enable the teachers to support the student more successfully.

The joint counseling commences with a painstaking collection and systematic analysis of all available information. Although I do not get to see the student directly, he or she thus provisionally becomes a "case" of *intervention*. Only occasionally does the intervention extend to my having to advise that the student should be presented to myself or other professionals outside of the school.

The result of the joint discussions is more frequently that the student's adult partners use their own abilities to counter the growth or fixation of the student's difficulties. This should return the student to the status of a student like all the rest and no longer a case. This procedure and its result then correspond to a *secondary prevention*. In fact, the effect extends beyond the student who is provisionally identified as a case. The new possibilities of perception and understanding and the extension of the action scope that the teacher group have worked out with expert guidance also influence how the teachers cope with difficulties in other students. Through this, the teachers concerned go beyond intervention and secondary prevention and become mediators of a *general prevention*.

The particular willingness to learn that has grown out of the crisis, and which led those concerned to seek advice is essential for the effectiveness of such a prevention growing out of an intervention. This precondition is the essential difference between such a procedure and theoretical teaching in seminars and courses (cf. Uchtenhagen, 1980).

I have mentioned the intervention character of preventive procedures as the other side of this first complex of questions. That which is defined as *secondary* and *tertiary* prevention basically corresponds to an intervention or interference that is triggered by the disorders of a specific, single child or adolescent. This produces constellations and forms of action that are largely in agreement with those of intervention. The child or the child's family are assigned specific measures in which the expert classification of the "case" and the expert selection of methods are decisive. The meaning of preventive thereby corresponds with the intent to "anticipate", that is, the intent to prevent the increase and fixation of disorders or their reoccurence. However, this produces the same problems as those found in interventions.

However, this is not the case in all those preventive activities that do not relate to single persons who have already been identified as needing help but are aimed at more favorably shaping the relation between stress and coping in children and adolescents through *mediators, explanation,* and *political action*. It may therefore be useful to discriminate conceptually particularly between those measures that are used to respond to risks that have become evident *individually* and measures that are directed at the change of *generally* effective influences and conditions.

3. What Relationships Exist Between Prevention, Self–Help, Counseling, and Treatment and Which Persons or Groups of Persons are Reached Through Prevention and Intervention?

The relationships between the different possibilities of intervention can be illustrated in a diagram.

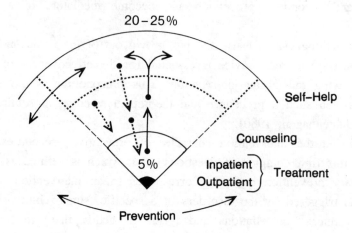

Fig. 1:   Relationships between the Different Possibilities of Intervention

We can conceptually extend the sector illustrated to form a complete circle. This would represent the total of all children and adolescents. The sector presented here covers the portion of children and adolescents whose behavior or mental condition is regarded as disordered at a certain point in time either within their social system or by persons who are significant for them, and this has led to worry, concern, or disapproval. For some of these children and adolescents, either their behavior or mental condition, or its evaluation changes without professional interference, that is, through *self-help*. For a further portion, *counseling* proves to be necessary but also sufficient to effect such changes. Long-term therapeutic interventions are only necessary for a small portion. Finally, such interventions only require separation from the family, that is, a shorter or longer inpatient treatment, for a very small portion. In the diagram, the surfaces of the sector are only partially assigned numerical percentages for self-help, counseling, and treatment. However, their interrelation roughly corresponds to the dimensions found in various epidemiological surveys (cf. Castell et al., 1981; Esser and Schmidt, 1987; Rutter et al., 1977).

The composition of persons in each actual cross-section changes over time. The fluctuation should decrease from the outside to the inside in the sector illustrated. The children and adolescents who do not require counseling or treatment change most frequently. Those who need treatment because of more marked or persistent disorders and handicaps remain the longest.

However, we should not expect *general prevention* to decisively reduce the portion of children and adolescents who at some time − illustratively speaking − end up in the sector presented here (Fig. 1). Confrontation with difficulties can always express itself in disordered behavior or mental conditions. A certain degree of stress and problems cannot be avoided in any development, and successful coping with difficulties is also a favorable experience. For this reason, general prevention must particularly see how children and adolescents can leave the field of disordered problem−indicating behavior before consolidation occurs. This particularly involves providing as many adults as possible with the capability to understand the problem behavior of children and adolescents and to strengthen and support their coping abilities. Whether this is really effective in the single case does not just depend on the extent of actual disorders and impairments, but also on a series of social variables. Therefore counseling at least is necessary for a portion of children and adolescents, and the size of this portion can hardly be changed.

By counseling I mean institutionalized counseling. As with treatment, there are a variety of different kinds of organization providing this. In West Germany, assistance for children and adolescents whose mental development is threatened, disturbed, or impaired is provided by several systems: youth welfare, social health, social welfare, and education. In addition to doctors with their own practices (child psychiatrists, neurologists, and pediatricians), psychologists, and child psychotherapists, the 800 educational and family counseling centers and outpatient child psychiatric services are also particularly important institutions. A clear separation is made between counseling and treatment in Fig. 1 in order to illustrate the demand for treatment. However, there is not such a clear discrimination between the two forms of intervention in actual practice. In particular, counseling and treatment are often interlinked and one can follow the other during the course of interventions.

The border between the area labeled self−help and interventions raises completely different problems. Those who are in particular need of help only partially, or with a delay, reach the professional and institutional services. This only partially explains why the services available for children and adolescents nowhere correspond to the epidemiologically recorded demand and why rural areas are particularly handicapped. It has been shown that it is far more the case that many parents are completely unaware of counseling and treatment services, or that they are unable to conceive in what way they could be helped (cf. Rutter et al., 1977).

Tab. 1:   Knowledge of Availability of Assistance

Nonexistent or low ⟵	Knowledge of availability of assistance	⟶ Thorough
Larger field of tolerance for diversity	Favorable effects	Timely, limited interventions
Failure to take advantage of timely assistance	Unfavorable effects	Unnecessary "self-diagnoses" of therapy

Tab. 1 summarizes the consequences of inadequate or extensive knowledge of available assistance. A lack of knowledge may imply that appropriate counseling or treatment is not used. The lack of knowledge may, however, also mean that parents consider that they have to mobilize their own powers, and that they also see themselves as being obliged to be more tolerant of the characteristics and particularly of their children. Parents with an extensive knowledge of the possibilities and forms of intervention assistance quickly take advantage of them when they have problems with their children. This increases the chances that intervention can be limited to counseling. More complete knowledge can, however, lead to the parents diagnosing syndromes with lists of characteristics and demanding the corresponding treatment without such a self-diagnosis being actually justified. This is, for example, the case when attention is drawn to particular developmental disorders in the media. Thus at present we frequently have to deal with incorrectly self-diagnosed hyperkinetic syndromes.

The tolerance field for diversity also presents a variable and a problem.

Tab. 2:   Field of Tolerance for Diversity

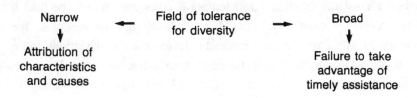

From the preventive point of view, a broad field of tolerance for diversity is desired. With a broad field of tolerance, children with, for example, light general developmental retardation or higher vegative reactivity are faced with a lower risk of being exposed to reactions from reference persons that will make them insecure and consolidate their disorders. When, in contrast, the opinions of adults set very narrow limits on the diversity of children, particularities in development and characteristics of behavior can too quickly and unjustifiably lead to the attribution of permanent properties and causal relationships. On the other hand, a field of tolerance that is too broad has the disadvantage that in a number of children the significance of deviations in development that require intervention is belittled and supportive assistance is not given.

This shows that concepts of prevention and the needs for intervention can run into clear conflict with one another.

Knowledge of the possibilities of assistance and the effects of narrow or broad fields of tolerance form a kind of filter that only lets a proportion of the necessary interventions take place. Even when the availability of assistance is known and help is needed, the decision to seek professional help undergoes evaluation and weighting processes. The extent and duration of the problem–indicating behavior and whether it will become known and recognized outside of the family are significant here. However, the parents' social status, ability to cope with stress, concepts of autonomy, and particularly their subjective theories on problem load play an essential role (cf. e.g., Höger, 1986). Middle-class parents appear to be more capable of reconciling the use of professional services with their concepts of autonomy than parents who feel themselves to be placed in an inferior position and do not anticipate any understanding for their environment and life-style. Frequently, the contact with experts is feared, and is labeled as an expropriation or a parceling out of the problems (cf. Steiner, 1985). In addition, the *advantages* to be expected from professional help are weighed against the emotional and temporal *costs* that have to be paid for it.

Thus, prevention cannot limit itself to forestalling interventions. When it is necessary to avoid or reduce permanent developmental deviations, then prevention should also simultaneously facilitate timely interventions. Examples of this are particularly to be found in educational and family counseling centers, a great number of which attempt to bring about an increase in contacts with mediators while at the same time they try to reduce access thresholds through presence in institutions and more publicity. This is a result of fundamental considerations and is not just intended to tie more families to counseling centers. However, previous observations indicate that the reduction of the access threshold through knowledge and trust toward the center leads on the one hand to an increase in the number of timely and consequently short-term interventions in low problem loads but on the other hand decreases the reservations of some families with serious loads and correspondingly leads to an increased frequency of costly interventions. It remains to be seen to what extent this will lead to a new relationship between preventive activities and intervention and above all a more informal link between the two.

4. To What Extent Can Preventive Measures be Justified, and What Should be Their Orientation?

It is difficult to record the long-term effectiveness of single positive or negative effects on the course of development in *prospective* studies. That which appears to clarify the relationships in single cases retrospectively does not permit any conclusions about the general significance of the single factors thus detected.

Prevention means both the reduction of avoidable risks and loads, and perhaps more importantly, the strengthening of the ability to withstand risks and loads.

In recent times, doubt has been cast on, among others, the long- term effect of stressors in early childhood, which had previously been considered very significant on the basis of many single-case histories (cf. Ernst and von Luckner, 1985). Nevertheless, hardly anyone would consider that the institutionalized mass care of infants should be called good and reintroduced. The statistical relevance of single factors is apparently not equivalent to their causal relevance in interaction processes. In the somatic field, we know we have to differentiate between the statistical and biological relevance of single factors, and we orient at their biological relevance.

When it is true for unfavorable effects that their influences on development depend on the addition of further unfavorable effects *or* on the lack of protective and strengthening conditions, this must similarly apply to planned positive interventions, that is, for general preventive measures, for secondary and tertiary prevention, and for corresponding early interventions in problematic courses of development. The findings from comparative longitudinal studies on the effectiveness of timely interventions in risk-loaded children are sometimes discouraging. Conclusions from comparisons between intervention groups and nonintervention controls can only be made when all the major, unplanned conditions of the further course of development are also recorded and taken into account with configural analysis.

Those studies that point to conditions under which the children's abilities to resist and cope can grow so that they are able to withstand unfavorable effects and events without permanent damage to their development are even more important. To recognize such protective conditions and their preconditions, to retain them, and to support their effectiveness both generally and individually could prove to be the decisive task of prevention.

In preparation for the 7th Jugendbericht der Deutschen Bundesregierung (Youth Report of the West German Government), Bubert (1987) has evaluated publications on such strengthening and protective conditions. Tab. 3 summarizes the major conditions and experiences.

Tab. 3:   Experiences with protective effects

Constant interest in the child as a person

The experience of being important for others and being respected by them

Possibilities of successfully influencing one's own situation

Sufficient support in attaining self-sufficiency and acquiring communication abilities

---

Even if we are dealing with simplified statements removed from concrete preconditions, it is exactly against such criteria that preventive proposals can also be measured. Measures with preventive goals should continually be checked for side-effects that could counter such goals. In fact there have been a sufficient number of very contradictory proposals and suggestions for prevention. In a lecture to parents, the following comment during the discussion received much applause: "Everything leads up to the fact that we parents never do it right and are always to blame for everything. Even when we follow advice, this is wrong because the same advice is considered wrong on the next day."

Many proposals and counsels that are assigned a preventive effectiveness in fact refer to ideologies and prejudgments. I shall conclude with a quotation from one of my earlier publications:

Each ideology makes it possible to assign a preventive effectiveness to certain behaviors and actions. In an almost random manner, interventions or noninterventions can be justified if they are not related to the present reality but to one that first has to be constructed. It is certainly questionable whether prevention can be kept at all free from ideology, as social reality in any case continually undergoes actual changes. Without doubt, assumptions refering to this enter into all preventive proposals. Accordingly, criteria are necessary to prevent the change in ideologies and the exchange of prejudgments leading to disorientation, contradictory procedures, and finally also to resignation or a wholesale disavowal of preventive ppoposals and efforts (Specht, 1979).

References

Bubert, R. (1987): Erkennung und Kennzeichnung schützender und stützender Bedingungen für Kinder und Jugendliche in der Familie und ihrem Umfeld. In Materialien zum 7. Jugendbericht, Bd. 4: Soziale Netzwerke und Gesundheitsförderung. München: Juventa.

Castell, R., Biener, A., Artner, K., Dilling, H. (1981): Häufigkeiten von psychischen Störungen und Verhaltensauffälligkeiten bei Kindern und ihre psychiatrische Versorgung. Zeitschrift für Kinder- und Jugendpsychiatrie 9, 115-125.

Ernst, C., von Luckner, N. (1985): Stellt die Frühkindheit die Weichen? Eine Kritik an der Lehre von der schicksalhaften Bedeutung erster Erlebnisse. Stuttgart: Enke.

Esser, G., Schmidt, M. (1987): Epidemiologie und Verlauf kinderpsychiatrischer Störungen im Schulalter — Ergebnisse einer Längsschnittstudie. Nervenheilkunde 6, 27-53.

Höger, Ch. (1986): Zur Bedeutung von subjektiven Theorien von Eltern für die Inanspruchnahme psychosozialer Dienste durch Grundschulkinder. Unveröffentl. Manuskript.

Rutter, M., Tizard, J., Yule, W., Graham, P.J., Whitmore, E. (1977): Epidemiologie in der
Kinderpsychiatrie — die Isle of Wight Studien 1964 1974. Zeitschrift für Kinder- und
Jugendpsychiatrie 5, 238–279.

Specht, F. (1979): Was bedeuten Prävention und seelische Gesundheit im Kindesalter? In K.
Schütt (Ed.): Wie ist die seelische Gesundheit im Kindesalter praktisch zu fördern?
Deutsches Nationalkomitee für Seelische Gesundheit, Hamburg.

Steiner, H. (1985): "Enteignung der Konflikte" — Analyse eines Typs von Gesellschaftskritik.
In Bundeskonferenz für Erziehungsberatung (Ed.): Bedingungen und Einflußmöglichkei-
ten instituioneller Erziehungs- und Familienberatung, 1. Arbeitsgemeinschaft. Fürth:
Eigenverlag.

Uchtenhagen, A. (1980): Intervention und Prävention. In K. Gerlicher (Ed.): Prävention –
Vorbeugende Tätigkeiten in Erziehungs— und Familienberatungsstellen. Göttingen:
Vandenhoeck & Ruprecht.

Early Mobility Training of Children Born Blind — Needs and Prerequisites

Gunnar Jansson

1. Introduction

An often observed difference between the blind adults who were born blind and those who have some sighted history concerns their locomotory performance. Those who have never seen appear to have more problems with their independent travel. However, no detailed description of these problems seems to be available. Several of them are certainly the same as those encountered by any blind adult, but it seems probable that there are problems that have their origin in the fact that these people have never been sighted. What are these special problems? Have they been the same from childhood on, or are there kinds of problems that appear and disappear during the growing up of these people? Are there problems that persist throughout life and that are not compensated for? In sum, very little is known about the special locomotory problems of adult blind people who were born blind, as compared with those of other blind adults.

However, it seems reasonable to assume that as the difference in experience between the two groups of blind people is that the most unfavorable group did not have certain perceptual information available during their childhood, the special problems may be decreased by suitable intervention during the growing up of the blind children; especially, maybe, during their very first year when so much of the perceptual–motor development takes place. Again, however, our present knowledge about which measures might be effective is fragmentary. Further, the research that has been done has often reported mean results over a large age range, and the preschool years, so important for the training in mobility, have a relatively low representation in research (cf. Warren, 1984). This means that we do not get much guidance from earlier research with regard to what measures are appropriate and at what age they should be applied.

The aim of this paper is to present the background for a research project in progress on needs concerning mobility, as indicated by problems remaining in adult age for people born blind, and, further, on the prerequisites of early mobility training of children blind from birth as an intervention aiming toward the elimination of these problems. A general background for the project, to be presented first, is an analysis of the perceptual information needed for the guidance of locomotion with special attention to nonvisual information. After that, a background for the study of early mobility training will be given.

2. A General Model for the Perceptual Guidance of Locomotion

The model consists of three parts: (1) the most important features of the environment from a locomotion point of view, (2) the perceptual–motor tasks the pedestrian has to perform when moving around in this environment, and (3) the perceptual information needed in order to perform these tasks. In the latter case it will also be discussed what nonvisual information is available and useful. I have presented this model in more detail elsewhere, most recently in Jansson (in press), and only an outline will be given here.

2.1   The Most Important Features of the Environment

The basis for the analysis of the environment is the description given by Gibson (1979) with some minor modifications to suit the present context. The most important features are the following: the *ground* upon which locomotion is performed; the *places* where the pedestrian as well as the relevant features of the environment are located; *objects* that may be goals to be approached, obstacles to be avoided, or landmarks to refer to; *openings* between objects indicating possible passage; and *elongated features*, such as barriers or margins between different kinds of surfaces.

2.2   The Perceptual–Motor Tasks of the Pedestrian

In many contexts in which the locomotion of blind people is discussed it is assumed that obstacle detection is the main task. That is, for instance, the task studied in the classical experiments by Dallenbach and his associates (e.g., Supa, Cotzin, and Dallenbach, 1944). This task seems also to be considered as the main problem for blind mobility by constructors of travel aids for the blind (cf. Jansson, 1985). Even if this is an important task, there are three other main perceptual–motor tasks that are, I think, at least as significant: finding support, walking toward, and walking along. Further, obstacle detection is part of a larger task that can be called "walking around" which in turn can be analyzed in terms of walking toward and walking along (cf. Jansson, in press).

Finding support. In order to move successfully over the ground it is necessary to find support for one's feet. In natural environments with their many uneven and slanted ground surfaces this may be very problematic; in artificial contexts with their more plane and horizontal surfaces it is less so. However, in both natural and artificial environments the adjustment to steps is very important; stairs, for example, being a main hazard indoors.

Walking toward. This kind of task is applicable when there is a perceivable goal available in the environment. It may be an object to reach or an opening to pass through. In the context of locomotion without sight it is important to stress that the goal must be perceivable, as it often is the case that a feature in the environment is easily observed by sight but otherwise not detectable, for instance, because of its being silent, out of reach of the hands, or having no smell. This kind of task is much less applicable for blind persons than for the sighted.

Walking along. Pedestrians can apply walking along when there is some elongated feature in the environment, a barrier or a margin that can be followed in a desired direction. The elongated feature may be followed until it ends, or until the appearance of some landmark suggests that the walking along should be terminated. This kind of task is the main task applied by visually impaired pedestrians for locomotion as the short range available for them is often sufficient. However, it may sometimes mean awkward detours as compared with direct routes that may be detected by a sighted person.

2.3   Perceptual Information for These Tasks

For each of the three main tasks, the perceptual information needed – nonspecific concerning sense involved – will be discussed, followed by a review of nonvisual information that is available and useful for the visually impaired.

Finding support. Every sighted person knows from his/her own experience that it is, in most cases, possible to see — directly — if the ground is "walk-upon--able" (cf. Gibson, 1979, especially chapter 8 on affordances). Even if it may be difficult to specify for each piece of information what visual information is available and useful, it is usually apparent that there is such information. The situation is highly different for a person having to rely on nonvisual information. Especially newly blinded persons may have difficulty in finding useful nonvisual information in this respect, which is probably one of the main reasons for their commonly felt fear of independent walking. On the other hand, the confidence of a well- trained long cane user or guide dog owner may be assumed to depend very much on the information about the ground provided by these aids (cf., e.g., Schenkman, 1986).

Walking toward. When walking toward a perceptible goal, the pedestrian needs information about the following aspects (continuously changing during walking): (1) the direction from his/her present position to the goal, (2) his/her direction of walking, and (3) the distance to the goal, which is especially important during the final approach when the necessary information is probably best defined in temporal terms, time-to-contact, as Lee (e.g., 1980) has suggested. Again, vision provides an abundance of information useful for the guidance of this task, while the nonvisual information is quite restricted. Especially, the range of space covered nonvisually is very much limited, for haptics to the length of the arms. Hearing may cover somewhat larger space by echolocation, at least a few meters (cf. Schenkman, 1985), and sound sources may be detected over longer distances. However, in most situations there is hardly any information about the space further away than a few meters, even if an electronic travel aid is used; the aid with the longest range so far, the Sonicguide, can work up to 7-8 meters, but the other aids work typically over 1-2 meters. This short range available to the blind is a plausible reason for walking toward being so relatively seldom applied by them.

Walking along. For this task the pedestrian needs information about the following aspects of his/her relation to features of the surroundings: (1) the distance between his/her present position and the guiding feature (to follow along), especially changes in this distance; and (2) the termination of the guiding feature (e.g., the end of the margin/barrier or the appearance of anything that serves as a landmark). The perceptual information needed for this task is more easily provided nonvisually as a long range is not necessary. In fact, when following along you have, in most cases, a rather short distance to the guiding feature. Touching with the hand, using echolocation, and tapping with a long cane are examples of common ways of getting the information needed. Electronic travel aids may be useful for this task, too; one advantage being that there does not need to be any physical contact with the guiding feature. It is not surprising that walking along is more common among blind people than walking toward.

The temporal precedence of perception. One important aspect of the perceptual information necessary for walking is that it has to be picked up some time before it is needed for action. This principle may be given in terms of preview or anticipation. Jansson and Schenkman (1977) demonstrated the increase in detection of objects when the range of an electronic travel aid was augmented, and Barth and Foulke (1979) showed the deleterious effects of restricted preview on several aspects of walking. An increased range is a main demand for future travel aids (Jansson, 1987).

Detection and identification of relevant features. It should be noted that there are some prerequisites for the perceptual tasks mentioned above. The relevant features must, of course, be detected. They must be discriminated from the irrelevant ones and identified as the feature wanted for guidance. The pedestrians must be able to determine which of the many features of the environment are a goal to walk toward, an elongated feature to walk along, an obstacle to walk around, a landmark to take account of, or a feature to ignore. This is very difficult without vision. Within the range of space covered, perception without vision is often restricted to the detection of an object or an opening at best, while the identification of the detected feature is much more difficult. Most electronic travel aids do not add anything to the detection of the mere existence of a feature; at most its position and form, and, in some cases, properties of its surface may be perceived.

2.4   A Summary of the Present Situation for Locomotion Without Vision

The present situation for a blind pedestrian is characterized by limitations, but also by possibilities. A realistic analysis must provide both aspects and also remind us of the loss in redundancy of information which may be the most important drawback of a lack of vision in this context (cf. Leonard, 1971).

Above, mainly problems and shortcomings have been indicated. However, it should be remembered that blind persons with all their other senses intact have much information available that is important for locomotion via these other senses: auditory, tactual, and vestibular information as well as information picked up by the sensors in the joints, tendons, and muscles. This information is also available for sighted people, even if they often, because of the dominance of vision, do not make use of it as much as the blind have to do.

It is also the case that blind people may use kinds of information ordinarily not used at all by sighted people, especially the well-known capacity of echolocation which, according to many anecdotal reports, may appear suddenly after some time of blindness. It is an important capacity, but, again, its limitations should be observed: it is mainly restricted to localization, it does not have the precision of vision, and there are visually impaired people who do not seem to be able to use it, at least not effectively (cf. Schenkman, 1985; Schenkman and Jansson, 1986).

The introduction several decades ago of the traditional aids, the guide dog and the long cane, was a major improvement but did not solve all the problems. A further effort to solve some of the problems of blind mobility was the development of electronic travel aids. But these have not been too successful, probably because of their additions to the traditional aids being so limited (for a more detailed discussion, see Jansson, 1985). Thus, many of the problems that blind pedestrians encounter still remain.

Also, the large individual differences should be noted. There are blind individuals who perform well, but most of the blind have great problems; many of them cannot walk alone at all. Furthermore, those who do so typically visit only areas they know well and mainly in man-made environments indoors or in townscapes. Walking in natural surroundings that are more complex is much less common.

3. Mobility Training of Blind Infants

According to the analysis above, blind persons manage relatively well to find support for their walking and to guide themselves along some elongated feature in their environment. The main difference between blind and sighted mobility, at least with the travel aids available today, is the reduced possibilities, for nonvisual guidance, of walking toward a goal at a distance greater than a few meters. This is a disadvantage common to all the blind, irrespective of age and history as a blind person. However, this reduction of a main kind of loco-motory task because of the restriction of the perceptual space that is simultane-ously available may have especially profound effects on many aspects of the perceptual and cognitive development of blind children, as it makes them much less motivated to move around and explore the environment.

My research project in this problem area is divided into two parts. The first part intends to study in some detail the differences concerning locomotory performance between adults who have been blind all their life and blind adults who have seen during some period. This part of the project is directed toward the special needs of those born blind, as indicated by the problems remaining in adulthood. The two groups of blind adults are compared by (1) interviews on travel habits, techniques used during travel, problems experienced, accidents, and near–accidents; (2) video–recordings of travel in well–known environments analysed in a series of parameters; and (3) objective measures in simplified situations (concerning the latter methods, see Jansson, 1985, 1986, in press). The expected results from this part of the project are a more detailed know-ledge about the locomotory deficits specific to adults born blind. On the basis of this knowledge, hypotheses about suitable measures during childhood will be formulated.

The second part intends to investigate the prerequisites for such measures during childhood. Most of this part of the project has to await the results of the first part, but earlier research indicates the importance of some measures that, it seems to me, should be included. Some aspects will be dealt with below, especially the very early gross motor development.

3.1   The Start of Spontaneous Mobility Training

The start of spontaneous mobility training of blind infants was studied by Fraiberg and her co-workers (Fraiberg, 1977; Fraiberg, Siegel, & Gibson, 1966; Fraiberg, Smith, and Adelson, 1969; Adelson and Fraiberg, 1974). They found blind children to be considerably delayed, in comparison with sighted children, in using their motor system for mobility, in spite of the maturity of this system being similar in the two groups. The largest difference, a delay of 7 months (a median age of 19 months for the blind and 12 for the sighted children) was found for walking alone across a room. I think this kind of locomotion corresponds to what I have called walking toward a goal.

In their experiments, Fraiberg and her co-workers studied in more detail the potential of hearing to replace vision in its role of starting locomotion toward an object at a distance. Their conclusion was that hearing did not seem to be able to replace vision as a starter of locomotion because of the sound not being perceived by the blind infant as originating from an object.

However, there are important restrictions in Fraiberg's experiments, one of them being pointed out by herself with regret, namely that they were concerned with midline reach only. This means that under all conditions the sound source was located only directly in front of the child, not, as in real life, in any direction. Thus, the sound was presented such that the children did not have to make any orienting movement in order to direct themselves towards it.

When vision is used, there is usually, immediately after the first detection of the object (often by peripheral vision), an eye movement which brings objects into the view of the part of the retina with the best acuity. This first movement is usually followed by more movements of the eye, the head, and/or the whole body, making a closer examination of the object possible.

In a similar way, when a sound is detected under natural conditions, the observer adjusts by orienting toward the sound source (cf. Gibson, 1966, p. 83). This may be such a basic condition for listening that Fraiberg's pessimistic conclusion can be called in question. If we tried closer–to–life conditions including sound sources in many directions, it might very well be that sound can serve as an initiator of locomotion. Schwarz (1984) has developed the theoretical differences between Fraiberg's and Gibson's approaches in more detail and advocated a related, ecologically based view.

In another context, experiments with the Sonicguide used by infants (Bower, 1977; Aitken and Bower, 1982), there was such an exploratory activity with an auditory stimulation. These investigators concluded that very young children can use hearing for the detection of objects and the starting of at least grasping movements toward these objects. It might very well be that hearing can be much more useful for the blind than is generally assumed, especially if exploratory activities are stimulated. In his extensive review, Warren (1984, pp. 17–26) also discussed other reasons for relatively optimistic expectations.

3.2   A Note on the Potentials of Hearing

Vision is such a dominating sense that people with sight often forget about the possibilities of hearing. For the blind themselves and people in their neighborhood, the contributions of hearing are quite apparent. Consequently, training in the use of the rich auditory information available in the environment is an important part of the rehabilitation of newly blinded people. It is very clear that it is possible, especially after proper training, to use hearing much more also for the purpose of orientation and mobility than the sighted do. But the research on the use of audition by blind children is very scanty (cf. Warren, 1984).

It should be noted that the usefulness of hearing in this context also goes far beyond the localization of sound sources. It is often possible to identify sounds very precisely. For instance, sound may inform about what kinds of surfaces a long cane has touched (cf. Schenkman, 1986), or about which person is talking. The sound waves contain enormous amounts of information which we have only just begun to understand. Research, especially on what has been called ecological acoustics (cf. Jenkins, 1985), can be expected to be important also for training in the use of audition for the purpose of orientation and mobility.

4. An Example of an Experiment to Get Blind Infants Started in Their Exploration of the Environment

This example was inspired by the experiments of Fraiberg and her co-workers referred to above, and it is included in my project in progress. The experiment concerns itself with the possibilities of using sound for starting spontaneous locomotion by infants.

An infrared transmitter, similar to those used for television control, is attached to the infant's head. When the transmitter, as a result of the infant's own head movements, is directed toward an object in the environment, it starts a tape recorder placed in the same location as the object. The sounds produced are the same as those normally made by the object when it is moved in some way. If the child has had earlier positive tactual and auditory experience of the object, it is predicted that the sound, indicating the existence of this object in the neighborhood, should motivate the child to approach it. This use of the sound from an object known to the child will, hopefully, circumvent the problem indicated by Fraiberg (1968) that auditory information may not be identified by the blind infant as originating from an object. (The use of a technical device instead of a human manipulator is motivated partly by the more precise timing of the perceptual–motor relations, and partly by the patience expected from the device.)

By a carefully planned series of situations starting with the object within reaching distance and continuing with increasing distances, the expectation is that it will be possible to train the infant to start moving toward sound sources on its own. Hopefully, the child will later generalize this behavior to other situations and other objects, thus using sound as a starter of locomotion more generally.

4.1   Final Comment

It should be remembered that the presented discussion here is mainly the background of a project in progress. The final empirical results of the project are not yet available. Therefore, this article has the character of a status report.

Acknowledgement

This project on early mobility training of children born blind is being funded by the Swedish Ministry of Health and Social Affairs: Delegation for Social Research.

References

Adelson, E. and Fraiberg, S. (1974): Gross motor development in infants blind from birth. Child development, 45, 114–126.

Aitken, S., and Bower, T.G.R. (1982): The use of sonicguide in infancy. Journal of Visual Impairment and Blindness, 76, 91–100.

Barth, J.L. and Foulke, E. (1979): Preview: A neglected variable in orientation and mobility. Journal of Visual Impairment and Blindness, 73, 41–48.

Bower, T.G.R. (1977): Blind babies see with their ears. New Scientist, 73, 255–257.

Fraiberg, S. (1968): Parallel and divergent patterns in blind and sighted infants. Psychoanalytic Study of the Child, 23, 264–300.

Fraiberg, S. (1977): Insights from the blind. Comparative studies of blind and sighted children. New York: Basic Books.

Fraiberg, S., Siegel, B.L. and Gibson, R. (1966): The role of sound in the search behavior of a blind infant. Psychoanalytic Study of the Child, 21, 327–351.

Fraiberg, S., Smith, M., and Adelson, E. (1969): An educational program for blind infants. Journal of Special Education, 3, 121–139.

Gibson, J.J. (1966): The senses considered as perceptual systems. Boston: Houghton Mifflin.

Gibson, J.J. (1979): The ecological approach to perception. Boston: Houghton Mifflin.

Jansson, G. (1985): Implications of perceptual theory for the development of non–visual travel aids for the visually handicapped. In D.H. Warren and E.R.Strelow (Eds.): Electronic spatial sensing for the blind. Contributions from perception, rehabilitation, and computer vision (pp. 403–419). Dordrecht, Holland: Nijhoff.

Jansson, G. (1986): Development and evaluation of mobility aids for the visually handicapped. In P.L. Emiliani (Ed.): Development of electronic aids for the visually handicapped (pp. 297–303). Dordrecht, Holland: Nijhoff/Junk.

Jansson, G. (1987): Theoretical reasons for increasing the range of the next generation of electronic travel aids for the visually impaired. In E. Foulke (Ed.): Proceedings of the Louisville Space Conference, April 13–14, 1984 (pp. 25–30). Louisville, Kentucky: University of Louisville, College of Arts and Sciences.

Jansson, G. (in press): Non–visual guidance of locomotion. In R. Warren and A.H. Wertheim (Eds.): Perception and Control of Egomotion (Chapter 19). Hillsdale, New Jersey: Erlbaum.

Jansson, G., and Schenkman, B. (1977): The effect of the range of a laser cane on the detection of objects by the blind (Report No. 211). Uppsala, Sweden: University of Uppsala, Department of Psychology.

Jenkins, J.J. (1985): Acoustic information for objects, places, and events. In W.H. Warren and R.E. Shaw (Eds.): Persistence and change (pp. 115–138). Hillsdale, New Jersey: Erlbaum.

Lee, D.N. (1980): Visuo–motor coordination in space–time. In G.E. Stelmach and J. Requin, (Eds.): Tutorials in motor behavior (pp. 281–295). Amsterdam: North-Holland.

Leonard, J.A. (1971): The concept of minimal information required for effective mobility and suggestions for future non–visual displays. Mimeographed report. Nottingham, England: University of Nottingham, Department of Psychology.

Schenkman, B.N. (1985): Human Echolocation: The detection of obstacles by the blind. Acta Universitatis Upsalienses. Abstracts of Uppsala Dissertations from the Faculty of Social Sciences, No. 36.

Schenkman, B.N. (1986): Identification of ground materials with the aid of tapping sounds and vibrations of long canes for the blind. Ergonomics, 29, 985–998.

Schenkman, B.N., and Jansson, G. (1986): The detection and localization of objects by the blind with the aid of long cane tapping sounds. Human Factors, 28, 607–618.

Schwartz, M. (1984): The role of sound for space and object perception in the congenitally blind infant. Advances in Infancy Research, 3, 23–56.

Supa, M., Cotzin, M., and Dallenbach, D.M. (1944): "Facial vision": the perception of obstacles by the blind. American Journal of Psychology, 57, 133–183.

Warren, D.H. (1984): Blindness and early childhood development (2nd ed., revised). New York: American Foundation for the Blind.

Particle Versus Wave Theories of Learning to Read and Write. Toward a Field Model of Success and Failure in Literacy Acquisition

Hans Brügelmann

This paper reports on the planning of PLUS, a study in our project *Kinder auf dem Weg zur Schrift (Children's Routes to Literacy)*. PLUS is the acronomyn for *Progress in Literacy Understanding and Skills*. This is only a brief account of some of our basic assumptions that are relevant to the topic of the conference (cf. for a more detailed description of the project: Brügelmann, 1987; an English summary of the main principles of our educational approach can be found in Brügelmann, 1986).

1. Two Philosophies of Psychological and Educational Thinking

At the present time, two philosophies of psychological and educational thinking have to be distinguished when looking at the different attempts to explain children's failure in reading and writing. Not without any ulterior motive, I have named them after sets of theories that competed for recognition in physics some time ago.

The first comprises what I call "particle" theories of learning. They adopt an atomistic view, assuming that learning takes place by adding bits and pieces of knowledge (skills, etc.) together step by step. These are seen as intact modules that eventually will build up a functioning system (of reading and writing, for instance). This is a rather mechanistic view that seems to make it easy, however, to plan instruction, to measure progress, and to define failure.

"Wave" theories, on the other hand, start from the opposite view. They assume that children display imperfect, but comprehensive forms of reading and writing even before school (e.g., scribbling and mock reading). Learning, then, is seen

as gradually refining these rough forms through experimenting with approxima-
tions. Children, from this point of view, are active constructors of their own
thinking, trying to make sense from their experience (of print, for example) in
more holistic, but also in more divergent terms than assumed by the particle
theories (v. Glasersfeld, 1987). Learning is thus interpreted as the continuous
replacement of "waves" of theories and strategies developed by the child one
after the other.

What are the implications of this controversy for our topic *Children at risk* and
the prevention of school failure?

The first issue concerns our interpretation of what children do or do not bring
to school, that is, the definition of so-called *prerequisites* of literacy acquisition.

Are we interested in *general functions* such as "memory", "visual perception"
and "motor skills", that is, prerequisites in domains other than reading and
writing? Such a module view of the psychological system implies that important
conditions for success and failure in the acquisition of literacy are not related to
print as the object of learning. The consequence for instructional planning
would be first to repair missing or deficient prerequisites and only afterwards to
confront the child with print.

Our project adopts the opposite perspective on the acquisition of literacy and
views it as a *continuous process* rooted in and gradually emerging from everyday experiences of print before and outside (as well as in) school. Differences
in progress are assumed to be due to developmental lags in such experiences
and the concepts built from them. Thus, children differ not only in the number
of letters they can name, sight-words, they can read, or words they can write;
they also have different ideas about the use of print and, which has often been
overlooked, about the technical relationship between written and spoken language (cf., e.g., Ferreiro and Teberosky, 1982). In educational terms, this view
demands rich and diverse encounters with print as the best means for over-
coming difficulties in reading and writing.

The second issue focuses more narrowly on the notion of *difficulties:* How are
mistakes interpreted in the two respective frameworks?

Atomistic models of learning generally imply a *deficit interpretation* of errors.
They are seen as signals of something going wrong. Problems children have

with understanding and using print are seen as "disturbances" of the learning process. The causes of such disturbances are not located in the complexity of the object, but in individual "defects" (e.g., of perception, memory, concentration). Thus, particle didactics try to avoid or minimize the occurrence of errors through systematic instructional planning (e.g., controlling the vocabulary of texts, highly focused drill-and-practice).

Wave models, however, see errors as indicators of *developmental stages*. Early forms of reading and writing, of course, are "defective" in comparison to the more elaborated performance of experienced readers and writers. Yet, there is nothing "disturbing" about these deficiencies. Again, it is primarily the amount and the quality of experience with print that explains differences. Different types and proportions of errors are characteristic of intermediate stages that are *necessary transitional steps* in the acquisition process (cf. the sketch in Fig. 2 below).

Variation of performance is natural. Faster and slower learning are just one dimension of human differences. Slow learners demand attention and special resources, but mistakes (and difficulties in learning in general) should not and cannot be "prevented". They rather should be recognized as necessary features of the individual construction of knowledge. If we try to suppress their emergence, or if we do not respond to them as constructive attempts of the child, difficulties can indeed become "disturbances" and eventually consolidate as individual "deficiencies".

This is not to deny that some children need more help; often considerably more help than others. This help, however, has to be focused on the child's active exploration of print and its specific features. It should understand and support the child's attempts to make sense of this medium and to gradually expand and differentiate her/his repertoire of using it effectively.

As will have become apparent to the reader, I personally strongly favor the wave interpretation of learning (cf. for further evidence, the contributions in: Balhorn and Brügelmann, 1987). Nevertheless, I acknowledge that in certain cases, at least, the atomistic view has stimulated successful educational practice. It would be arrogant to neglect the fact that it is not only the children who construct their theories. Our theories, too, are just models that approximate reality by emphasizing certain features and deliberately neglecting others. Thus, different, even contradictory theories can coexist. Just this has happened with the particle and the wave explanation of light in physics over the past decades. And the great physicist *Niels Bohr* has argued that such *complementarity* is unavoidable because of the limitations of our thinking, and that it generally can serve as a useful epistemological principle (cf. Fischer, 1987).

If this argument holds up to the reader's scrutiny, one conclusion is apparent: Psychologists explaining learning difficulties, and even more so, educationists trying to intervene, have to be very modest in claiming expert control over the children's idiosyncratic attempts to use print (which may be a reasonable approximation that fits their individual possibilities).

It seems to be easier for the "wave" school of thinking to accomodate this charge within their framework than for the "particle" approach. In addition, historically we also have a lot of catching up to do in the wave mode of understanding children's acquisition of literacy. Much has to be done in theory as well as in the classroom to strengthen the holistic view of children's learning as a complement to traditional "particle" thinking.

Thus, I personally would limit the particle model to a pragmatic use within the context and on the basis of the wave theory. A particle analysis could help, for example, to investigate and define more clearly the processes of reading and writing *at different stages*. Then, however, such component skills would have to be (1) directly related to print, (2) integrated in a process model of reading and writing, and (3) interpreted developmentally.

2. Implications of the Wave Theory

In our project, we have developed a "didactic map" of eight learning areas (cf. Fig. 1) linked to a four-stage model of development (cf. Fig. 2) that together provide such a framework (cf. for more details Brügelmann et al., 1986). Thus, our pragmatic conclusion from the complementarity principle is to encourage and to support teachers to broaden and to consciously vary their methodical options, that is, to provide ample scope, rich materials, and diverse activities for discovering print *side by side* with focused instruction and carefully selected and limited, but steady drill–and–practice exercises.

Analysis of oral language and distinction of phonemes	Understanding different types and functions of symbols	Using written language in and for different contexts and purposes
	Understanding the structure of print and the technical role of its elements	
Knowledge of letters in different fonts and writings	Grouping of letters and segmentation of words in frequent morphemes, syllables, etc.	Extending and automatic mastery of a personal sight word vocabulary
	Production and comprehension of different types of text	

Fig. 1: Eight areas within which beginning reading experience can be offered to children (Brügelmann, 1986)

Handwriting	Spelling	Reading
From aimless to directed scribbling	From analogous drawings to arbitrary symbols	From telling stories to mock reading
From scribbling to imitating shapes and experimenting with them	From arbitrary letter combinations to a sound-oriented shorthand	From mock reading to context oriented calling or naming
From single letters to letter rows	From sound skeleton to phonetic spelling	From context guessing to deciphering text
From rows of separate letters to connected movements ("melodies")	From sound analysis to orthographic patterns and finally specific orthographies of individual words	From conscious decoding to automatic decoding and comprehension guided by context and personal experience

Fig. 2: Four critical steps in the development of handwriting, spelling, and reading (Brügelmann, 1986)

Nevertheless, the issue of "prevention" remains a serious one in a school system that is organized according to age. Most curricula assume a high degree of homogeneity in the way children learn. And from a very early age on, school presupposes the ability to read and write as a means for participating successfully in school activities.

Two shifts in theoretical attention and research design are needed.

Firstly, we have to broaden the range of variables to be included in our re-search. To a much greater extent, we have to change the quality of describing and analyzing what is called "variable" in the psychometric tradition.

In our project PLUS, we use a set of "Reading and Writing Tasks for School

Beginners" (Brügelmann et al., 1988) that demand the use of print in a meaningful way. Following Clay, Downing, Ferreiro and Teberosky, and others, we use material that enables children to express their individual concepts and to use strategies, as we are interested in the development of their *thinking* and not only in isolated skills and elements of knowledge.

One example is the "marked memory" game with picture card pairs. The name of the object depicted on the bottom of the card is printed on the visible top. Thus, we can see if the child attends to print at all or if she/he turns up the cards in a random order. Children attending to print have realized that print can serve as sign in a one–to–one relationship to objects. By using words that are similar in different respects (such as: *Boote/Boot/Brot/Brote; Kirche/Kirsche; Stop/Post*) we can challenge the child's strategy and check if she/he is able to learn that all letters as well as their order is relevant for the identification of a word. Thus, among all the children who cannot yet read, some turn the cards in random order, others perhaps need as many attempts as the first group but display a great number of "similar" mistakes (such as *Kirsche/Kirche*), and a third group does not need more attempts than the number of pairs available. Moreover, we can observe whether children learn from the practical consequences of their strategy.

The basic assumption of PLUS is the hypothesis that there is a logic in the ways children conceptualize and use print as well as in the order through which they acquire different patterns of reading and writing. The key theoretical constructs in our study are:

1. cognitive clarity of the task (Downing, 1979; Clay, 1979)
2. (meta–)linguistic awareness (Lundberg, 1978, 1989; Bradley, and Bryant, 1985; Downing, and Valtin, 1984)
3. learning as personal and active construction (Piaget, 1959; Bergk, 1980)
4. qualitative stages of acquisition (Ferreiro and Teberosky, 1982; Frith, 1985; Henderson, 1985)
5. developmental matching of experience (Vygotski, 1962; Mason, 1981).

Beyond this "constructionist" shift, a second change in the focus of attention is called for.

We have not only to enlighten the "black box child" by trying to better understand (and not just: "cognitively" explain) his/her thinking about print, its functions, and technical logic. We also have to clear the theoretically rather foggy context within which the child gathers his/her personal experiences and tries to make sense of them. An ecological and more dynamic interpretation of the acquisition of literacy and its difficulties is needed. We have to replace, or at least to complement, the static and highly individualistic model of "defects" as causes of school failure by an analysis of the social "cultures" of print (and of learning) the child encounters at home, in kindergarten, in the street, and at school (cf., e.g., Goelman et al., 1984, Part I; Teale and Sulzby (1986); and also the work of Heinrich Bauersfeld (1982, 1983, in press) in the area of mathematics learning).

3. Predicting the Acquisition of Literacy and the Design of PLUS

Psychologists aiming at "prevention and intervention" in coping with learning difficulties tend to look for individual "predictors" of school failure. They have been puzzled, however, by the number of significant (but mostly moderate) correlations. This variety cannot be interpreted consistently in a theoretical model. Such a great number and broad range of variables can serve as indicators of school failure (if we take low enough values on the respective test) that the result can be summarized as follows: Children who are in bad shape today run a high risk of being in bad shape tomorrow. Thus, these variables can only serve as "warning lamps". They do not explain why children have difficulties and what to do about them. This is the help, however, that parents, kindergarteners, and teachers need.

Moreover, the correlations reported vary considerably in different studies (cf., e.g., Weinert and Schneider, 1987, pp. 151–152; Ayers and Downing, 1982). We have to acknowledge that predictions of school failure from individual characteristics only hold under certain conditions. To put the case more strongly: Individual predictors are not signs of personal "defects"; they are indicators of the school's ability to respond appropriately to the diverse needs of children. When children come to school, they are at different levels of development; each of them being a useful intermediary step. Learning "disturbances" result from the mismatch between the average curriculum the school offers and what the child brings with him/her.

Thus, not only do we have to complement the particle model of knowledge and skill components by a wave model of concept development and meaningful understanding of print, but we have to embed both interpretations in a *field model* of literacy acquisition that relates this development to the milieus within which the child collects his/her experiences. As Heinrich Bauersfeld (in press) puts it: We need a theory of the child not only as an active, but as an *interactive* learner.

The consequence for PLUS is not only to broaden the range and to reinterpret the quality of variables, but also to develop a research strategy that elaborates the simplistic pre-/posttest control-group design by also investigating and deliberately influencing the context of learning.

PLUS has been conceived of as:

1. *a longitudinal study*, that is, over two years (from K through 2);
2. *an intervention study* exploiting the full range of methodical ideas that can be accommodated in the "didactic map" (not just implementing and evaluating one specific program) and documenting these activities as well as their effects in:
3. *detailed descriptions* of the learning and interaction history of selected children and their classes leading to:
4. *individual learning biographies* of so-called "children at risk" identified according to criteria from the predictive individual prerequisite model, but followed up and supported
5. *within the individual milieu* of ·educationally-relevant situations and contexts that provide significant experiences with print for the child.

Fig. 3 gives an overview of the features we want to study, clarifying how we want to relate the developmental aspect to a field interpretation of learning. The interaction between the child as an active constructor of his experience and the environment as the stimulator of such experience can be sketched out in the following spiral model.

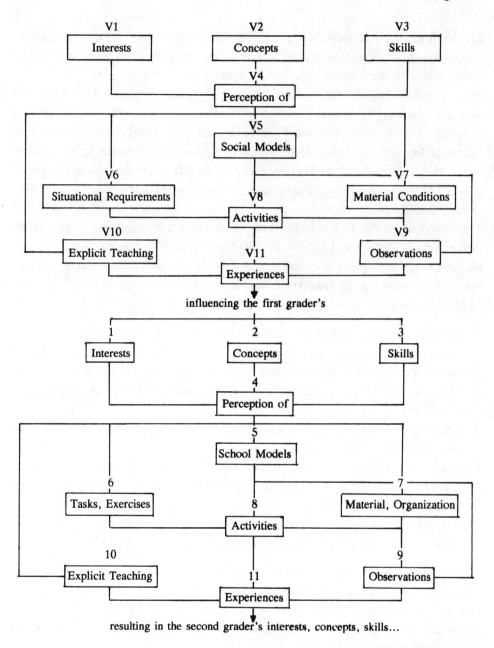

Fig. 3: A Spiral Field Model of Literacy Development emerging from the preschool Child's encounters of print

Individual interests, concepts, and skills (V1–V3) already built from earlier experience influence how the preschool child perceives (V4):

1. (missing) social models of reading and writing (V5),
2. situational requirements (not) to use print (V6), and
3. material conditions (V7) supporting/hindering such attempts.

Depending on these objective conditions, their social interpretation in the (sub)culture the child lives in, and how they both are perceived by the child from his personal experience, she/he will embark on certain activities (V8) or not do so. These activities, together with explicit teaching attempts by others (V10) and with observations the child can collect in this specific environment (V9), will shape the experiences the first grader brings to school.

From these preschool experiences (V11), in turn, a more differentiated set of interests, concepts, and skills (1–3) emerges that are moulded in similar ways in the classroom context. Here, again, we have to be careful not to equate "teaching" with "learning". The curriculum, the material, the exercises, the behavior of others, and so forth are not perceived passively, but interpreted by the child in a field of two further forces: firstly, reflected through the normative interpretation by the teacher, by his/her classmates, and by parents (i.e., by socially "significant others"), and, secondly, reconstructed through the cognitive and emotional filters resulting from his/her personal biography. Thus, we have to learn about the values of the child and the subcultures she/he lives in if we want to understand motives and cognitive constructs.

Field theories in physics still have their problems. In education the situation is even more complex. Thus, we have a long way to go from the programmatic declaration in our project proposal. Without such an orientation, however, we would continue this Winnie-the-Pooh sort of tracking of artificial phenomena by studying one's own footprints going round in a circle (it really is worth rereading Chapter 3 of A.A. Milne's book "In which Pooh and Piglet go hunting and nearly catch a Woozle" from this perspective). "Prediction" and "prevention" are very delicate notions that may mislead educational research and classroom practice if we are not very careful in clarifying their theoretical implications beforehand.

References

Ayers, D., and Downing, J. (1982): Testing children's concepts of reading. Educational Research, 24, 277–283.

Balhorn, H. and Brügelmann, H. (Eds.)(1987): Welten der Schrift in der Erfahrung der Kinder. Jahrbuch "Lesen und Schreiben" Bd. 2. Konstanz: Ekkehard Faude.

Bauersfeld, H. (in press): Interaction, construction, and knowledge: Alternative perspectives for mathematics education. In T. Cooney, and D. Grows (Eds.): Effective mathematics teaching. Reston, Virginia: N.C.T.M.

Bauersfeld, H., et al. (Eds.)(1982): Analysen zum Unterrichtshandeln. IDM-Reihe Bd. 5. Köln: Aulis.

Bauersfeld, H., et al. (Eds.)(1983): Lernen und Lehren von Mathematik. IDM-Reihe Bd. 6. Köln: Aulis.

Bergk, M. (1980): Leselernprozeß und Erstlesewerke. Bochum: Kamp.

Bradley, L. and Bryant, P. (1985): Rhyme and reason in reading and spelling. Ann Arbor, Mich.: University of Michigan Press.

Brügelmann, H. (1986): Discovering print – a process approach to initial reading and writing in West Germany. In The Reading Teacher, 40, 294–298.

Brügelmann, H. (1987): Kinder auf dem Weg zur Schrift: PLUS. (Projekt Lese- und Schreibfortschritte). Forschungsantrag an die DFG. Bericht No. 38b. Projekt "Kinder auf dem Weg zur Schrift", FB 12, Universität Bremen, West Germany.

Brügelmann, H., et al. (1986): Die Schrift entdecken – Beobachtungshilfen und methodische Ideen für einen offenen Anfangsunterricht im Lesen und Schreiben. Konstanz: Ekkehard Faude.

Brügelmann, H., et al. (1988): Lese- und Schreibaufgaben für Schulanfänger. Bericht No. 33e. Projekt "Kinder auf dem Wege zur Schrift", FB 12, Universität Bremen, West Germany.

Clay, M.M. (1979): Early detection of reading difficulties. Heinemann: London.

Downing, J. (1979): Reading and reasoning. Edinburgh: Chambers.

Downing, J., et al. (1983): Linguistic awareness in reading readiness (LARR) test. Windsor: NFER–Nelson.

Downing, J., and Valtin, R. (Eds.)(1984): Language awareness and learning to read. New York: Springer.

Ferreiro, E. and Teberosky, A. (1982): Literacy before schooling. Portsmouth: Heinemann.

Fischer, E.P. (1987): Sowohl als auch – Denkerfahrungen der Naturwissenschaften. Hamburg: Rasch & Röhring.

Frith, U. (1985): Beneath the surface of developmental dyslexia. In K. Patterson et al. (Eds.): Surface Dyslexia: Neuropsychological and cognitive studies of phonological reading. Hove: Lawrence Erlbaum.

Glasersfeld, E.v. (1987): Wissen, Sprache und Wirklichkeit. Braunschweig: Vieweg.

Goelman, H., et al. (Eds.)(1984): Awakening to Literacy. London: Heinemann Educational.

Henderson, E.H. (1985): Teaching spelling. Boston: Houghton Mifflin.

Lundberg, I. (1978): Aspects of linguistic awareness related to reading. In A. Sinclair et al. (Eds.): The child's conception of language. New York: Springer.

Mason, J.M. (1981): Prereading: A developmental perspective. Technical Report No. 298. Center for the Study of Reading, University: Urbana–Champaign, Ill.

Mason, J.M., and McCormick, C. (1981): An investigation of prereading instruction from a developmental perspective. Technical Report No. 224. Center for the Study of Reading, University: Urbana–Champaign, Ill.

Piaget, J. (1959): The language and thought of the child. 3rd ed. London: Routledge & Kegan Paul.

Teale, W.H., and Sulzby, E. (Eds.) (1986): Emerging literacy: Writing and reading. Norwood, NJ.: Ablex.

Vygotski, L.S. (1962): Thought and language. M.I.T. Press: Cambridge, and Mass.

Weinert, F.E., and Schneider, W. (1987): Documentation of assessment procedures used in waves one to three. Report No. 2 from The Munich Longitudinal Study on the Genesis of Individual Competencies (LOGIC). Max–Planck–Institut für Psychologische Forschung: München.

Family Variables as Predictors of Differential Effectiveness in Child Therapy*

Fritz Mattejat and Helmut Remschmidt

1. Introduction

The investigation reported here deals with the general question whether and to what extent prognoses can be made about the outcome of child and adolescent psychiatric treatment: Which factors are favorable for a positive development during the treatment, and which factors impede therapeutic progress in children and adolescents with psychiatric disturbances?

In this report, we want to refer to one particular aspect: the influence of family variables on the treatment outcome.

The practical background of these questions is evident: More detailed findings in this field might enable us to improve the therapeutic possibilities for children and adolescents with psychiatric disturbances and their families.

2. Method

2.1 Patient Sample

Our data refer to a therapy evaluation study of all consecutive patients who underwent treatment in the Marburg University Clinic for Child and Adolescent Psychiatry and who fulfilled the following criterion:

"An outpatient treatment is not sufficient, on the contrary, an inpatient treat-

*) The data were assessed by Dr. F. Braun and H.G. Heinscher. The text of this paper was translated by E. Le Guillarme; the statistical analyses were carried out by G. Albrecht. The authors express their gratitude to these colleagues.

ment or, alternatively, an intensive home treatment is necessary."

Thus, the study comprises only such patients in whom (according to the clinical indication) both treatment modalities were likewise possible: inpatient treatment and home treatment: That is, those patients were excluded for whom only an inpatient treatment could be justified (in whom, following the clinical indication, a home treatment was out of the question). Furthermore, patients were excluded for whom a normal outpatient treatment would have been sufficient. Thus, the evaluation study comprised a rather specific group of patients. Further criteria for inclusion in the evaluation study were: diagnosis, age, and intelligence: The patients should be of normal intelligence, aged between 6 and 18 years, and only the following diagnostic groups were admitted: neuroses, anorexia, enuresis, enkopresis, obesity, social conduct disorders, specific emotional disorders, and hyperkinetic syndrome.

A total of 54 patients who fulfilled these criteria were admitted to the Marburg study, while another study was run parallel in the Mannheim Institute for Mental Health with the additional possibility (besides inpatient and home treatment) of a day clinic treatment.

In the following, however, we only refer to the Marburg data.

The main question in the investigation was the comparison of the treatment modalities. The patients were thus randomly assigned to the two therapy modalities "inpatient treatment" versus "home treatment". Half of the 54 patients were treated as inpatients, half of them underwent home treatment.

2.2   Assessment Methods

Before the beginning of the treatment, at the end of the treatment, and continuously during the course of the treatment, the patients underwent detailed diagnostic measures. After the end of the treatment, the assessed data were summed up in an evaluation report.

This evaluation report did not reveal in which treatment modality the patient had been treated. The evaluation reports were presented to independent evaluators (colleagues of other clinics) who rated the outcome of the treatment on a number of scales. These evaluators' ratings represented for us the standard measure for the therapy outcome.

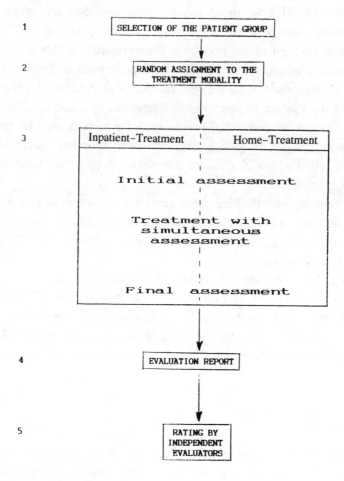

Fig. 1: Course of the Investigation

The two groups "inpatient treatment" and "home treatment" did not differ with regard to the therapy outcome.
Thus, an important conclusion that can be drawn from this investigation is that inpatient treatment can be replaced by home treatment for a specific group of patients. Detailed information concerning these results is given in Remschmidt

and Schmidt (1988). But here we want to discuss another aspect of our study, the question of therapy prognosis.

With regard to this question, we can consider the group of all 54 patients together, regardless of whether they underwent inpatient or home treatment.

2.3   Data Analysis

For our question, we selected one rating of the independent evaluators as our criterion variable, namely the rating "Therapy outcome regarding symptomatology (improvement of symptomatology)".

In principle, all data assessed before the beginning of the therapy may serve as predictor variables. For data analysis, we chose the method of hierarchic classification used in the CART-programs by Breiman et al. (1984). CART is an abbreviation for "Classification And Regression Trees".

The hierarchical classification solves discrimination problems. Given is a variable vector with prognostically relevant characteristics of the patients (in our case variables from the initial assessment), and further given is a criterion variable (in our case the therapy outcome). We are looking for information about the predictive value for the criterion variable of the variables of the initial assessment. For this purpose, the CART procedure uses binary decision trees. At the start of the procedure all investigated objects (in our case all patients) are members of the same group. In the first step the program looks for a split of this whole group into two subgroups that are as different as possible on the criterion variable. Thus the procedure looks for a split which resembles the distribution on the criterion variable. For this purpose the list of predictor variables is screened to find the best predictor for such a grouping. Additionally, the program looks for the value of the predictor variable at which this split should be made. For example, when the age of the patient is important for the therapy outcome, the variable age may be the decision variable of the first node in the tree, and the value "40 years" may be the best split point. The subgroups of patients younger than 40 years would then be classified as the group with a good prognosis, the patients older than 40 years as the group with an unfavorable prognosis.

In the next step the two subgroups are separately analyzed in the same way and so on. In the two branches of the tree, different predictor variables may have the best predictive value.

A procedure which produces binary decision trees has the advantage that the structure of automatic classification can be demonstrated easily in a diagram and directly interpreted.

Further advantages of this method lie in the fact that continuous and categorical variables can be included at the same time in the analysis. Finally, the continuous variables do not have to be scaled on an interval level; an ordinal scale level is sufficient.

Several methodological problems have to be solved in the implementation of this procedure. Here, we want to refer to just *one* aspect:

The decision procedure can theoretically be continued until all objects of a node have identical values in the criterion variable. In the extreme case, every terminal node has only one element in its group. In this way, we get a very large decision tree with a minimal rate of misclassifications.

The application of this decision structure to another sample, however, results in a higher rate of misclassifications, because − especially in a further differentiation of a small number of objects random effects of the investigated sample take effect which do not represent real connections. Thus, it is necessary to keep the decision tree so small that only real contingencies are included. The obvious choice for reaching this goal is to investigate a separate validation sample that may be gained − if the original sample is large enough − by random selection from the investigated sample. This procedure implies a loss of information that may, however, be kept relatively slight by using internal cross validation. This crossvalidation procedure uses in exchange 9/10 of the sample at a time as a so−called learning sample; the classification obtained is verified on the remaining 10%. In this way, we can obtain a realistic estimation of the misclassification rate. And we can use this cross−validation procedure to determine the optimal size of the decision tree. While the misclassifications in the apparent structure decrease continuously the more differentiations are made, in the cross validation, in contrast, the misclassification rate increases when random effects of the learning sample cannot be reproduced in the validation sample.

Our analysis was carried out with the CART–program on the SPERRY–computer of the University Statistical Center in Marburg.

3. Results

3.1 Results of the Analysis Taking Into Account All Prognostic Variables

These results can be summarized as follows:

1. Taking into account all the variables gained in the initial assessment, prognoses could be made that proved to be valid in the cross validation.
2. The results were complex: Variables often masked each other. To a large extent, individual symptom variables and variables of psychosocial stress could replace one another.
3. On the whole, the psychosocial variables (e.g., psychosocial stress) were to a certain degree more important for the prognosis than the individual variables.
4. In most of the analyses, the diagnosis on Axis 1 played an important role, that is, the diagnosis was an important prognostic factor.

The relations between diagnosis and therapy outcome were statistically significant (Craddock–Flood $p < 0.05$). Our results agreed with the already known connections: Neuroses had a relatively good prognosis, the same was true for specific emotional disturbances and for enuresis, whereas social conduct disorders showed a bad prognosis.

3.2 Results of Specific Analyses of the Predictive Value of Psychosocial Stress Factors

Furthermore, we investigated the following more specific questions:
"Is a prognosis of therapy outcome possible, if we presume *only* psychosocial stress factors (as they are fixed in our 'Profile of psychosocial stress factors')

as known quantities"; and "Which psychosocial variables are particularly relevant for the prognosis?"

The "Profile of Psychosocial Stress Factors" is a further development of Axis 5 of the multiaxial classification system (Rutter et al., 1976) which was introduced and adapted for the German speaking countries by Remschmidt and Schmidt (1977). In comparison with Axis 5 of the MAS, the profile introduced a couple of new criteria, whereas other criteria which were rarely present were combined to one new variable. The profile consisted of 16 rating scales, representing essentially family diagnostic criteria. These 16 variables of the profile of psychosocial stress factors were integrated into the analysis as predictor variables.

Psychological stress variables:
(Profile of psychosocial stress factors − experimental form)

PSV1   Psychosocial stress factors outside the family
PSV3   Abnormal psychosocial circumstances
PSV4   Insufficient living conditions
PSV5   Insufficient stimulation
PSV6   Psychiatric disturbances in parents or siblings
PSV7   Disharmony between parents and patient
PSV8   Disharmony between parents (marital problems)
PSV9   Disharmony between patient and siblings (sibling rivalry)
PSV10 Lack of emotional warmth
PSV11 Extremely close family relationships
PSV12 Insufficient or inconsistent parental control
PSV13 Excessive parental control
PSV14 Lack of communication
PSV15 Problem− or conflict−denying communication
PSV16 Distorted or displaced communication

Before the beginning of treatment, each one of these variables was rated by the responsible therapist on a 5−point scale ranging from *no stress present* (0) to *extreme stress* (4).

As criterion variable, we used the therapy outcome regarding the symptomatology as rated by the independent evaluators. Originally the therapy outcome was rated by the evaluators on a 5-point scale. (As each case was rated by four evaluators, we assumed an averaged outcome value by partializing out the individual rater tendencies of each rater, cf. Remschmidt and Schmidt, 1988). As the original variable did not apply directly to the CART-analysis, we reduced this 5-point scale to two respectively three outcome groups, as shown in Fig. 2.

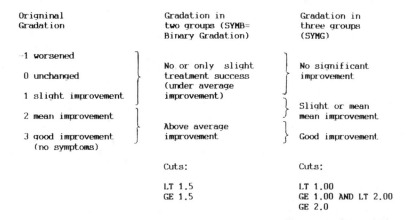

Fig. 2: Evaluators's Rating "Therapy Success Regarding Symptomatology (Symptomatic Improvement)": Gradation of the Variable

That is, we used two different groupings of the same variable "Improvement regarding psychiatric symptoms". For our first analysis, we classified the patients in the two groups: (1) therapy outcome below average, and (2) therapy outcome above average. Whereas for the second analysis, we classified them in three groups: (1) no improvement, (2) slight to mean improvement, and (3) marked improvement.

In both analyses the resulting prognostic structures retained their validity in a cross validation.

Let us first have a look at the results of our first analysis:

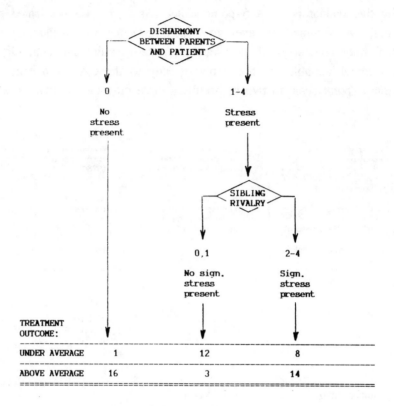

Fig. 3:   Decision-Tree: Prediction of Symptomatic Improvement (Symb = Two Outcome
Groups) on the Basis of Psychosocial Stress

Fig. 3 can be interpreted as follows: The variable "disharmony parents–patient" was the absolutely best variable for prognosis; it discriminated best between the patients with a good therapy prognosis and those with a bad one. The
patients with the stress factor "disharmony parents–patient" generally showed a
worse therapy prognosis than the patients without this stress factor.

By inspecting only the patients *with* this stress factor ("disharmony parents–patient") more closely, we found that the patients with sibling difficulties (rivalry,
etc.) showed a better prognosis than those without sibling difficulties.

This result seems, at first glance, rather strange. Why should quarrels or rivalry between the patient and his siblings be a good prognostical criterion? Here one has to consider that "sibling rivalry" in isolation is, of course, in no way a good prognostic criterion. It must, however, be noted that only those patients were taken into account who showed the adversity factor "disharmony between parents and patient", and that this group was being differentiated further.

The results thus indicated that disharmony between parents and patient had, on the whole, an unfavorable effect on the prognosis. However, this factor was prognostically not so unfavorable when associated with sibling rivalry.

That is, "disharmony parents–patient" *lost* − to a certain degree −its negative prognostic value if it was associated with the criterion "sibling rivalry". Or, vice versa: "Disharmony between parents and patient" *only* had a bad prognosis if it occured as an isolated criterion and not together with sibling problems.

In order to understand such a result, we can look at the so–called surrogate-variables of the CART–analysis. Surrogates are variables which − at the same node of the decision tree − may produce a similar split as the variable which was included in the decision tree.

In our exploratory analysis, in which we used all variables of the initial assessment, the variable "sibling rivalry" had the same functional role, as here; furthermore we found strong surrogates for this variable. These surrogates for "sibling rivalry" were

1. "Family conflicts" (a sum score of disharmony, quarreling, rivalry, conflicts in the family)

The circumstance that the variable "familial conflicts" might produce a similar split as the variable "sibling rivalry" allows the following conclusion:

"Disharmony between parents and patient" implies an *especially* bad prognosis if it represents the *only* disharmony within the family; whereas its prognostic effect is not as bad if it is associated with other disharmonies (between both parents or between the patient and his siblings). Therefore the disharmony between parents and patient has a bad prognosis if it proves to be a *specific drop–out criterion within the family*, that is, if only the patient is specially concerned by this disharmony. If the disharmony between parents and patient, however, is associated with other similar conflicts, or if the family, on the

whole, proves to be a "struggle family", then the criterion "disharmony parents–patient" loses its prognostically unfavorable value. From the psychological
point of view, a clear interpretation is possible: If, in an otherwise conflict-
avoiding family, the expulsive tendencies particularly and exclusively concern
the patient, that is, if the patient holds the role of a scapegoat within the
family, then we have a prognostically bad situation.

2. "Familial deficits" (a sum score of variables which indicated that basic
    needs of nurturance, stimulation, and so on could not be fulfilled in the
    family because of, e.g., insufficient familial conditions)

The circumstance that the variable "family deficits" might produce a similar
distribution as the variable "sibling rivalry" allows the following conclusion:
"Disharmony between parents and patient" has a specially bad prognostic effect
on children and adolescents of deficitary families. That is, if the relationship
between parents and children is deficitary, if the parents neglect the patient, and
so forth, then disharmony between parents and patient has an unfavorable
effect. If, in contrast, sufficient stimulation, emotional warmth, control, and
communication are present, the effect of the disharmony "parents–patient" is
not as bad.

3. "Age of the patient"

The circumstances that the variable "age of patient" might produce a similar
distribution as the variable "sibling rivalry" leads us to the following conclusion:
"Disharmony between parents and patient" has a prognostically bad effect on
older children and adolescents, whereas it does not lead to a bad prognosis for
younger children (who, on the whole, use to have more sibling problems). That
is, the factor "disharmony between parents and patient" gives an unfavorable
prognosis, especially for older children and adolescents, but not for younger
children. Younger children with "disharmony between parents and patient"
show a better prognosis for therapy outcome than older children and adolescents with the same criterion.
We see that an at first glance simple decision tree may require rather complex
further analyses and interpretations.

Our second analysis showed that the interpretation of binary decision trees is not always as difficult. In this analysis, we divided the patients into three outcome groups according to the criterion variables (1) no significant improvement, (2) slight to mean improvement, and (3) good (marked) improvement. Here too, the result proved to be valid in the cross validation.

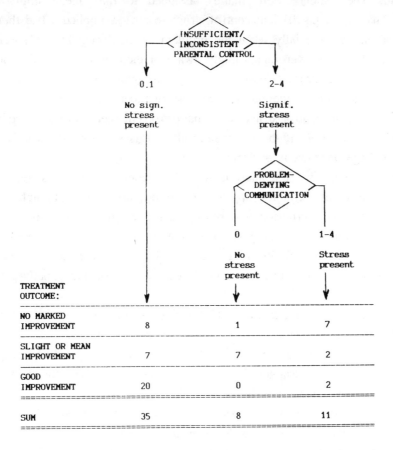

Fig. 4:   Decision-Tree: Prediction of Symptomatic Improvement (Symb = Three Outcome Groups) on the Basis of Psychosocial Stress

Here, the criterion "insufficient or inconsistent parental control" produced the absolutely best discrimination between the groups. If there was no significant stress regarding the criterion, the prognosis was relatively good. If, however, this stress factor was present, the prognosis was rather bad. This result is already known from similar investigations.

The decision tree showed the variable "problem–denying family communication" as a second criterion. Stress on this factor led to especially bad prognoses, whereas the prognosis was somewhat better if there was no stress in this field: The patients were mainly assigned to the "mean improvement group". That is, an insufficient control structure always implied a bad therapeutic prognosis, but especially when the problems were denied by the parents. If the parents, however, were accordingly aware of their problems (and supposedly suffered from them), at least an average progress could be attained. This attracts our attention to the question of the therapeutical alliance: In families with an insufficient control structure, a main problem seems to be to establish a meaningful cooperation; if the therapeutic alliance is successfully established, at least an average progress is possible.

If we now compare the first analysis with the second one, we first realize that completely different variables appear in the decision tree, although we are referring to the same criterion variable (once in two groups and once in three groups). One might think that just the definition of the outcome groups would lead to totally different findings. Thus, one ought to come to the conclusion that the results are very unstable and dependent on voluntary methodological decisions.

This conclusion, however, is false. This can be shown by inspecting not only the finally resulting decision trees, but also the analysis process. This inspection involves looking at the surrogate variables and also the so–called competitor variables, that is, the variables that could produce a different split at this node that, however, has a similar differential quality.

On each node, all variables "compete" for admission to the decision tree; it is often the case that several variables can produce a split of similar quality. Which variable is to "make the running" may depend on insignificant sample characteristics or methodological decisions. For this reason, it would be risky to rely only on the produced decision tree; on the contrary, it is necessary to consider the competitor variables in the interpretation. The following figure compares the variables in the produced decision tree and the competitor variables of our two analyses.

```
ANALYSIS 1: RATING OF THERAPY SUCCESS REGARDING SYMPTOMATOLOGY / SYMPTOMATIC
            IMPROVEMENT   (SYMB = TWO GROUPS):

NODE        VARIABLE IN THE            COMPETITOR VARIABLE*
NR.         DECISION TREE

1.          Disharmony              -  Insufficient/inconsistent
            parents-patient            parental control
                                   -  Insufficient living conditions
                                   -  Disharmony between the parents
                                      (marital conflicts)

2.          Sibling                -  Disharmony parents - patient
            rivalry                -  communications deficits
                                   -  Insufficient/inconsistent
                                      parental control


ANALYSIS 2: RATING OF THERAPY SUCCESS REGARDING SYMPTOMATOLOGY / SYMPTOMATIC
            IMPROVEMENT   (SYMG = THREE GROUPS):

NODE        VARIABLE IN THE            COMPETITOR VARIABLE*
NR.         DECISION TREE

1.          Insufficient/          -  Disharmony between parents
            inconsistent              (marital conflicts)
            parental control       -  Disharmony parents - patient
                                   -  Insufficient stimulation

2.          Problem-               -  Disharmony between parents
            denying                   (marital conflicts)
            communication          -  Disharmony parents - patient
                                   -  Insufficient living conditions
================================================================================
*The three best Competitors are named.
================================================================================
```

Fig. 5:   Prediction on the Basis of Psychosocial Stresses: Comparison of the two Analyses

Fig. 5 shows that although in Analysis 1 the variable "insufficient parental control" did not appear in the decision tree, it proved to be an important competitor variable, and vice versa, in the second analysis, the variable "insufficient parental control" was in the decision tree, but the variable "disharmony between parents and patient" was an important competitor. Both variables, of course, correlated; which one of two correlating variables is finally incorporated in the decision tree can depend on relatively slight shifts. Correlating variables may mask one another in the CART-analysis; thus, it seems a meaningful procedure to compare several analyses with each other to obtain a reliable interpretation.

The comparison of the two analyses regarding the competitor variables showed another result: The criterion "marital problems" appeared several times as a competitor, was thus of distinct prognostic value, but was not "successful" in any of the decision trees.

4. Summary and Discussion

Our results can be summarized as follows:

1. A cross-validated prognosis of therapy outcome (symptomatic improvement) is already possible with relatively few family variables.

2. One has to differentiate clearly between absolute and relative prognostic factors:

   By far the most important absolute factors are: (1) disharmony between parents and patient, and (2) inconsistent/insufficient parental control.

   An independent (absolute) importance of, however, somewhat less relevance is also found for the factor: (3) disharmony between parents (marital problems).

   Absolute factors of, however, clearly less relevance are criteria which indicate objective or interactional deficits such as: (4) insufficient stimulation, and (5) insufficient living conditions.

3. The most important relative prognostic factors (relative to the absolute prognostic factors "disharmony parents–patient" and "inconsistent/insufficient parental control") in our analyses are: (6) sibling rivalry, and (7) problem- or conflict–denying communication.

The importance of the variable "sibling rivalry" leads us to the hypothesis that disharmony between parents and patient is a prognostically unfavorable factor if:

(1) it is a specific family characteristic ("scapegoat hypothesis"),
(2) it concerns older children and adolescents, or
(3) it is associated with deficitary familiy conditions.

The importance of the criterion "problem- or conflict-denying communication" leads us to the hypothesis that in families with insufficient control structure the awareness of the problems and, on this basis, the establishment of a therapeutical alliance play a central role in the therapeutic process.

From a methodological point of view, we come to the following conclusions:

1. The classification analysis in which binary decision trees are produced is an appropriate complement for the well-known methods, such as multiple regression or discriminant analysis. In addition to the fact that binary decision trees (in contrast to, e.g., complicated regression equations) are directly intelligible and adapted to clinical thinking, a considerable advantage of analysis using binary decision trees lies in the fact that relative or dependent factors can be identified. By means of these relative prognostic factors, the effect of the absolute factors can be specified in a more detailed way or also relativized. Thus, one can come to more specific hypotheses.

2. When interpreting binary decision trees, one has to pay attention to whether possibly important variables that do not appear in the decision tree are masked by the analysis. This is especially true if the prognostic variables correlate. For this reason, comparative analyses are important to gain hints about the stability of the results. From this point of view, the CART-analysis does not differ from similar or alternative statistical methods.

The results presented are, of course, nothing more than very tentative hypotheses. The sample is relatively small; 54 patients with different psychiatric diagnoses. Furthermore, it is a quite specific group of relatively severe cases for whom outpatient treatment was not sufficient. It is questionable whether these results can be generalized to other groups. Other questions follow, for example, how the prognostical structures differ in different psychiatric diagnoses, and so forth.

We are at present investigating these questions in a larger project in which we can refer to more extensive and methodologically improved assessment methods (e.g., reliability, independence of the ratings, more precise outcome measures). We will see whether we are able to replicate our results and to specificate our hypotheses. We hope that these investigations will lead us to results that have direct practical relevance for treatment indication and treatment planning.

References

Breiman, L., Friedman, J.H., Olshen, R.A., and Stone, C.J. (1984): Classification and regression trees (CART). Wadsworth International Group Belmont, Cal.

Remschmidt, H., and Schmidt, M. (Eds.) (1977): Multiaxiales Klassifikationsschema für psychiatrische Erkrankungen im Kindes- und Jugendalter nach Rutter, Shaffer und Sturge. Huber, Bern.

Remschmidt, H., and Schmidt, M. (Eds.) (1988): Alternative Behandlungsformen in der Kinder- und Jugendpsychiatrie. Stationäre Behandlung, tagesklinische Behandlung und Home-treatment im Vergleich. Stuttgart: Enke.

Rutter, M., Shaffer, D., and Shepherd, M. (1976): An evaluation of a proposal for a multiaxial classification of child psychiatric disorders. Geneva: WHO Organization Monograph.

Problem Intensity and the Disposition of Adolescents to Take Therapeutic Advice

Inge Seiffge-Krenke

1. Introduction

Whether mental disorders and deviant behavior occur more frequently during adolescence than at other times of life is controversial. Various authors point out that certain behavioral problems do increase at this age: There are reports of a rise in the accident and suicide rate (Garfinkel et al., 1982) and of increased drug and alcohol abuse (Bergeret, 1981; Jessor,1982). Manifest psychotic behavior comparable to adult schizophrenia tends to emerge after puberty (Achenbach and Edelbrock, 1978), whilst delinquent behavior is observed now for the first time (Lösel, 1982; Farrington, Ohlin and Wilson, 1986). On the other hand, large-scale epidemiological surveys, such as those by Rutter et al. (1977) or Achenbach (1982), contradict such conclusions: They found that the mean frequency of disorders in general remained constant throughout the periods studied, although the nature of the symptoms was age-related.

But even those young people who manage the transition from childhood to adulthood without manifest difficulties are still confronted with a series of complex developmental tasks, partly interrelated, which have to be mastered within the relatively short period of 5 to 10 years. In coping with these demands the parents are often not particularly helpful; this is partly because, historically, they grew up in a different generation but also because of their own ambivalence toward their children's need for detachment (Seiffge-Krenke, 1984a).

Nevertheless, offers of professional help in case of particular problems are rarely taken up (Specht et al., 1979). According to the review by Wittchen and Fichter (1980) of psychotherapeutic care in West Germany, 90% of treatments carried out by German psychotherapists involved adults and 60% children. Adolescents appeared in only 40% of treatments. Even allowing for the great

individual differences in the attitude of adults toward psychotherapy or counseling, the "counseling aversion" amongst adolescents is striking in comparison
with other age groups and has resulted in adolescents being stigmatized as
"unmotivated patients" (Rogers, 1970). Even in those centers which specialize
in helping young people, adolescents are usually underrepresented. In our own
investigation of the clienteles of various therapeutic or counseling institutions we
found that adolescents made up the following proportions of those in treatment:
55% in a childrens' psychiatric department, 33% in a counseling center, 23%
in the outpatient department of a psychotherapy unit, and only 3% in a private
psychotherapeutic practice (Seiffge–Krenke, 1985).

In the following we shall try to answer the question of why so few adolescents
are willing to take up existing offers of therapeutic help in dealing with
pressing problems. To this end, we shall present some empirical findings which
demonstrate the strong influence of developmental dynamics on the attitude of
this age group toward psychotherapy.

2. Diagnostic Problems in Measuring Problem Intensity and Manifest Disorders

The more recent diagnostic procedures, such as the Child Behavior Profile
(Edelbrock and Achenbach, 1980) and DSM III (Rutter et al., 1977), represent
a considerable step forward in this field in that they take a multidimensional
approach and make allowances for interactions between various disorders, so
that more complex assessments can be made. If, like Achenbach and his colleagues, one further takes into account various reference persons such as
parents and teachers, they may also be assumed to be more valid than earlier
methods. It is thus all the more surprising, analyzing the assessment procedures
employed by most therapists working with adolescents, how unreliable their
diagnoses are. For no other age group does the diagnosis "nonspecific transitional disorder" occur so frequently. Weiner and Del Gaudio (1976) found this
diagnosis applied to 36% of adolescent patients, as compared with 5% of
adults. Similar results are reported by Rosen et al. (1965), who analyzed the
diagnoses of 41496 adolescent patients. Our own research revealed that 20% of
disturbed adolescents were diagnosed as having unspecified disorders (Seiffge–Krenke, 1986a).

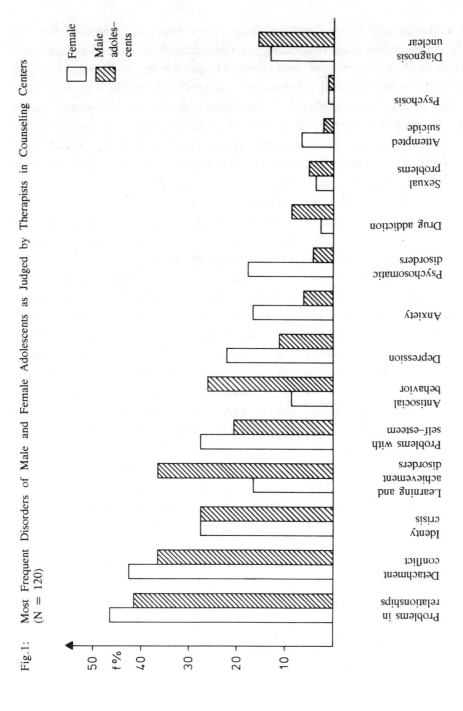

Fig.1:   Most Frequent Disorders of Male and Female Adolescents as Judged by Therapists in Counseling Centers (N = 120)

In this inquiry 120 psychotherapists from a representative sample of the 748 family counseling centers (Erziehungsberatungsstellen) in West-Germany were asked about their diagnosis of adolescents. On the whole, the therapists named disturbances in interpersonal relationships and separation conflicts as the central problems of both sexes at this age. The comparatively heavy emphasis placed by the therapists on the concept of identity crisis as a form of disorder corresponds to the general assumption widespread among therapists, regardless of their therapeutic approach, that adolescence is a period of crisis. With regard to sex-related differences, our findings correspond to the distribution generally described by other authors (cf. Rutter, Tizard, Yule, Graham, and Whitmore, 1977). Delinquency and antisocial behavior, drug abuse, and learning disorders are diagnosed far more frequently for male adolescents, whereas depression, anxiety, and attempted suicide are more typical of females.

We may assume that the insecurity amongst therapists in diagnosing adolescent disorders has its origin largely in the fact that, especially at the beginning of adolescence, developmental changes exercise a strong influence on the behavior and feelings of their young clients. As has been shown by Hamburg (1974), early adolescence in particular is a phase of rapid physical development accompanied by a variety of transitional psychological changes, such as temporary drops in positive self-esteem (Simmons, Rosenberg, and Rosenberg, 1973). This knowledge has led those in psychological practice to be cautious in their diagnoses, to avoid stigmatizing their young patients through over-hasty labeling. Where diagnoses are made, they often prove unreliable. In less than half of the cases analyzed by Kelly et al. (1977) and Langen (1965), could one speak of a stable diagnosis. As Anna Freud already pointed out in 1960, this has to do with the fact that developmental changes not only cause disturbances, but can also bring about spontaneous remissions and the solution of old conflicts.

In order to be able to reach a reasonably reliable assessment of the severity of a problem, several diagnostic sessions are necessary. The symptoms often vary; making it difficult to distinguish the rather more extreme forms of "typical adolescent behavior" from a serious pathological development. Matters are complicated still further by the fact that young people going through this developmental phase typically have strong inhibitions about disclosing personal information to an adult therapist. By about the age of 15 a change in disclosure partner has usually taken place (Rivenbark, 1971; Seiffge-Krenke, 1987a); adolescents are no longer as willing to accept their parents as disclosure partners, preferring to share intimacies with their peers. At the same time, the capacity to distinguish between private and public information becomes fully developed, and adolescents are increasingly reluctant to talk about personal and/or private matters with adults (Laufer and Wolfe, 1974). In their self-presentations they now differentiate between an inner "true self" and an external "facade" (Broughton, 1981).

Knowledge of such complex dynamics makes it easy to underestimate the real degree of stress oppressing an individual adolescent. Thus, in the studies by Offer (1984) on the development of self-concept, we find that self-descriptions remain on the whole consistently positive, but that depressive moods are also in evidence. *"I sometimes feel sad and lonely"*, for example, was answered in the affirmative by 45% of his sample.

The discrepancies found between the way in which adolescent symptoms are evaluated by parents or therapists and by the adolescents themselves can probably be interpreted in a similar light. In the study by Pierce and Klein (1982), for example, parents and adolescents agreed on only 7 of the 52 items presented on a Behavior Rating Scale. Only in items referring to conspicuous behavioral disturbances such as enuresis, stealing, or eating disorders did the adolescents describe themselves in the same way as their parents. By and large, they experienced themselves as more anxious and depressed than their parents did, which stands in direct contradiction to the findings of Adelman et al. (1979), whose young subjects tended to regard their problems as *less* serious than did their parents and teachers. These studies lead one to doubt whether parents should be taken as reliable sources of information in assessing the problem intensity and manifest disturbances of their adolescent offspring, although when dealing with children their assistance is indispensable (Achenbach, 1982). On the other hand, it is also questionable how much one can rely on self-evaluations by the adolescents themselves. As was shown by Mechanic as early as 1962, disturbances can in their turn affect illness perception, and if one further relates this to what we know about age-specific difficulties in self-perception and self-presentation, the diagnostic insecurity plaguing therapists in their dealings with adolescents becomes easier to understand. Under such circumstances, criteria such as the degree of personal suffering, insight into the nature of illness, and treatment motivation take on particular significance when it comes to the diagnosis and treatment of troubled adolescents.

3. Coping and Defending: Different Approaches to Solving Age-Specific Problems

The coping skills of young people in dealing with age-specific problems such as detachment from parents, heterosexual relationships, building up an occupational identity have so far been considerably underestimated. This is at least partly due to the clinical orientation which was predominant in what little research has been done on adolescent coping. Compared with adults, adolescents have been sadly neglected by most researchers: Only 7% of the studies on coping carried out in the past 20 years have dealt specifically with adolescence. Within this limited scope, interest in responses to extremely stressful events has steadily increased and currently comprises two-thirds of research activity on adolescent coping (cf. summary in Seiffge-Krenke, 1986b). Usually, small, homogeneous groups of adolescents who have experienced extremely stressful, nonnormative events, are analyzed. As a result of this one-sided trend, a great many defence strategies have been assessed but very little actual coping behavior. Thus, high defence rates and withdrawal have been reported in studies investigating adolescents who have had to cope with kidnapping (Terr, 1979), rape (McCombie, 1976), or serious illnesses like cancer (Kikuchi, 1977). Because of this orientation, the operational definition and measurement of "coping"[1] have been heavily dominated by defence aspects; they comprise roughly half of the items in the questionnaires by Haan (1974) and Weinstock (1977). Eleven of the 12 "coping dimensions" in the instrument developed by Houston (1977) are in fact classical defence mechanisms in the sense described by A. Freud (1936), such as denial, suppression, or reaction formation.

At present, a change can be observed which is probably due to recent trends in

---

1) Lazarus et al. (1974, p.250) defined coping as "problem-solving efforts made by an individual, when the demands he/she faces are highly relevant ...and tax his/her adaptive resources."

the theory of adolescence (Coleman, 1978; Lerner and Busch-Rossnagel, 1981). Coping with normative events, with everyday problems and developmental tasks, is coming into focus. Research with nonclinical adolescent groups has revealed that their responses to developmental tasks in fields such as peer groups, school, or future, can be described as involving three main modes of coping (Seiffge-Krenke, 1984b), as shown in Fig. 2.

Fig. 2:   Modes of coping[1] in adolescence

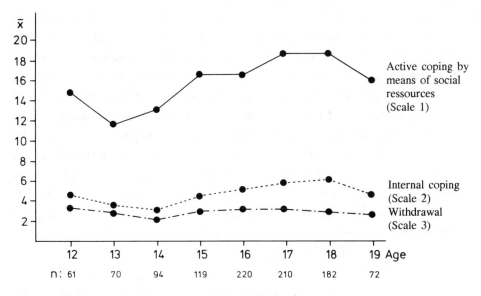

1) Coping-Questionnaire by Seiffge–Krenke (in press)

In this study, coping was measured by a two-dimensional matrix consisting of 20 coping strategies (e.g., *"I discuss the problem with my parents"*) applied to eight problem fields (e.g., school: *"bad marks"*; parents: *"quarrel with parents"*). For each problem, the subjects could choose any number of coping strategies. On the basis of their responses, the 20 coping strategies, taken across all problem situations, could be reduced to three major dimensions. The first dimension involves activities such as information-seeking or taking advice (Scale 1, Fig. 2), the second one emphasizes the adolescent's appraisal of the

situation and internal reflection on possible solutions (Scale 2), and the third —
which may be regarded as dysfunctional — includes defences such as denial
and repression, entailing a fatalistic attitude that ultimately leads to withdrawal
(Scale 3). The Cronbach alphas for these dimensions were .80, .77, and .73
respectively (Seiffge–Krenke, in press).

A similar three-dimensional structure was reported by Frankel (1986) for a
sample of nonclinical adolescent girls. He found that functional coping included
strategies such as support-seeking and cognitive coping, whereas dysfunctional
strategies were mostly characterized by emotional catharsis.

As can be seen in Fig. 2, the 12- to 19-year-olds in our study tended to
present themselves as competent copers, well able to deal with problems arising
in developmental fields such as school, parents, peers, opposite sex, and so
forth. Functional coping modi dominated; dysfunctional coping being employed
very rarely and only for certain types of problems. We found that such behavior occurred particularly frequently with "self-related problems" (such as "dis-
contented with oneself"), in which about a third of responses involved withdrawal (Seiffge–Krenke, 1987c). The general proportion of functional to dysfunctional coping was highly stable over time (Seiffge–Krenke, 1984b) and
cross-culturally comparable (Seiffge–Krenke and Shulman, in press). The
tendency to apply dysfunctional coping across all situations was generally low
and similar for both German and Israeli samples (21% and 16% respectively).

However, whereas the functional approach would thus seem to be characteristic
for the problem-solving behavior of nonclinical subjects, defence mechanisms
are far more prominent in all studies with clinical groups. Dysfunctional
coping, operationalized in our research as responding with defence mechanisms
such as withdrawal, includes the inability to reach an adequate solution to the
problem. Nevertheless, withdrawal can be a meaningful way of coping with
situations of extreme stress or where direct action is inhibited by external barriers (Lazarus and Launier, 1978). In our studies, the withdrawal dimension
proved especially effective for discriminating between different clinical groups.
Adolescents with high problem intensity but not yet referred to counseling
(N = 43), adolescents in psychotherapy (diagnosed as suffering from depression
or problems in interpersonal relationships, N = 37) and adolescent drug abusers
(N = 28) can be adequately identified through their tendency to withdrawal.

Scores on this dimension were high amongst adolescents with high problem intensity and drug abusers, whereas the scores of those referred to treatment did not differ from those of the normal group (N = 266).

Tab. 1: Separating Clinical Groups by Discriminant Analysis

Level 1	Variable	Wilks Lamda	Significance
1	Coping Scale 3: Withdrawal	.84	.00
2	OFFER Scale 1: Generally content with oneself and the world	.79	.00
3	OFFER Scale 3: Confidence in one's own abilities	.67	.00
4	Sex	.60	.00
5	"Do you know someone personally who is mentally ill?" (Item)	.58	.00
6	Chances of recovery from mental Illness (Item)	.49	.00
7	Schmitz Scale 1: Sceptical toward therapists	.45	.00

As can be seen in Tab. 1, Coping Scale 3 ("Withdrawal") made the largest contribution to group discrimination, followed by self-concept dimensions. Confidence in their own abilities is particularly low amongst drug abusers, whilst adolescents referred to treatment are distinguished by their low self-esteem. It is worth noting that the clinical groups differ neither with respect to active coping and support-seeking nor to internal reflection of possible solutions. In these ways their approach is as functional as that of their nonclinical peers.

Fig. 3: Differences in Coping Strategies across Clinical and Normal Groups of Adolescents

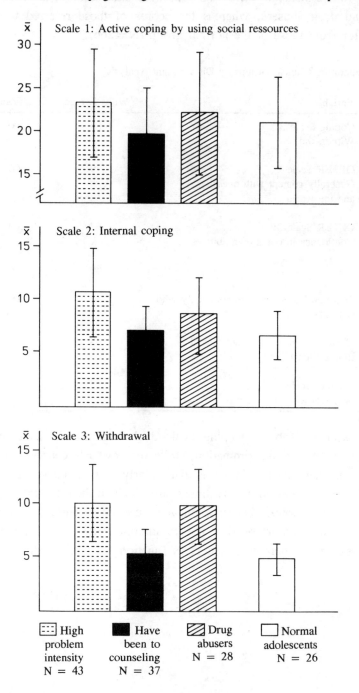

The use of defence mechanisms in combination with certain self-concept dimensions is not only a powerful factor for discriminating between clinical groups but seems also to be the most significant predictor for deviant or anti-social behavior and drug abuse (Seiffge-Krenke, 1986a).

Tab. 2:   Prediction of Drug Abuse

Step	Variable	F-Value	Significance	Multiple R
1	Coping Scale 3: Withdrawal	17.6	.000	.37
2	FPI Scale Aggressiveness	8.9	.003	.41
3	Problem Scale 4: Problems with peers	4.6	.034	.44
4	Problem Scale 3: Problems with parents	3.8	.046	.49
5	OFFER Scale 3: Self-confidence in own ability	3.4	.052	.55

Self-concept variables ranked lower in predictive validity, after personality variables such as aggressiveness and problems in interpersonal relations. It is remarkable that adolescents in treatment have particularly high coping and low defence scores (cf. Fig. 3); a combination judged by Gomes-Schwartz (1978) to be one of the conditions for therapeutic success. Closer analysis will have to clarify whether this can be taken as a sign of therapeutic progress in the sense that more normal behavior patterns have been adopted, or whether the low defence scores in combination with high functional coping were themselves necessary preconditions for taking up treatment.

Typical of all those adolescents who are burdened by considerable problem intensity are simultaneously high scores in both coping and defending (Seiffge-Krenke, 1984a). This was confirmed by a further investigation analyzing the relationship between personality type and coping behavior (Seiffge-Krenke, Lipp, and Brath, 1989). 15- to 19-year-old adolescents were grouped by cluster analysis on the basis of their scores in a personality questionnaire (FPI by Fahrenberg and Selg, 1970).

Tab. 3: Withdrawal (Coping Scale 3) by Adolescents with Three Personality Types, Differentiated for Eight Problem Areas

	Personality type				
Problem area	Cluster 1 Sociable/ extravert N = 115	Cluster 2 Emotionally in- stable/depressed N = 127	Cluster 3 Normal/ controlled N = 111	Test of Significance overall F ANOVA	Scheffé
School	.09	.17	.07	$F (2,350) = 8.72; p = .001$	2 > 1.3
Teachers	.03	.12	.07	$F (2,350) = 8.55; p = .0001$	2 > 1
Parents	.05	.10	.04	$F (2,350) = 5.29; p = .005$	2 > 3
Peers	.06	.14	.06	$F (2,350) = 7.82; p = .0001$	2 > 1.3
Opposite Sex	.07	.18	.10	$F (2,350) = 10.74; p = .0001$	2 > 1.3
Self–Related Problems	.07	.19	.06	$F (2,350) = 19.94; p = .0001$	2 > 1.3
Leisure Time	.05	.11	.04	$F (2,350) = 5.83; p = .088$	2 > 1.3
Future	.05	.15	.07	$F (2,350) = 4.62; p = 0.12$	2 > 1.3

The groups of adolescents with different personality structures did not differ with respect to active coping and support seeking, nor in internal reflection of possible solutions; where they did differ was in their withdrawal scores. Adolescents from Cluster 2 (high emotional lability and depression) had the highest scores for withdrawal, which proved to be a generalized response to problems from all eight developmental fields. It appears that adolescents in this group adjust their behavior very little according to situational demands but tend rather, as described by Averill (1973), to employ the same strategy consistently, regardless of the controllability of the situation in question.

This situationally invariant tendency to withdrawal is strongly influenced by family climate (Shulman, Seiffge–Krenke and Samet, 1987), whereas the functional approach is less dependent on family influences. In terms of the classic distinction between coping and defending drawn by Norma Haan (1974), it seems inappropriate to classify such adolescents as "defenders" because of their simultaneously high scores in functional coping. It would appear rather to be a matter of a continuous oscillation between approach and avoidance (Roth and Cohen, 1986), which in a way is characteristic for this developmental period in general. Adolescents with high problem intensity and partially inadequate coping behavior (e.g., drug abuse) thus show a more pronounced "adolescent pattern" than nonclinical subjects. Perhaps we should regard this behavior pattern as a preventive strategy that protects the adolescent from physical symptoms or from a more serious neurotic or antisocial development.

4. The Dilemma Between the Desire for Privacy and the Need for Therapeutic Help

As indicated above, accepting therapeutic help is a coping strategy chosen relatively rarely by adolescents — only 9% of those in our study saw it as an acceptable alternative (Seiffge–Krenke, 1984a). The tendency to accept or reject psychotherapy is clearly not simply a function of problem pressure, for as problem pressure increases, so does the disinclination to talk about it. As we found in a study comparing adolescents with high and low problem intensity[1], they are often caught up in a dilemma between their desire to give expression to their worries and a strong inhibition preventing them from doing just that.

---

1) The criterium chosen was the upper and lower 25% in the Problem Test by Seiffge–Krenke (1984b).

Tab. 4:   Differences in Attitudes to Psychotherapy[1] Between Adolescents with High and Low
          Problem Intensity

| | Problem intensity | | | | | |
| | High (N = 43) | | Low (N = 42) | | | |
	x	s	x	s	t	p
1. Scepticism toward psychotherapy	33.9	7.0	32.4	5.6	1.1	.27
2. Readiness to accept help	64.1	12.0	59.7	10.9	1.7	.08
3. Need for privacy	29.9	7.1	23.0	5.7	4.8	.00
4. Attitudes toward illness	25.5	6.4	24.8	9.2	.63	.71

1) Psychotherapy-Questionnaire by Schmitz (1981)

The adolescents with high problem intensity included in this study had so far shown no evidence of manifest disturbance. They had a very negative self-concept and reported a great many problems with parents, peers, the opposite sex, and self. They showed a strong tendency to employ withdrawal and other problem-avoiding behavior, which was generalized across different problem situations. They did not differ from their less stressed agemates with regard to their use of active or internal coping, except for an increased tendency to turn to "neutral" sources of help (books, magazines, etc.).

It is striking that these adolescents, who were so very oppressed by their personal difficulties, showed only slightly more willingness to seek professional help, whilst their need for privacy was so great that their subjective sense of suffering and their disinclination to talk about it were about equally balanced. This led us to assume that their extremely difficult relations with their families were at least partly responsible for their highly ambivalent attitude toward offers coming from other adults, in this case therapists or counselors.

Further research has shown that adolescents with a high proportion of dysfunctional coping often come from a special family type, namely from unstructured and conflict-oriented families (Shulman, Seiffge-Krenke, and Samet,

1987). These families are characterized by a high degree of conflict in their interactions and by their lack of mutual support; they have a low level of organization and little intrafamilial control. Personality growth and individuality are not encouraged except in the field of achievement, the emphasis on which is often an additional source of conflict and stress in such families.

This makes it understandable that adolescents who have grown up against such a background hesitate to take up offers of therapeutic advice, quite apart from their general developmental orientation toward autonomy and away from parents or adults in general. Should they nevertheless find themselves in treatment, they appear to be manifestly unmotivated (Rogers, 1970) and withdrawn (Argelander, 1970), even though they may well be latently quite keen to accept treatment.

This brings us to the question of what sort of adolescents come to treatment at all, since both the developmental dynamics typical of their age group in general (detachment/self–disclosure behavior) and the special features of the family backgrounds of many disturbed adolescents would seem to combine to prevent them from accepting this sort of help.

We attempted to answer this question with the help of the data from 266 non-clinical and 108 clinical adolescent subjects. A multiple regression analysis was carried out using the self–concept, coping behavior, and problem intensity scores of these samples, as well as their answers on their attitude toward psychotherapy.

As can be seen in Tab. 5, high psychotherapy motivation, high scores in school–related problems, and a positive attitude toward the efficacy of psycho-therapy are important factors contributing to a fundamental willingness to accept offers of therapeutic assistance. Further important predictors are: quality of relations with parents, the neuroticism score on the FPI, and the subjects' actual experiences with the mentally ill or relevant institutions.

From these results we can conclude that it is not so much the pressure of special problems that drives an adolescent to seek therapeutic help but rather a combination of his or her basic willingness to take advice at all, confidence in and familiarity with therapeutic procedures, and especially a reasonably good relationship with parents.

Tab. 5: Results of Multiple Regression of the Question: "If you had a very serious problem, can you imagine yourself going to a psychotherapist or counseling centre, or doing psychotherapy?"

	F	Significance	Multiple R	Simple R
1. SCHMITZ Scale 2: Psychotherapy motivation	64.5	.01	.44	.44
2. Problem Scale 1: school–related problems	10.9	.03	.47	.18
3. Effectiveness of Psycho–therapy (item)	8.0	.04	.48	.18
4. OFFER Scale 2: good relations with parents	6.3	.05	.50	.11
5. FPI Scale 11: neuroticism	6.0	.05	.51	.21
6. Problem Scale 6: problems with the opposite sex	5.9	.08	.52	.09
7. Do you know someone who is mentally ill (item)	3.5	.09	.53	.11
8. Active experience with counseling (item)	2.8	.11	.54	.12

5. Conclusions

The above review of research has been undertaken in an attempt to answer the question of why adolescents have so little inclination to take up offers of thera-peutic assistance in case of pressing problems. It turned out that certain impor-tant developmental changes peculiar to this age group, such as, the process of detachment from parents and shifts in disclosure partner, are vital in explaining this phenomenon. Analyzing nonclinical and mildly disturbed adolescents, we were surprised by the great competence and mastery they showed in solving age–specific problems. Even the excessively stressed adolescents had, besides a psychologically understandable tendency to resort more often to defences, similarly high scores in active and internal coping to those of clinically normal adolescents. These findings lend support to the assumptions of Lazarus et al. (1974) that both approaches (coping and defending) can be adequate responses to a particular situation, and speak against Norma Haan's conception (1977) that a person is either a coper or a defender. The simultaneously high scores in both coping *and* defending found for clinically disturbed adolescents not yet in treatment, could be interpreted as attempts to develop preventive strategies. Of relevance here is the useful distinction drawn by Laufer and Laufer (1984) between two forms of defensive functioning: that which allows some progressive development to take place and affects only some specific areas, and that which appears to dominate the whole of adolescent functioning so that the adolescent becomes progressively unable to adapt.

This indeed represents a further complication in reaching a diagnostic decision already impeded by the age–related unwillingness of many adolescents to disclose personal information at all, as well as by the general instability of symptoms at this age. Assessment must include an estimate of the sort of normal developmental progression that has been disturbed, which can be used as a basis for decisions about the focus and intensity of subsequent therapeutic efforts. Diagnostically speaking, adolescence is a period when we may be able to detect early signs of potentially serious trouble that could arise later, offering us a unique opportunity to intervene in a way that may preclude pathological solutions to the age–related developmental tasks confronting every adolescent.

Diagnostic systems such as that suggested by Achenbach (1985) can be of great assistance here, since they are able to assess not only problems but also competencies, and because they also allow for very exact comparisons between clinical and nonclinical samples. In his studies, as in ours, the age- and sex–dependency of symptoms came out clearly. As we were able to demonstrate (Seiffge–Krenke, 1986a), it is not only the disturbances themselves that differ with age and sex, but also the rates of accepting offers of therapeutic help and the nature of the offers themselves. Thus, whereas we find far more boys than girls amongst the children attending counseling centers, this relationship is reversed around the age of 15: from then on considerably more girls than boys seek institutional help. A stronger tendency to use informal sources of help, as well as greater openness in expressing feelings and discussing problems, are the most striking sex-related criteria which distinguish female from male coping behavior at this age (Seiffge-Krenke, 1984b), and these in turn lead to corresponding differences in the inclination to accept therapeutic help from an institution.

The therapists themselves are apparently acutely aware of the special problems attached to this developmental phase. This shows, for example, their hesitation to commit themselves to a definite diagnosis, and their individually planned, problem- and sex-related offers to help.

In our studies, we found that the way in which the process of detachment from parents has taken place influences an adolescent's attitude toward psychotherapy. A poor relationship with parents increases the already ambivalent attitude of many young people toward adults. One may ask whether new approaches such as peer counseling would not be more suited to the increasing orientation toward extrafamilial settings typically found amongst this age group. Peers play a crucial role for issues and concerns of immediate relevance to the adolescent's life, such as heterosexual behavior and drug-involvement (Kandel, 1986). Nevertheless, especially our studies on the effect of family climate on coping style have shown that parental influences are especially strong in the development of defensive behavior and tend to lead to a generalized pattern of withdrawal applied indiscriminately to all problem situations. This is a poor starting point for many traditional forms of therapeutic intervention that were originally developed for highly motivated adults.

References

Achenbach, T.M. (1982): Developmental psychopathology. New York: Wiley.

Achenbach, T.M. (1985): Assessment and taxonomy of child and adolescent psychology. Beverly Hills: Sage.

Achenbach, T.M. and Edelbrock, C.S. (1978): The classification of child psychopathology: A review and analysis of empirical efforts. Psychological Bulletin 85, 1275–1301.

Achenbach, T.M. and Edelbrock, C.S. (1981): Behavioral problems and competencies reported by parents of normal and disturbed children aged four through sixteen. Monographs of the Society for Research in Child Development 46, No.1.

Adelman, H., Taylor, L., Fuller, W., and Nelson, P. (1979): Discrepancies among student, parent, and teacher ratings of the severity of a student's problems. American Educational Research Journal 16, 38–41.

Argelander, H. (1970): Das Erstinterview in der Psychoanalyse. Darmstadt: Wissenschaftliche Buchgesellschaft.

Averill, J.R. (1973): Personal control over aversive stimuli and it's relationship to stress. Psychological Bulletin 80, 286–303.

Bergeret, J. (1981): Young people, drugs ... and others. Bulletin on Narcotics 33, 1–14.

Broughton, J.M. (1981): The divided self in adolescence. Human Development 24, 13–32.

Coleman, J.C. (1978): Current contradictions in adolescent theory. Journal of Youth and Adolescence 7, 11–34.

Edelbrock, C.S., and Achenbach, T.M. (1980): A typology of child behavior profile patterns: Distribution and correlates in disturbed children aged 6 to 16. Journal of Abnormal Child Psychology 8, 441–470.

Fahrenberg, H., and Selg, H. (1970): Das Freiburger Persönlichkeitsinventar. Göttingen: Hogrefe.

Farrington, D.P., Ohlin, L.E., and Wilson, J.K. (1986): Understanding and controlling crime. New York: Springer.

Frankel, K. (1986): The relationship of coping and social milieu perception to self-reported depression in middle school girls. Paper presented at the First Biennial Meeting of the Society for Research in Adolescence. Madison, Wisconsin.

Freud, A. (1936): The ego and the mechanism of defence. London: Hogarth Press.

Freud, A. (1960): Probleme der Pubertät. Psyche 14, 1–23.

Garfinkel, B.D., Froese, A., and Hood, J. (1982): Suicide attempts in children and adolescents. American Journal of Psychiatry 139, 1257–1261.

Gomes–Schwartz, B. (1978): Effective ingredients in psychotherapy: Prediction of outcome from process variables. Journal of Consulting and clinical psychology 46, 1023–1035.

Haan, N. (1974): The adolescent's ego model of coping and defense and comparison with Q–sorted ideal personalities. Genetic Psychology Monographs 89, 273–306.

Haan, N. (1977): Coping and defending. Processes of self–environment organization. New York: Academic Press.

Hamburg, B.A. (1974): Early adolescence: A specific and stressful stage of the life cycle. In Coelho, G.V., Hamburg, D.A., and Adams, J.E.: Coping and adaption. New York: Basic Books, 101–124.

Houston, B.K. (1977): Open ended and structural questionnaires to elicit information concerning coping behavior. Unpublished manuscript. Psychological Clinic, University of Kansas.

Jessor, R. (1982): Problem behavior and development transition in adolescence. Journal of School Health 52, 295–300.

Kandel, D.B. (1986): Processes of peer influences in adolescence. In Silbereisen, R.K., Eyferth, K, and Rudinger, G.: Development as action in context: Berlin–Heidelberg–New York–Tokyo: Springer, 203–228.

Kelly, J.G., Snowden, L.R., and Mumoz, R.F. (1977): Social and community interventions. Annual Review of Psychology 28, 232–261.

Kikuchi, J. (1977): An adolescent boy's adjustment to leukemia. Maternal Child Nursing Journal 6, 37–49.

Langen, D. (1965): Die Psychotherapie der Pubertätskrisen unter dem Blickwinkel ihrer Weiterentwicklung. Medizinische Welt 16, 2917–2920.

Laufer, M., and Laufer, M.E. (1984): Adolescence and developmental breakdown. New Haven and London: Yale University Press.

Laufer, R.W., and Wolfe, M. (1974): The concept of privacy in childhood and adolescence. In Larson, D.H. (Ed.): Man–environment interactions (Proceedings of EDRA). Washington, D.C.: Environmental Design Research Association, 29–54.

Lazarus, R.S., and Launier, R. (1978): Stress–related transactions between person and environment. In Pervon, L., and Lewis, M. (Eds.): Perspectives in interactional psychology. New York: Plenum, 287–327.

Lazarus, R.S., Averill, J., and Opton, E. (1974): The psychology of coping. In Coelho, G.V., Hamburg, D.A., and Adams, J.E. (Eds.): Coping and Adaptation. New York: Basic Books, 249–315.

Lerner, R.M., and Busch-Rossnagel, N.A. (1981): Individuals as producers of their own development. In Lerner, R.M., and Rossnagel, N.A. (Eds.): Individuals as producers of their own development: A life-span perspective. New York: Academic Press.

Lösel, F. (1982): Prognose und Prävention von Delinquenzproblemen. In Brandstädter, J., and van Eye, A. (Eds.): Psychologische Prävention. Bern: Huber, 197–238.

McCombie, E.L. (1976): Characteristics of rape victims seen in crisis intervention. Smith College Studies in Social Work 46, 137–158.

Mechanic, D. (1962): Some factors in identifying and defending mental illness. Mental Hygiene 46, 66–74.

Offer, D. (1984): Das Selbstbild normaler Jugendlicher. In Olbrich, E., and Todt, E. (Eds.): Probleme des Jugendalters. Neuere Perspektive. Berlin: Springer, 111–113.

Pierce, L., and Klein, H. (1982): A comparison of parent and child perception of the child's behavior. Behavioral Disorders 7, 69–74.

Rivenbark, W. (1971): Self-disclosure among adolescents. Psychological Reports 28, 35–42.

Rogers, R. (1970): The "unmotivated" adolescent patient who wants psychotherapy. American Journal of Psychotherapy 24, 411–418.

Rosen, B.M., Bahn, A., Shellow, R., and Bower, E.M. (1965): Adolescent patients served in outpatient psychiatric clinics. American Journal of Public Health 55, 1563–1577.

Roth, S., and Cohen, J.J. (1986): Approach avoidance and coping with stress. American Psychologist 47, 813–819.

Rutter, M., Shaffer, D., and Shepherd, M. (1977): An evaluation of the proposal for a multiaxial classification of child psychiatric disorders. Psychological Medicine 3, 244–250.

Rutter, M., Tizard, J., Yule, W., Graham, P., and Whitmore, K. (1977): Epidemiologie in der Kinderpsychiatrie – die Isle of Whight Studien 1964–1974. Zeitschrift für Kinder- und Jugendpsychiatrie 5, 238–279.

Schmitz, B. (1981): Ein Fragebogen zur Erfassung von Einstellungen zur Inanspruchnahme therapeutischer Hilfe. Unveröffentlichte Dissertation. Tübingen.

Seiffge-Krenke, I. (1984a): Formen der Problembewältigung bei besonders belasteten Jugendlichen. In Olbrich, E., and Todt, E. (Eds.): Probleme des Jugendalters: Neuere Sichtweisen. Berlin-Heidelberg-New York-Tokyo: Springer, 353–386.

Seiffge-Krenke, I. (1984b): Problembewältigung im Jugendalter. Thesis submitted for the certificate of habilitation. Gießen.

Seiffge-Krenke, I. (1985): Psychische Gesundheit bzw. Krankheit in der Adoleszenz: Ergebnisse von Untersuchungen an Jugendlichen und ihren Therapeuten. In Stiksrud, A., and Wobitt, F.: Adoleszenz und Postadoleszenz. Frankfurt: Klotz.

Seiffge-Krenke, I. (1986a): Psychoanalytische Therapie bei Jugendlichen. Stuttgart: Kohlhammer.

Seiffge-Krenke, I. (1986b): Problembewältigung im Jugendalter: (Übersichtsreferat). Zeitschrift für Entwicklungspsychologie und Pädagogische Psychologie 18, 122–252.

Seiffge-Krenke, I. (1987a): Disclosure behavior in adolescence. In Spitznagel, A. (Ed.): Recent developments in psychology. Berlin-New York-Tokyo: Springer.

Seiffge-Krenke, I. (in press): Der Coping-Fragebogen für Jugendliche. Zeitschrift für Diagnostische und Differentielle Psychologie.

Seiffge-Krenke, I. (1987c): Development of self-concept in adolescence. In Jackson, S., and Bosma, H. (Eds.): Coping and self-concept in adolescence. New York: Springer.

Seiffge-Krenke, I., Lipp, O., and Brath, K. (1989): Persönlichkeitsstruktur und Bewältigungsverhalten bei Jugendlichen. Zeitschrift für klinische Psychologie, 3.

Seiffge-Krenke, I., and Shulman, S. (in press): Cross-cultural comparison in coping-styles of adolescents. International Journal of Cross-cultural Psychology.

Shulman, S., Seiffge-Krenke, I., and Samet, N. (1987): Adolescent coping style as a function of perceived family climate. Journal of Adolescent Research 2, 367–381.

Simmons, R., Rosenberg, F., and Rosenberg, M. (1973): Disturbance in the self-image at adolescence. American Sociological Review 38, 553–568.

Specht, F., Gerlicher, K., and Schütt, K. (1979): Beratungsarbeit mit Jugendlichen. Göttingen: Vandenhoeck und Ruprecht.

Terr, L.C. (1979): Children of chowchilla: A study of psychic trauma. Psychoanalytic Study of the Child 34, 547–632.

Weiner, I.B., and Del Gaudio, A.C. (1976): Psychopathology in adolescence. Archives of General Psychiatry 33, 187–193.

Wittchen, H.U., and Fichter, M.M. (1980): Psychotherapie in der Bundesrepublik. Weinheim und Basel: Beltz.

Author Index

Subject Index